HEALTH
94/95

Fifteenth Edition

Editor

Richard Yarian
Towson State University

Richard Yarian is a health educator with extensive training in the area of biomedical health. He received his B.A. in biology from Ball State University. Before leaving Ball State University he also received both an M.A. and an Ed.S. in the area of health education. He continued his academic training at the University of Maryland where he received his Ph.D. in biomedical health. Following completion of his doctoral program, he became an assistant professor at the University of Maryland and taught courses in the areas of personal health, stress management, drug abuse, medical physiology, and cardiovascular disease.

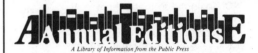

A Library of Information from the Public Press

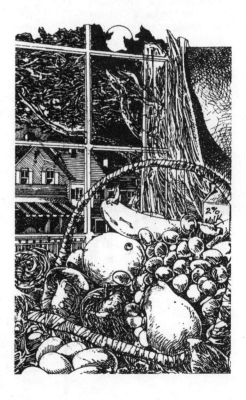

The Dushkin Publishing Group, Inc.
Sluice Dock, Guilford, Connecticut 06437

Cover illustration by Mike Eagle

The Annual Editions Series

Annual Editions is a series of over 60 volumes designed to provide the reader with convenient, low-cost access to a wide range of current, carefully selected articles from some of the most important magazines, newspapers, and journals published today. Annual Editions are updated on an annual basis through a continuous monitoring of over 300 periodical sources. All Annual Editions have a number of features designed to make them particularly useful, including topic guides, annotated tables of contents, unit overviews, and indexes. For the teacher using Annual Editions in the classroom, an Instructor's Resource Guide with test questions is available for each volume.

VOLUMES AVAILABLE

Africa
Aging
American Foreign Policy
American Government
American History, Pre-Civil War
American History, Post-Civil War
Anthropology
Biology
Business Ethics
Canadian Politics
Child Growth and Development
China
Comparative Politics
Computers in Education
Computers in Business
Computers in Society
Criminal Justice
Drugs, Society, and Behavior
Dying, Death, and Bereavement
Early Childhood Education
Economics
Educating Exceptional Children
Education
Educational Psychology
Environment
Geography
Global Issues
Health
Human Development
Human Resources
Human Sexuality
India and South Asia
International Business
Japan and the Pacific Rim

Latin America
Life Management
Macroeconomics
Management
Marketing
Marriage and Family
Mass Media
Microeconomics
Middle East and the Islamic World
Money and Banking
Multicultural Education
Nutrition
Personal Growth and Behavior
Physical Anthropology
Psychology
Public Administration
Race and Ethnic Relations
Russia, Eurasia, and Central/Eastern Europe
Social Problems
Sociology
State and Local Government
Third World
Urban Society
Violence and Terrorism
Western Civilization, Pre-Reformation
Western Civilization, Post-Reformation
Western Europe
World History, Pre-Modern
World History, Modern
World Politics

Library of Congress Cataloging in Publication Data
Main entry under title: Annual editions: Health. 1994/95.
      1. Hygiene—Periodicals. I. Yarian, Richard, *comp.* II. Title: Health.
613'.05   81–643582   ISBN: 1–56134–277–7

Fifteenth Edition

Printed in the United States of America

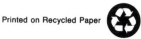

Printed on Recycled Paper

To the Reader

In publishing ANNUAL EDITIONS we recognize the enormous role played by the magazines, newspapers, and journals of the *public press* in providing current, first-rate educational information in a broad spectrum of interest areas. Within the articles, the best scientists, practitioners, researchers, and commentators draw issues into new perspective as accepted theories and viewpoints are called into account by new events, recent discoveries change old facts, and fresh debate breaks out over important controversies.

Many of the articles resulting from this enormous editorial effort are appropriate for students, researchers, and professionals seeking accurate, current material to help bridge the gap between principles and theories and the real world. These articles, however, become more useful for study when those of lasting value are carefully *collected, organized, indexed,* and *reproduced* in a *low-cost format*, which provides easy and permanent access when the material is needed. That is the role played by *Annual Editions.* Under the direction of each volume's *Editor*, who is an expert in the subject area, and with the guidance of an *Advisory Board*, we seek each year to provide in each *ANNUAL EDITION* a current, well-balanced, carefully selected collection of the best of the public press for your study and enjoyment. We think you'll find this volume useful, and we hope you'll take a moment to let us know what you think.

America is in the midst of a health revolution that is changing the way millions of people view their health. Traditionally, most people delegated responsibility for their health to their physicians and hoped that medical science would be able to cure whatever ailed them. This approach to health care emphasized the role of medical technology and funneled billions of dollars into medical research. The net result of all this spending is the most technically advanced and expensive health care system in the world. Unfortunately, health care costs have risen so high that millions of Americans can no longer afford health care, and even among those who can, there is limited accessibility to many of the new technologies, because the cost is prohibitive. Despite all the technological advances, the medical community has been unable to reverse the damage associated with society's unhealthy lifestyle. This fact, coupled with rapidly rising health care costs, has prompted millions of individuals to assume a more active role in safeguarding their own health. Evidence of this change in attitude can be seen in the growing interest in nutrition, physical fitness, and stress management. If we as a nation are to capitalize on this new health consciousness, then we must devote more time and energy to educating Americans in the health sciences so they will be better able to make informed choices about their health.

Health is such a complex and dynamic subject that it is practically impossible for anyone to stay abreast of all the current research findings. For this reason, Americans have generally come to rely on the public press for information on major health issues. Unfortunately, the quality of information presented in some health articles is questionable at best, and in many cases it is totally inaccurate. If consumers are to make wise decisions about their health based on information such as this, then they must possess the skills necessary to sort out fact from conjecture. *Annual Editions: Health 94/95* was designed to aid in this task. It presents a sampling of quality articles that represent current thinking on a variety of health issues, and it serves as a tool for developing critical thinking skills.

The articles in this volume were carefully chosen on the basis of their quality and timeliness. Because this book is revised and updated annually, it contains information that is not currently available in any standard textbook. Thus, it serves as a valuable resource for both teachers and students. The book itself is divided into topical areas that are commonly covered in introductory health courses. These nine areas are *America's Health and the Health Care System, Contemporary Health Hazards, Stress and Mental Health, Drugs and Health, Nutritional Health, Exercise and Weight Control, Current Killers, Human Sexuality,* and *Consumer Health.* Because of the interdependence of the various elements that constitute health, the articles selected were written by naturalists, environmentalists, psychologists, economists, sociologists, nutritionists, consumer advocates, and traditional health practitioners. The diversity of these selections provides the reader with a variety of points of view regarding health and the complexity of the issues involved.

Annual Editions: Health 94/95 is one of the most useful and up-to-date publications currently available in the area of health. Please let us know what you think of it by filling out and returning the postage-paid article rating form on the last page of this book. Any anthology can be improved. This one will be—annually.

Richard Yarian

Richard Yarian
Editor

Contents

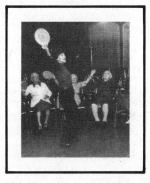

Unit 1

America's Health and the Health Care System

Six selections discuss the current state of health care in today's society by focusing on self-care, health care costs, and the health care industry.

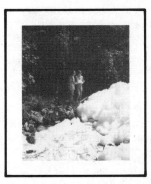

Unit 2

Contemporary Health Hazards

Six articles examine hazards that affect our health and are encountered in today's world.

The concepts in bold italics are developed in the article. For further expansion please refer to the Topic Guide and the Index.

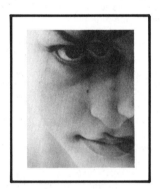

Unit

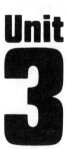

Stress and Mental Health

Five selections consider the impact of stress and emotions on mental health.

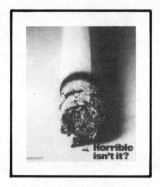

Unit 4

Drugs and Health

Seven articles examine how drugs affect our lives. Subjects discussed include the dangers of tobacco, alcohol, and the potential hazards of over-the-counter medications.

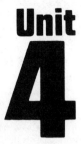

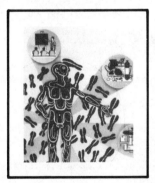

Unit 5

Nutritional Health

Five articles discuss the effects of diet and nutrition on a person's well-being. The topics include the link between diet and disease, fat in the diet, and latest recommended dietary allowances.

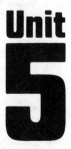

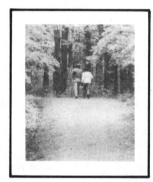

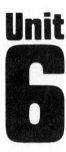

Unit

6

Exercise and Weight Control

Five articles examine the influence of exercise and diet on health. Topics discussed include walking as the latest form of exercise, how to stay with an exercise program, eating disorders, and dieting myths.

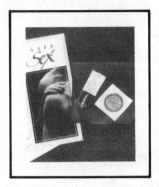
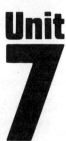

Unit 7

Current Killers

Eight selections examine the major causes of death in the Western world. Heart attack, stroke, cancer, and AIDS are discussed.

The concepts in bold italics are developed in the article. For further expansion please refer to the Topic Guide and the Index.

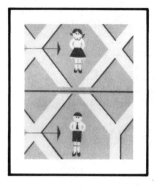

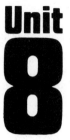

Unit 8

Human Sexuality

Five articles discuss the most recent research on human reproduction and sexuality. The selections consider sex differences, sexual violence, birth control, and sexual myths.

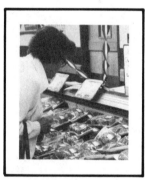

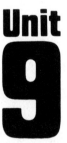

Unit 9

Consumer Health

Seven selections examine how food labeling, cholesterol testing, and food and drug interactions relate to consumer health.

The concepts in bold italics are developed in the article. For further expansion please refer to the Topic Guide and the Index.

The concepts in bold italics are developed in the article. For further expansion please refer to the Topic Guide and the Index.

Topic Guide

This topic guide suggests how the selections in this book relate to topics of traditional concern to health students and professionals. It is very useful for locating articles that relate to each other for reading and research. The guide is arranged alphabetically according to topic. Articles may, of course, treat topics that do not appear in the topic guide. In turn, entries in the topic guide do not necessarily constitute a comprehensive listing of all the contents of each selection.

TOPIC AREA	TREATED IN:	TOPIC AREA	TREATED IN:
Abortion	45. New, Improved and Ready for Battle	**Consumer Health (cont'd)**	19. Food and Drugs That Don't Mix 20. Rx to OTC 48. 'Nutrition Facts' 49. 'Daily Values' 50. Full Sun Protection 51. Purist's Guide to Tap Water 52. Patient, Treat Thyself 53. Preventing STDs 54. Top Medical Centers
Addiction	17. Mindset of Health 23. Alcohol and Tobacco 24. Alcohol in Perspective		
AIDS (Acquired Immune Deficiency Syndrome)	4. Unclogging the Drug Pipeline 10. Sleeping with the Enemy 41. Confronting the AIDS Pandemic 42. Long Shot 44. Female Condom 46. It's Not Just AIDS	**Depression**	47. How Do You Know If It's PMS?
		Dietary Fat	25. How's Your Diet? 26. Eating Right 28. New Thinking About Fats 29. Snack Attack 36. Cholesterol 37. "Diseasing" of Risk Factors 40. Eat to Beat Cancer 49. 'Daily Values'
Alcohol	17. Mindset of Health 23. Alcohol and Tobacco 24. Alcohol in Perspective 26. Eating Right 40. Eat to Beat Cancer		
Anti-Oxidants	36. Cholesterol 40. Eat to Beat Cancer	**Dietary Fiber**	25. How's Your Diet? 26. Eating Right 40. Eat to Beat Cancer 49. 'Daily Values'
Birth Control/ Contraception	44. Female Condom 46. It's Not Just AIDS 53. Preventing STDs	**Dietary Minerals**	26. Eating Right 27. To Salt or Not to Salt 48. 'Nutrition Facts' 49. 'Daily Values'
Birth Defects	24. Alcohol in Perspective		
Blood Fats/ Serum Cholesterol	36. Cholesterol 37. "Diseasing" of Risk Factors	**Dietary Salt**	25. How's Your Diet? 27. To Salt or Not to Salt
Cancer	4. Unclogging the Drug Pipeline 7. Beach Bummer 9. Dangerous Liaison 10. Sleeping with the Enemy 15. Mind Over Malady 17. Mindset of Health 23. Alcohol and Tobacco 24. Alcohol in Perspective 26. Eating Right 28. New Thinking About Fats 35. Your Health History 39. From Here to Immunity 40. Eat to Beat Cancer 45. New, Improved and Ready for Battle 50. Full Sun Protection 51. Purist's Guide to Tap Water	**Drugs**	4. Unclogging the Drug Pipeline 18. Ordinary Medicines 19. Food and Drugs That Don't Mix 20. Rx to OTC 21. Placebo Effect 22. Saying Goodbye to an Old Flame 23. Alcohol and Tobacco
		Environmental Health Hazards	7. Beach Bummer 8. Gut Reactions 50. Full Sun Protection 51. Purist's Guide to Tap Water
		Exercise	30. To Be Active or Not to Be Active 31. Exercise Without Injury 32. Walk Off Calories and Get Fit 33. Losing Weight 36. Cholesterol 38. Pressure Treatment 39. From Here to Immunity 40. Eat to Beat Cancer
Cardiovascular Disease	13. Stress 16. How Anger Affects Your Health 24. Alcohol in Perspective 26. Eating Right 30. To Be Active or Not to Be Active 33. Losing Weight 36. Cholesterol 37. "Diseasing" of Risk Factors 38. Pressure Treatment		
		Food Labeling	48. 'Nutrition Facts' 49. 'Daily Values'
Consumer Health	7. Beach Bummer 18. Ordinary Medicines	**Genetics**	33. Losing Weight 35. Your Health History

TOPIC AREA	TREATED IN:	TOPIC AREA	TREATED IN:
Health Behavior	22. Saying Goodbye to an Old Flame	**Mental Health and Stress**	6. Mainstreaming of Alternative Medicine 13. Stress 14. Slow Down, You Breath Too Fast 15. Mind Over Malady 16. How Anger Affects Your Health 17. Mindset of Health 30. To Be Active or Not to Be Active 34. Chemistry and Craving 36. Cholesterol 47. How Do You Know If It's PMS?
Health Care Costs	1. Wasted Health Care Dollars 2. Clinton Cure 3. Healthtown, U.S.A. 4. Unclogging the Drug Pipeline 5. Keeping Score 6. Mainstreaming of Alternative Medicine 41. Confronting the AIDS Pandemic 52. Patient, Treat Thyself 54. Top Medical Centers		
		Nutrition	26. Eating Right 28. New Thinking About Fats 29. Snack Attack 33. Losing Weight 36. Cholesterol 48. 'Nutrition Facts' 49. 'Daily Values'
Health Promotion and Preventative Medicine	13. Stress 25. How's Your Diet? 37. "Diseasing" of Risk Factors 39. From Here to Immunity 41. Confronting the AIDS Pandemic		
		Osteoporosis	26. Eating Right 30. To Be Active or Not to Be Active
Health Risk Analysis	33. Losing Weight 35. Your Health History 36. Cholesterol 37. "Diseasing" of Risk Factors	**Personality and Disease/Type A Personality**	13. Stress 16. How Anger Affects Your Health
Health Statistics	5. Keeping Score 31. Exercise Without Injury 41. Confronting the AIDS Pandemic	**Radiation**	7. Beach Bummer 50. Full Sun Protection
Hypertension	24. Alcohol in Perspective 27. To Salt or Not to Salt 30. To Be Active or Not to Be Active 36. Cholesterol 37. "Diseasing" of Risk Factors 38. Pressure Treatment	**Rape**	12. What Every Woman Needs to Know
		Sexual Behavior	10. Sleeping with the Enemy 43. Mating Game 44. Female Condom 46. It's Not Just AIDS 53. Preventing STDs
Immunity	6. Mainstreaming of Alternative Medicine 13. Stress 15. Mind Over Malady 39. From Here to Immunity 42. Long Shot	**Sexually Transmitted Diseases (STDs)**	9. Dangerous Liaison 10. Sleeping with the Enemy 11. ABC's of Hepatitis 41. Confronting the AIDS Pandemic 42. Long Shot 44. Female Condom 46. It's Not Just AIDS 53. Preventing STDs
Infectious Illness	8. Gut Reactions 9. Dangerous Liaison 10. Sleeping with the Enemy 11. ABC's of Hepatitis 39. From Here to Immunity 41. Confronting the AIDS Pandemic 42. Long Shot		
		Tobacco and Health	17. Mindset of Health 22. Saying Goodbye to an Old Flame 23. Alcohol and Tobacco 30. To Be Active or Not to Be Active 36. Cholesterol
Longevity	33. Losing Weight 35. Your Health History 37. "Diseasing" of Risk Factors		
Medical Concerns and Ethics	1. Wasted Health Care Dollars 5. Keeping Score 6. Mainstreaming of Alternative Medicine 18. Ordinary Medicines 19. Food and Drugs That Don't Mix 20. Rx to OTC 21. Placebo Effect 37. "Diseasing" of Risk Factors 42. Long Shot 52. Patient, Treat Thyself 54. Top Medical Centers	**Vitamins**	25. How's Your Diet? 26. Eating Right 28. New Thinking About Fats 36. Cholesterol 40. Eat to Beat Cancer 48. 'Nutrition Facts' 49. 'Daily Values'
		Weight Control	26. Eating Right 29. Snack Attack 30. To Be Active or Not to Be Active 32. Walk Off Calories and Get Fit 33. Losing Weight 34. Chemistry and Craving 36. Cholesterol 38. Pressure Treatment

America's Health and the Health Care System

Americans are healthier today than at any time in this nation's history. Americans suffer more illness today than at any time in this nation's history. Which statement is true? They both are, depending on the statistics you quote. According to longevity statistics, Americans are living longer today and, therefore, must be healthier. Still other statistics indicate that Americans of today report twice as many acute illnesses as did our ancestors 60 years ago. They now also report that their pains last longer. Unfortunately, this combination of living longer and feeling sicker places additional demands on a health care system that, according to experts, is already in a state of crisis. How severe is the health care crisis? What has caused it? Who is responsible? What can and should be done to solve it? This unit will attempt to explore these questions and present some possible solutions along the way.

From the discovery of the smallpox vaccine and penicillin to the first heart transplant, the marriage of modern medicine and science has seemed a perfect match. Over the last 30 years, Americans have witnessed some remarkable scientific breakthroughs that have revolutionized the diagnosis and treatment of a variety of illnesses. While these advances have established America as the leader in medical technology, waste, inefficiency, and greed have so corrupted the system that despite the advances, millions of Americans can no longer afford basic health care.

To better understand the gravity of the problem consider this: Americans spent over $817 billion on health care in 1992 (approximately 14 percent of the GNP). If health care costs continue to grow at this rate for the next 40 years, they will account for 37 percent of the GNP by the year 2030. Despite spending all this money, 28 percent of Americans have no health care insurance, and over 35 million Americans are underinsured. Albeit spending more than twice as much per capita on health care as the average for industrialized nations, the United States ranks 21st in infant mortality, 17th in male life expectancy, and 16th in female life expectancy.

Why have health care costs risen so high? The answer to this question is multifaceted, and includes such factors as hospital costs, physician's fees, insurance costs, pharmaceutical costs, and health fraud. While these factors operate within any health care system, in the United States these components of health care are compartmentalized to protect their own individual needs, rather than integrated into a system promoting quality and economy. Clearly any organizational system for health care is bound to have a certain amount of waste and inefficiency, but amounts as high as 20 percent are outrageous and the United States has the distinction of having the most wasteful and inefficient health care system among industrialized nations.

Physician's fees account for approximately 19 percent of the total amount spent on health care. While this figure may not appear excessive, it is a multidimensional factor that involves much more than simply the cost of the service rendered by a doctor. The fee-for-service that doctors charge has risen in response to reimbursement through third-party payments plans such as Medicare and private health insurance.

The third-party payment plan has not only reduced incentives to keep prices affordable, but it also changed the very nature of medicine itself. Today, private physicians must spend increasing amounts of time and money on the business aspect of their practice just to keep up with the increasing demands of third-party reviews, regulations, and paperwork. Many private physicians' clerical staff outnumber their clinical staff. This cost is passed on as fee-for-service, but contributes nothing to the quality of health care. Another expense incurred by the private physician that is passed along in the fee-for-service is the cost of malpractice insurance. The threat of malpractice suits has also led to wasted health care dollars through the practice of defensive medicine, in which physicians order unnecessary medical tests for their patients as a hedge against litigation. In addition to wasting billions of dollars, this subjects patients to additional risks. Malpractice claims have become so common in certain areas of medicine that many doctors have terminated their practice in these areas for fear of litigation.

Hospitals also contribute to the high cost of health care in the United States. They account for approximately 38 percent of all health care expenditures, so reducing hospital costs could significantly reduce the cost of health care. The concept of supply and demand normally dictates that as supply exceeds demand, the price drops. Unfortunately, the reverse is true in the case of hospitals. Studies have found that as the number of hospitals increases in a given region, the cost of hospitalization rises. It has been estimated that 15 to 30 percent of hospitalization is unwarranted and merely wastes health care dollars. Also, approximately 20 percent of a hospital's budget is spent on billing, and this figure might be cut substantially if the United States were to adopt nationalized health care.

One area of health care costs that is often considered immutable is the cost of medical technology and pharmaceuticals. Americans pay substantially higher prices for pharmaceuticals and diagnostic tests than do people in any other industrialized country. The manufacturers argue that these prices are necessary if they are to continue to pour large sums of money into research and development in order to satisfy the stringent guidelines established by the FDA. Perhaps it is time to let the rest of the world contribute their fair share to the research and development costs. Recent changes by the FDA regarding the approval and licensing of new drugs should significantly reduce the cost of bringing them to market. The pharmaceutical companies could respond by lowering their prices. Jon Hamilton's article "Unclogging the Drug Pipeline" discusses how and why changes in the FDA's approval program will significantly shorten the time needed to get new drugs approved, while maintaining high quality standards.

For years, researchers and health care officials believed that high-tech medicine would reduce medical care costs by providing safer, less expensive procedures. While some new procedures may be safer, they have not always replaced existing ones, and instead they are often used in conjunction with them. The result is a compounding of health care costs, with marginal gains in therapeutic effectiveness. In other cases, new technologies have provided doctors with a means to treat disorders that were previously untreatable. These cases have a twofold effect on raising medical costs: First, the cost of the life-saving procedure, and second, the cost of the additional health care that will be needed by these patients, since they will live longer.

Despite all our technology, and the vast sums we spend on health care, health statistics such as infant mortality are disturbingly poor. Resources are devoted to advancing new technologies rather than primary prevention programs. While it is not desirable to eliminate high-tech medical care, we must carefully consider its role in our health care system. (Given the economic realities of today, some major changes in our approach to health care spending are necessary if we are to provide the American public with quality care at a reasonable cost.)

The United States now has a president who advocates health care reform, and there appears to be bipartisan congressional support for such reform. President Clinton has submitted a nationalized health care plan to Congress. The Clinton plan seeks to establish a base level of health care for all Americans, while attempting cost containment through reforms that would significantly reduce bureaucratic red tape, fraud, and greed. It is unlikely that the Clinton plan will be adopted in its original form, but at least it has started the reform ball rolling. The article "The Clinton Cure" discusses this plan. "Healthtown U.S.A." provides a graphical representation of the Clinton plan.

The real challenge is to find solutions that can control the costs and yet provide high quality health care for all. Critics of nationalized health care argue that it limits patients' choices and results in a rationing of services. While the rationing aspect may be true, it is already present in our current system. The article "Wasted Health Care Dollars" discusses why our health care is so expensive and suggests that perhaps the best solution is to scrap our current system and start anew. David Zinman's article "Keeping Score" discusses how outcomes accountability, in which doctors and hospitals are rated based on quality of services rendered, can have a positive impact on health care quality. At this time the exact nature of health care reform is uncertain, but one thing is clear, change is coming.

Looking Ahead: Challenge Questions

Is health care just another commodity? Should it be treated differently from other consumer services?

Is quality health care a right or a privilege?

How have third-party payments contributed to the rising cost of health care in America?

What can you as an individual do to help reduce health care costs? Give specific actions that can be taken.

How have hospitals contributed to the rising cost of health care?

What are the strengths and weaknesses of the Clinton plan for health care reform?

Is the FDA acting responsibly by instituting an accelerated approval program? Should this program be expanded to include all new drugs?

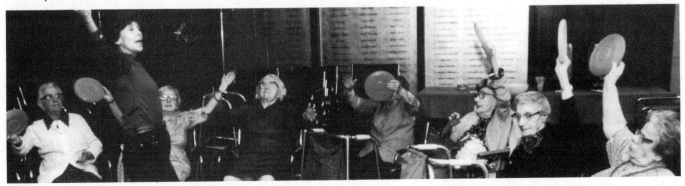

WASTED HEALTH CARE DOLLARS

The U.S. is spending enough to bring every citizen high-quality, high-tech medical care—if we stop squandering our resources.

Less waste, longer lives
"Look at the rest of the industrial world. On average, they spend half as much as we do on health care. They cover everyone and live longer. It's waste. There's no other explanation."
—Alan Sager, health economist, Boston University School of Public Health

Of the $817-billion that we will spend this year on health care, we will throw away at least $200-billion on overpriced, useless, even harmful treatments, and on a bloated bureaucracy. We are no healthier than the citizens of comparable developed countries that spend half what we do and provide health care for everybody. In fact, by important measures such as life expectancy and infant mortality, we are far down the list.

If the wasted money could be redirected, the U.S. could include those now shut out of the system—without increasing the total outlay for health care and without restricting the availability of $100,000 bone-marrow transplants or $40,000 heart operations to those relatively few who need them.

"I can't imagine a system that's more dysfunctional than the one we have now—more expensive, not doing the job, with more waste," says Dr. Philip Caper, an internist and medical policy analyst at Dartmouth Medical School. Although the total amount of waste in our health-care system is difficult to estimate, researchers have now examined many of the system's components, with consistent results. For a wide range of clinical procedures, on average, roughly 20 percent of the money we now spend could be saved with no loss in the quality of care. By restructuring the system, we could also save almost half of the huge amount we now spend on administrative costs (see "The $200-Billion Bottom Line"). A more efficient system would also make it much easier to detect health-care fraud—a problem that the U.S. General Accounting Office has estimated to cost tens of billions of dollars a year.

While these facts are well known to students of the health-care system, they've been remarkably absent from the debate that's developing over health care in this election year. Politicians and lobbyists for health-care providers have presented the public with a daunting choice: If we want to provide every American with access to health care, they say, we'll either have to pay much more into the system or accept lower-quality medical services.

However, such scenarios assume that the current price structure for medical care, and the current patterns of treatment and hospitalization, will remain fixed. They needn't, and they shouldn't. Our health-care system is so inherently wasteful and inefficient that a complete overhaul is an option worth contemplating. It may, in fact, be the only option that makes sense.

The waste in the system comes from many sources. We receive a great deal of care that we don't need at all. The care we do need is delivered inefficiently. And the futile effort to control a runaway system has created a huge bureaucracy that by itself sucks up more than a hundred billion dollars a year.

30 years of increases

By now, it's hardly news that health costs have spiraled out of control. Health care now consumes about 16 percent of state and local tax revenues. In the years since 1986, private businesses have spent about as much on health care as they earned in after-tax profits. For small businesses, insurance has become unaffordable; three of four concerns employing 10 or fewer people simply don't provide health bene-

---

This report [Part 1 of a 3-part series] examines the forces behind the current crisis in health-care costs. The next two reports in this special series will look at the possible solutions [see *Consumer Reports,* August and September, 1992].

One approach to cost control, pioneered by health maintenance organizations, is to "manage" medical care in detail. The management can include such practices as restricting patients to a single primary-care doctor who must approve all specialist referrals; penalizing doctors who order too many tests or procedures; and preapproving elective hospitalizations. In our next report, we'll rate HMOs and examine how well managed care actually contains costs.

Another approach is to set overall spending limits and stick to them, while otherwise leaving doctors and hospitals to practice as they see fit. That's what other industrialized countries, including Canada, do in various ways. Part three of our health-care series, [in] the September issue, will take a close look at the Canadian system, among others, and will analyze the criticisms that have been leveled against it by U.S. health-care providers and insurers.

Finally, we'll outline the health-care reform proposal that Consumers Union favors as providing the best combination of universal access, quality care, and cost containment.

fits. At any given time, roughly 35 million Americans—most of them employees of small businesses or their dependents—have no health coverage at all.

Over the last 10 years, Government and private business, appalled to see health care absorbing an ever-growing portion of their revenues, have tried to get a grip on its costs in various ways. But costs have risen as fast as ever. "As quickly as payers patch the system up, the providers find the spaces between the patches," says Maryann O'Sullivan, director of Health Access, a California consumer coalition.

Our health-care system doesn't just allow prices to rise—it practically demands that they do. Although some recent reforms have had a modest effect, the system has traditionally allowed doctors to order whatever procedures they want, and has paid both doctors and hospitals whatever they think they should get.

In both respects, the American system stands alone in the developed world. Though the particulars of their systems differ, Canada, Japan, and the Western European countries all have adopted universal, standard payment schedules set by direct negotiation with doctors and hospitals. In addition, most have set an overall ceiling on national medical expenditures. As a result, not a single developed country other than the U.S. devotes more than 10 percent of its gross national product to health care. The U.S. broke that barrier in 1985; this year, the nation will spend 14 percent of the GNP on health.

It wasn't always so. Back in 1960, the U.S. spent a modest 5.3 percent of its GNP on health care, about the same as other industrialized nations like Canada or Germany did at the time. What changed everything was the advent in 1965 of Medicare, which ultimately had implications far beyond the over-65 population it served.

Before Medicare, private insurance companies covered the population less extensively than they do today. All the insurers left treatment completely to the doctor's discretion and provided reimbursement for any test or treatment a physician ordered. But because a large percentage of people had only hospital coverage, and no insurance to cover doctors' bills, physicians tended to keep fees at affordable levels.

In 1965, Congress enacted Medicare, the vast, Government-financed

High-tech without high costs
Although they control health-care costs much more effectively than the U.S., other developed countries still provide high-tech care to those who need it. Between 1988 and 1990, Canada, France, Australia, and Israel all did more bone-marrow transplants per capita than the U.S.

THE $200-BILLION BOTTOM LINE

To date, no one has come up with a comprehensive price tag for the cost of unnecessary medical care, overpriced procedures, and inefficient administration in the U.S. health-care system. After extensive review of the literature, however, we believe that $200-billion is a conservative estimate of the amount the health-care system will waste this year. Here's why.

Of the $817-billion projected to be spent on health care this year, about one fifth—$163-billion—will go for administrative costs. Except for a fraction of a percent spent on research, the rest—roughly $650-billion—will go to actual patient care. Physician and hospital services together make up most of that total, with the rest going to dentists, nursing homes, drugs, and various other expenses.

By our estimates, at least 20 percent of that $650-billion, or $130-billion, will be spent on procedures and services that are clearly unnecessary.

Many researchers have now attempted to quantify the rate at which specific procedures are used unnecessarily. Twenty percent represents a rough average of the rates found in major studies, and is a figure that several leading researchers in this field told us was a good approximation for the rate of unnecessary care.

Twenty percent also seems to be a conservative estimate of the rate of unnecessary hospital days, even though changes in Medicare and private-insurance policies make it difficult to estimate that number precisely.

Finally, as Dr. John Wennberg of Dartmouth and his colleagues have demonstrated repeatedly, the rate at which physicians use a given procedure can vary four- or five-fold between one location and another. The supply of hospitals and physicians also varies greatly. Except in extreme cases where people lack access to basic medical care, people living in low-use or low-supply areas seem to be just as healthy as those in high-use or high-supply areas.

Dr. Wennberg and his colleagues argue that areas with abundant doctors and hospitals could provide significantly fewer health-care services without

harmful consequences. Similarly, the high rates of procedures done in many areas could be cut back without overall harm. This sort of adjustment happens automatically, they note, in industrialized countries that control costs by capping the amount of money available for health care.

If overuse of medical services wastes $130-billion a year, administrative inefficiency adds about $70-billion. Projecting from 1991 estimates by the General Accounting Office, the U.S. could save roughly $70-billion this year by switching from our fragmented and inefficient insurance system to a single-payer system—one in which all citizens receive health care from private doctors and hospitals that are paid by a single insurance entity. The savings would come roughly equally from insurance-company overhead and hospital and administrative costs.

Adding those two figures together—$130-billion plus $70-billion—gives an estimate of $200-billion for the annual waste in the U.S. health-care system. This estimate, however, leaves out several important elements: Physicians' fees and the cost of technology, drugs, and procedures. If those costs were brought into line with reimbursement standards in other countries, the savings would be greater.

Moreover, we have not added in the cost of outright fraud—a factor that the General Accounting Office estimates could eat up a full 10 percent of the total health-care budget.

Some physicians cheat the system by ordering unnecessary tests and procedures—a type of fraud that is included in our estimates of unnecessary care. Other types of fraud, however, would not have been caught in the studies of unnecessary care that have been done. These include billing for services never rendered, falsifying reimbursement codes to collect more than the usual payment for a service, and submitting inflated bills for supplies and medical devices.

Since we have not counted the cost of these fraudulent practices—or of the high price scale for health-care providers in the U.S.—our $200-billion figure is truly a minimum estimate.

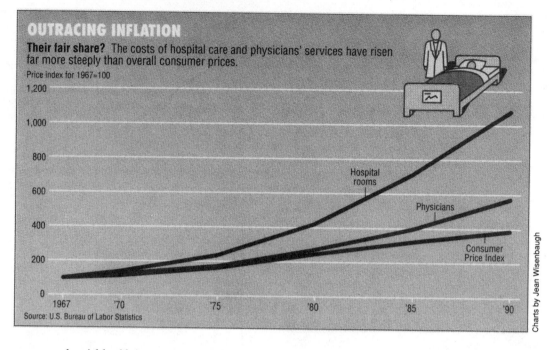

OUTRACING INFLATION

Their fair share? The costs of hospital care and physicians' services have risen far more steeply than overall consumer prices.

Price index for 1967=100

Hospital rooms

Physicians

Consumer Price Index

1967   '70   '75   '80   '85   '90

Source: U.S. Bureau of Labor Statistics

Charts by Jean Wisenbaugh

program of social health insurance for the elderly, along with the less extensive Medicaid program, in which the Federal Government shares costs with the states. In order to overcome the powerful, sustained opposition of doctors and hospitals to what they called "socialized medicine," Congress made a fateful—and, in retrospect, very expensive—decision. Under Medicare, all doctors were paid on the basis of their "usual and customary" fees for a given service (the system that Blue Shield was already using).

This approach, which allowed each individual physician to name his or her own price, soon became universal throughout the insurance industry. So as more and more employers began offering major-medical plans that covered doctors' bills, they bought into a system with no effective constraints on costs. Predictably, doctors' fees began a rapid upward climb.

Hospitals profited as well. Under Blue Cross, which had dominated hospital insurance, hospitals were paid only a daily room charge, plus additional fees for various services, tests, and supplies. Under Medicare, however, the hospitals were not only able to collect their actual charges; for the first time, they were allowed to build the cost of capital improvements into their rates. Hospitals, which had been receiving Federal subsidies for growth since the late 1940s, now got another incentive to expand.

After Medicare, U.S. health-care expenditures turned more sharply

upward. For a time—perhaps a decade or more—no one seemed to notice or care. But over the past 10 years or so, as costs have become truly staggering, the system has begun to change. Medicare has set limits on physicians' fees for several years, and private insurance companies have begun reviewing many procedures doctors perform before they will pay for them. Medicaid budgets have been steadily cut back, to the point where many states now pay doctors and hospitals less than the cost of delivering care.

Experience has shown, however, that attempts to manage the health-care system a piece at a time are likely to fail. Physicians and hospitals can charge their privately insured patients more to make up for Medicare's fee restrictions. And doctors and patients alike have resisted efforts by insurance companies to determine what is appropriate and necessary treatment, having grown used to a system that has provided as much medical care—to the insured population, that is—as anybody wants.

No sense of limits

Having operated for years under a system that sets virtually no limit on what can be done or what can be charged, both doctors and patients have been seduced by the idea that, when it comes to treating sickness, it's necessary to do "everything."

"We want more. We want more time with the doctor. We want more procedures. We want more pills," says Randall Bovbjerg, a health-

policy analyst at the Urban Institute in Washington, D.C. "We can't sit and watch the course of a cold; we go and buy tons of things we aren't even certain will make it better."

"Imagine if we sold auto-purchase insurance and said, go and buy whatever car you want and we'll pay 80 percent of it," says James C. Robinson, a health-care economist at the University of California, Berkeley. Under those conditions, a lot of people would go buy a Mercedes.

Much of the time, physicians will order more tests and procedures out of a genuine desire to do whatever they can for their patients. "Doctors look at one patient at a time and think, 'If I've done one thing, what else can I try?'" says Ann Lennarson Greer, a medical sociologist at the University of Wisconsin. "They're not inclined to think about overall costs." Several studies, in fact, have asked doctors if they knew the costs of hospital tests and services they routinely ordered—and found many had only a vague idea at best.

But while extra tests and treatments drive up the cost of medical care, they may do so with no real benefit to the patient. New diagnostic technologies, in particular, are especially likely to be overused; unlike surgery or invasive procedures, they "don't require the clinician to take any real risk," Greer says. Thus, the use of computerized tomography (CT) and magnetic resonance imaging (MRI) scans, two expensive, relatively new imaging technologies, has grown explosively in recent years. Yet no one has clearly defined when they are useful and when they are a waste of time and money.

"The original CT scanner proved to be an absolute revolution in the treatment of patients with head injury," says Dr. Mark Chassin, a physician who is senior vice president of Value Health Sciences, a private firm that analyzes the use of health-care services. "We produced hundreds of these things and they got out in the community. They were used for people with head trauma—terrific—but they also were used for people with headaches, dizziness, and all sorts of other vague symptoms." Diagnostic imaging, says Dr. Chassin, is a prime example of how "we continue to invest in technology in an absolutely irrational way."

The law of induced demand

Medical care is totally unlike services delivered by other professionals. When clients hire an architect or a lawyer, they generally know what they need and roughly how much it's going to cost. But in medicine, physicians make virtually all the decisions that determine the cost of care. The patient, ill and uninformed, is in no position to do comparison shopping—nor motivated to, if insurance is paying the bill.

And the more doctors do, the more they get paid—a situation that's tailor-made for cost escalation. "It's the easiest thing in the world to increase the volume [of things a doctor does]," says Dr. Philip Caper, the Dartmouth internist. "Just do a few more tests. There's always a rationale. Schedule three doctor visits instead of two, and reduce the time you spend on each visit."

The creation of medical "need" by those who then profit from it is called induced demand, and it's rampant. Most obvious is the problem of "self-referral," in which physicians will refer patients for treatment at facilities in which they have a financial interest. In Florida, where at least 40 percent of physicians have such investments, a study by professors at Florida State University found that physician-owned laboratories performed twice as many tests per patient as independent labs. Similarly, in a study of private health insurance claims records for more than 65,000 patients, University of Arizona researchers found that doctors who had diagnostic imaging equipment in their offices ordered four times more imaging exams than doctors who

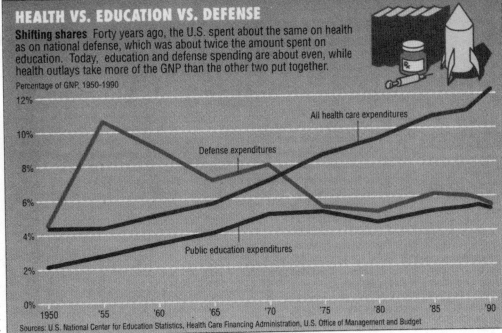

HEALTH VS. EDUCATION VS. DEFENSE

Shifting shares Forty years ago, the U.S. spent about the same on health as on national defense, which was about twice the amount spent on education. Today, education and defense spending are about even, while health outlays take more of the GNP than the other two put together.

Percentage of GNP, 1950-1990

All health care expenditures

Defense expenditures

Public education expenditures

12%
10%
8%
6%
4%
2%
0%

1950   '55   '60   '65   '70   '75   '80   '85   '90

Sources: U.S. National Center for Education Statistics, Health Care Financing Administration, U.S. Office of Management and Budget

referred patients elsewhere for the tests.

Occasionally, self-referral can turn into actual fraud. A recent report by the General Accounting Office—which estimated that fraud may account for as much as 10 percent of all health-care costs—cited several examples in which self-referral had been abused. In one California case, the owners of mobile medical laboratories allegedly gave kickbacks for referrals to physicians who sometimes used phony diagnoses. The case, which is still being investigated, involves an estimated $1-billion in fraudulent billings.

In other cases, however, physicians may increase the demand for their services without even being aware of it. When it comes to American medical care, supply seems to create demand almost automatically. Actuarial studies have shown that in areas with the greatest supply of physicians, people simply go to the doctor more often.

If more physicians create more demand for medical care, we can look forward to a flood of it in the near future. The per capita supply of practicing physicians is expected to increase 22 percent between now and the year 2000.

The phenomenon of induced demand applies to hospitals, too. Dr. John Wennberg, a physician who is professor of family and community medicine at Dartmouth Medical School, was curious as to why people in Boston went to the hospital more

frequently than people in New Haven. When he studied the problem, he found a simple answer: Boston has more hospital beds to be filled—one-third more than New Haven on a per capita basis.

Surprisingly, Dr. Wennberg found that physicians in Boston and New Haven were completely unaware of the discrepancy. When he asked doctors in New Haven whether they felt their area was short of hospital beds, they said they didn't. In fact, at any given time, about 85 percent of hospital beds in New Haven were filled—precisely the same percentage as in Boston.

The likely explanation, according to Dr. Wennberg, is that physicians almost unconsciously will refer their patients to the hospital if space is available, stopping only when the local hospitals' capacity is nearly used up. If many beds are empty, doctors will be more likely to refer patients with borderline conditions, such as gastroenteritis or acute low back pain, for which hospitalization is optional but not imperative. By doing so, of course, they drive up the cost of care.

An unnecessary burden

With so many incentives to overtreat patients, it seems inevitable that a sizable fraction of American medical care must be simply unnecessary, if not downright harmful. But how large a fraction? In the late 1970s and early 1980s, researchers at the Rand

Growth without limits
The Health Industry Manufacturers Association, a medical-equipment trade group, predicts a 7.4 percent annual growth rate for health technology throughout this decade—unless "negative scenarios," such as more safety regulation and cost containment, take effect.

MEDICAL RED FLAGS

IS THIS TREATMENT NECESSARY?

Over the past decade or so, an entire industry has sprung up to identify overused and unnecessary medical treatments. The players range from academic researchers to policy analysts to private entrepreneurs that have insurance companies as their clients.

Some treatments, by virtue of their cost or their ubiquity, have attracted particular attention from the watchdogs. These treatments, listed below, are hardly the only sources of unnecessary care in the system. Nor, of course, does a procedure's presence on the list mean that it is always used unnecessarily—or even that that is usually the case.

Nevertheless, if your physician does suggest that you have one of these procedures, you'd be well advised to think twice. You might want to seek a second opinion, if possible, or question your doctor closely on the possible alternatives to the suggested treatment.

Cesarean section. About one in four U.S. births is completed surgically, a rate that may be twice the ideal. In this country, obstetricians routinely perform cesareans when the baby is breech, or for the vaguely defined diagnoses of "prolonged labor" or "fetal distress." Hospitals that have systematically set out to eliminate unnecessary cesareans have cut their rate at least in half without any apparent risk to mothers or babies. (See CONSUMER REPORTS, February 1991.)

In recent years, the electronic fetal monitor, a device for tracking the fetal heart rate during labor, has come to be used routinely in American hospitals—and has contributed to the high cesarean-section rate. Since abnormal fetal heart rates

are associated with oxygen deprivation, it was assumed that prompt, automatic detection would enable doctors to intervene early enough to prevent fetal brain damage—for example, by performing a cesarean section on the mother.

But since the fetal monitor's introduction, no fewer than nine comparative studies, involving tens of thousands of women, have failed to demonstrate the hoped-for benefit. Monitored women do have a higher rate of cesarean sections and other costly interventions. But their babies fare no better than those of women monitored by the traditional means, in which a nurse simply checks the fetal heartbeat periodically with a stethoscope.

Hysterectomy. After cesarean section, this is the second most common major surgery in the U.S. Value Health Sciences, a firm that applies the Rand Corp.'s methodology for insurance-industry clients, calls 27 percent of hysterectomies unnecessary, the highest percentage of all procedures it evaluates. Rates of hysterectomy also vary greatly throughout the country, an indication that physician practice and preference play as much of a role as objective need in the decision to perform the operation. Many gynecologists still routinely recommend hysterectomy for fibroids, uterine prolapse, and heavy bleeding; alternative treatments are available for all three conditions. (See CONSUMER REPORTS, September 1990).

Back surgery. Value Health Sciences has reported that 14 percent of proposed laminectomies, the most common type of back surgery, are unnecessary. Occasionally, some material from a ruptured disc will press on spinal nerves and cause

disabling or painful symptoms that require surgical correction, says Dr. Charles Fager, a neurosurgeon at the Lahey Clinic in Burlington, Mass. But usually, back pain yields to bed rest, the passage of time, physical therapy, or a combination thereof. "I only operate on one out of every 25 or 30 people I see," says Dr. Fager. Some surgeons aren't so finicky. Dr. John Wennberg of Dartmouth Medical School has traced sudden "epidemics" of back surgery to the arrival of a new neurosurgeon in a locality.

Magnetic resonance imaging. This powerful new imaging technique, which produces detailed pictures of internal organs without exposing the patient to radiation, is still so new that doctors are working out its best uses. In the process, they'll inevitably use it when they don't need to. Some groups of physicians have invested in MRI machines, creating the added temptation to profit by referring their patients for the test. Also, because MRI is virtually risk-free, it's especially likely to be overused as a defensive measure.

Experts stress that MRI procedures, which cost about $1000 apiece, should be ordered only when a patient's symptoms suggest he or she may have a condition that cannot be diagnosed definitively in any other way.

Prostate surgery. Dr. Wennberg and his colleagues at Dartmouth have shown that surgery for non-cancerous enlargement of the prostate is among the most variable of procedures. They have also looked closely at what happens to men who get the surgery and those who don't. For many men, medical therapy can relieve symptoms. For

---

Redlined jobs
Many health-insurance companies won't sell policies to people working in barbershops, car washes, convenience stores, grocery stores, hospitals, nursing homes, doctors' offices, law offices, parking lots, or restaurants.

Corp., a think tank in Santa Monica, Calif., began to find out.

Using an elaborate process for developing a consensus among nationally recognized medical experts, the Rand team came up with an agreed-upon list of "indications" for various procedures. They then checked the actual medical records of thousands of patients who had

received the procedures, to see whether they had been treated appropriately. The definition of "appropriate" care was starkly simple: Based on the patient's condition and expert opinion, the likely benefit of the procedure must have been greater than the risk involved in doing it.

Even with their elaborate analysis,

the Rand researchers were not able to tell in every case whether a given procedure had been appropriate or not. They divided their cases into three groups: Those where the procedure had been "appropriate," those where it was "inappropriate," and those where its use was "equivocal," the largest group. Despite this degree of uncertainty, however,

others, putting off surgery isn't particularly dangerous, though the urinary obstruction caused by the condition can be uncomfortable.

When patients in a health maintenance organization were fully informed in advance of the risks and benefits of surgery, in a study that Dr. Wennberg designed, 80 percent of men with severe urinary symptoms chose to postpone the operation.

Clot-busting drugs. These drugs, when administered within four to six hours of the onset of a heart attack, can break up the blood clot blocking the coronary artery and thus greatly reduce the damage to the heart muscle. The largest comparative study done to date, of 41,000 patients worldwide, has found that all currently available clot-busting drugs are about equally effective in preventing fatal heart attacks—but one, streptokinase, has the lowest incidence of the most dangerous side effect, cerebral hemorrhage.

Of the two drugs used in the U.S., streptokinase also happens to be by far the cheaper—about $200 per dose compared to $2000 per dose for its genetically engineered competitor, tissue plasminogen activator (TPA). Nevertheless, TPA commands a majority of the U.S. market, apparently thanks to aggressive marketing by its manufacturer, Genentech.

For a person having a first heart attack, there's no reason to be treated with the more costly drug. Second treatments with streptokinase, however, are unsafe, since the first treatment can set up the mechanism for an allergic response to any future injection.

Rand found clear evidence of inappropriate overtreatment. Among the results:

▪ Of 1300 elderly patients who had an operation to remove atherosclerotic plaque from the carotid artery, nearly one-third—32 percent —didn't need it.

▪ Of 386 heart bypass operations, 14 percent were done unnecessarily.

▪ Of 1677 patients who had coronary angiography—an X-ray examination of blood flow in the arteries nourishing the heart—17 percent didn't need it.

So striking were the results that Rand's methods for determining appropriateness have since been put to commercial use. Value Health Sciences, which now employs some of the original Rand researchers, has extended the methodology to several dozen high-volume medical procedures. A number of major insurance companies and health maintenance organizations now use this program to flag unnecessary procedures.

Value Health's results confirm the original Rand findings. Its review system has found very high rates of unnecessary usage for certain procedures: hysterectomy, 27 percent unnecessary; surgery for an uncomfortable wrist ailment called carpal tunnel syndrome, 17 percent; tonsillectomy, 16 percent; laminectomy, a type of back surgery, 14 percent. Similar results have come out of studies done by other investigators, who have examined procedures from preoperative laboratory screening (60 percent unnecessary) to cesarean section (50 percent unnecessary) to upper gastrointestinal X-ray studies (30 percent unnecessary).

The uncertainty principle

Physicians can inadvertently contribute to the cost of unnecessary medicine even when they have only their patients' best interest in mind. Lay people tend to think of medical care as a straightforward proposition: For Disease A, prescribe Treatment B. That's not the way it is in real life. To practice medicine is to be afloat in a "sea of uncertainty," says Dartmouth's John Wennberg.

Every symptom can be investigated by a huge array of tests; for many diseases, physicians have a wide range of treatment choices. And doctors often base their choices as much on folklore and intuition as on science.

"Doctors really hate risks," says Ann Lennarson Greer, the Wisconsin sociologist. "They have certain procedures that seem to work for them, and they'd prefer to keep doing them, especially in areas where there's a lot of uncertainty."

This innate conservatism is reinforced by the isolation in which most doctors practice, says Greer, who has spent more than a decade studying why doctors and hospitals behave as they do. A physician can spend his or her entire career within a single referral network, based at a single hospital. These local colleagues, Greer has found, are the principal influence on a physician's decisions about how to diagnose and treat diseases or whether or not to adopt new technology. But they may not be the most reliable source.

A phenomenon called "small area variations," which was discovered by Dr. Wennberg early in his career, is a striking demonstration of just how unscientific medical practice really is. In the late 1960s, he had moved to Vermont to work as a health administrator and educator. Once there, he soon stumbled across a curious geographic pattern to a common operation, tonsillectomy.

"In Stowe, the probability of having a tonsillectomy by age 15 was about 70 percent," Dr. Wennberg recalls. "If you lived in Waterbury, over the hill from Stowe, it was about 10 percent." Indeed, there turned out to be a 13-fold difference in the local rates of tonsillectomy between the most and least surgery-happy Vermont communities he studied.

Medical uncertainty and the isolation of doctors largely explain those bizarre disparities. Dr. Wennberg discovered that doctors in Stowe, who talked mostly to each other, believed that if you didn't take tonsils out early, they'd become chronically infected and cause no end of trouble. Doctors in Waterbury, who didn't talk to the doctors in Stowe, held the opposite (and, as it turned out, correct) viewpoint: If left alone, most kids with frequent sore throats would eventually outgrow them.

This phenomenon turned out to be true of a lot more things than tonsillectomies. In Portland, Me., Dr. Wennberg found, 50 percent of men had prostate surgery by the age of 85; in Bangor, just 10 percent did. The rate of heart surgery was twice as high in Des Moines as it was in nearby Iowa City.

Subsequent studies by a number of researchers, working throughout the country, have shown that the use of all kinds of medical procedures varies dramatically from region to region. In fact, Dr. Wennberg has found the only procedures that *don't* show such variations are those few for which there is basically only one accepted treatment, such as hospitalization for heart attack or stroke.

Inefficiency experts

The waste in the system goes far beyond the provision of unnecessary

Serving the rich In 1988, Beverly Hills had one internist for every 566 people. Compton, a poor Los Angeles community, had one internist per 19,422 people.

care. Even when medical treatments are necessary, they're frequently done with no regard for efficiency.

Milliman and Robertson, a Seattle-based consulting firm, advises hospitals and other health-care organizations on ways to cut costs without compromising the quality of care. The firm's actuaries and physicians have examined thousands of individual medical records to develop guidelines on how long patients should stay in the hospital for such common conditions as childbirth or appendectomy—provided they're in generally good health and have no complications. Applying those guidelines to actual current records from a dozen urban areas across the country, the firm's actuaries concluded that 53 percent of all hospital days weren't necessary, including all the days spent in the hospital by the 24 percent of patients who didn't need to be there in the first place.

As a private, commercial firm, Milliman and Robertson is in business to identify overuse for its clients, and might have a bias in favor of finding what it's paid to find. However, other studies by academic researchers have also found high rates of inappropriate hospitalization. A recent Rand Corp. review of published studies, most of which used data from the early and mid-1980s, estimated that 15 to 30 percent of hospital use was unnecessary.

The current rates of unnecessary hospitalization are difficult to estimate, since the system is in flux. The overall number of hospital days per thousand Americans—a standard measure of hospital utilization—has dropped over the last decade, in response to efforts by Medicare, health maintenance organizations, and private insurers to contain costs. But there are still large regional variations in hospital use, suggesting that waste still exists in the system.

Past experience shows it's possible to lower the number of days people spend in the hospital with no ill effects. In 1984, Medicare created financial incentives for hospitals to discharge patients as soon as possible, and not to admit them at all unless strictly necessary. The incentives worked; in two years, the average number of in-patient days per Medicare recipient fell 22 percent.

That sharp decline apparently had no real impact on the health of the patients involved, according to several statistics. The rate at which discharged patients need to be re-admitted to the hospital shortly after

Where readers placed the blame Asked to name the biggest contributor to the cost of health care, 23 percent of our readers incorrectly picked malpractice suits (see the box at right). An equal number named hospital costs, which *are* the biggest factor. Doctors' fees and health-insurance companies came in third and fourth in the survey.

leaving—an important index of low-quality care—has actually gone down for Medicare patients since 1984. Some care that used to be provided in the hospital can now be done at home, at much lower cost.

A medical arms race

Despite the efforts over the past decade to keep the costs of hospitalization down—by limiting hospital admissions, length of stay, and in-patient costs—our national hospital bill continues to rise. In 1990, hospitals soaked up 38 percent of national health expenditures (twice as much as doctors) and collectively earned a profit of $7-billion. Hospital administrators have proven how nimble health-care providers can be in getting around virtually any effort to rein them in.

For many years, hospitals expanded at a rate well beyond the national need, with the Government's help. During the 1950s and into the 1960s, the Federal Government provided subsidies to build new hospitals, and a decade later, Medicare allowed hospitals to pay for their capital improvements by charging higher fees. The result was a spate of hospital-building that had little relationship to clear community needs. New facilities and new wings were built, beds needed to be filled, and the law of induced demand kept them occupied—imposing a high cost on the health-care system and providing a high profit for the hospitals themselves.

When Medicare started to crack down on costs in 1984—paying hospitals a fixed fee to take care of each patient, based on his or her diagnosis—the hospitals reacted swiftly. Fewer Medicare patients were admitted, and those that were admitted stayed in the hospital for a shorter time. But the hospitals compensated by boosting their outpatient, psychiatric, and rehabilitation services, for which Medicare had set no cost limits. Although charges for hospitalization dropped, the costs for those other services ate up those savings, and more.

Hospitals also stepped up their efforts to attract privately insured patients to make up for the money they were losing on Medicare and Medicaid. Having built the capacity for many more beds than the nation needs, hospitals now tried to fill them—and to fill them with patients who had generous insurance policies and needed lots of medical services. "Hospitals make money by deliver-

ing services," explains William Erwin, who is a spokesman for the American Hospital Association. "If you don't need much done to you, the hospital isn't going to make money on you."

Attracting patients to a hospital isn't the same as attracting customers to a new restaurant or hardware store. Consumers decide on their own when and where they want to eat out or buy some drill bits. When they're sick, their doctors decide when and where to hospitalize them. So hospitals must market on two fronts: They must appeal directly to privately insured patients, and they must keep their admitting doctors happy.

To induce physicians to admit patients, hospitals resort to everything from first-year guaranteed incomes to subsidies for initial practice expenses. The effort pays off. In 1990, according to an annual survey by Jackson and Coker, an Atlanta physician-recruiting firm, the average doctor generated $513,000 in in-patient hospital revenue.

Another way to keep doctors happy is to provide them with state-of-the-art medical equipment. As a bonus, hospitals can then tout their up-to-date technology directly to consumers. Uwe Reinhardt, a Princeton University health economist, likes to paint the following scenario in his lectures:

"Imagine that you're a young couple in Chicago, stuck in a traffic jam in the Loop, and you see a billboard that says: 'Mount Sinai: The Cheapest Place in Chicago, Have Your Baby Here.' Then you go on and you see another billboard that says, 'Holy Mercy: The Only Place with a Glandular Schlumpulator, Have Your Baby Here.' Where are you going to go?"

Some regulatory efforts were made in the 1960s and 1970s to restrain hospitals from acquiring excessive amounts of expensive technology, with mixed success. In any case, Federal support for that effort was discontinued during the Reagan years. The rationale was that "unleashing competition" among hospitals would allow the free market to operate and help keep the cost of medicine down.

The irony, though, is that competition actually drives costs *up* where hospitals are concerned. The hospitals gain no competitive advantage by controlling costs, since their customers—doctors and patients—don't pay for their services anyway. In-

THE 'CRISIS' THAT ISN'T

MALPRACTICE: A STRAW MAN

Ask physicians to explain why the cost of health care goes up continually, and you're likely to hear complaints that the U.S. malpractice system encourages unnecessary "defensive" medical care. The public seems to have bought this argument. In a recent survey, CONSUMER REPORTS subscribers guessed that malpractice tied with hospital costs as the biggest factor driving the cost of health care.

Is malpractice such a villain?

It's true that malpractice costs are higher in the U.S. than in other countries. And in the mid-1980s, malpractice claims—and, accordingly, insurance premiums—did take a sharp upward swing. There was much talk then of a malpractice "crisis." But that crisis now seems to have abated, as have previous ones. Malpractice is a cyclical phenomenon: Periodically, the incidence of claims rises, then falls back.

At the moment, malpractice claims have been in one such downswing. The rate of claims has declined steadily since the peak of the last "crisis" in 1985. So have malpractice insurance premiums. In 1990, according to Medical Economics magazine's annual survey of physicians, doctors' malpractice premiums on average consumed only 3.7 percent of their practice receipts—although the percentage may be double that for high-risk (and high-paid) specialties, such as obstetrics, surgery, and anesthesiology. The U.S. Department of Health and Human Ser-

vices puts the total cost of malpractice at less than 1 percent of total health outlays.

But then, no one argues that the direct cost of malpractice insurance is the main factor driving up the cost of care. Instead, it's assumed that physicians, fearing malpractice suits, are forced to practice "defensive medicine" just to protect themselves in the event of a lawsuit.

Defensive medicine undoubtedly exists, and doctors themselves feel that the threat of malpractice forces them to do more tests than are truly necessary. But quantifying the cost of defensive medicine is a slippery matter. The American Medical Association made a stab at it in the 1980s, and decided that the total cost of medical malpractice, including premiums and defensive medicine, was about 17 percent of physicians' earnings.

However, the AMA estimate was based on physicians' own reports of what they considered defensive practices, such as doing more diagnostic tests, sticking with the safest possible treatments, telling patients more about treatment risks, and keeping more complete records.

As that list suggests, one problem with defining defensive medicine—let alone measuring it—is that it's difficult to distinguish from care delivered for other reasons. Is a doctor doing an unnecessary test out of fear of a lawsuit, or because the medical culture values doing "everything," or simply to reassure an anxious patient? Did an obstetrician perform an

unnecessary cesarean for legal protection, for scheduling convenience, or to earn a higher fee?

"You mostly get anecdotes when you're talking about defensive medicine," says Randall Bovbjerg, an analyst at the Urban Institute in Washington, D.C., who has worked on several malpractice studies.

That's not to say there isn't a malpractice crisis, however. "The greatest single problem about malpractice is that there's a lot more of it out there than anyone is dealing with," says Bovbjerg. "Patients are getting avoidable injuries and no one is stopping it."

Documentation for Bovbjerg's claim comes from a study conducted by Harvard University researchers for the state of New York. The researchers reviewed a random sample of New York hospital records in 1984 and found that 3.7 percent of patients suffered "adverse events," slightly more than one-quarter of which could be attributed to actual negligence.

Of those who suffered negligent injuries, only about one-eighth ever filed malpractice claims, and only about one-sixteenth ever recovered any damages. Conversely, the study found many cases in which patients filed malpractice suits with no clear evidence of negligence.

Costs aside, the current malpractice system is at best only an imprecise means of controlling the quality of medical care.

stead, hospitals compete only on the basis of perceived quality, and end up vying to see which one can secure and promote the newest well reimbursed technology, whether the technology is needed or not. Several hospitals in an area may have their own neonatal intensive care units, MRI machines, or cardiac care centers, when only one would serve the population equally well (see "The Cardiac Money Machine"). This year, despite the recession, hospitals plan to increase spending on new equipment by 15 percent, according to a survey by Shearson Lehman Brothers.

To attract the well-insured population, hospitals also provide amenities that have nothing to do with actual health care but add to the bill, includ-

ing cable TV, private rooms and baths, gourmet menus, and the like. Baylor University Medical Center in Houston spent $18-million on the Tom Landry Sports Medicine and Research Center, complete with 7000-square-foot dressing rooms lined with oak lockers, and a 10-lane pool with underwater computerized video cameras used to analyze its patrons' swimming strokes.

Hospitals have also become more and more consciously concerned with projecting an upscale image that they hope will bring in an affluent clientele. Entries in a recent contest held by the Academy of Health Services Marketing, an organization of hospital marketing executives, reveal the new focus. For instance, the Southern Regional Medical Cen-

ter in suburban Atlanta got Rosalynn Carter to endorse its maternity service after her grandchild was born there—as part of a successful campaign "to increase gross revenue . . . by marketing to a target market of insured, higher-income women, ages 25-49," according to the contest submission.

The trend is troubling, because there's clear evidence that the total cost of health care rises in areas where many hospitals begin to compete for the same pool of well-insured patients. Health economists James C. Robinson and Harold S. Luft of the University of California, Berkeley, examined data from 5732 hospitals nationwide, and found that costs per admission were 26 percent higher in hospitals that had more

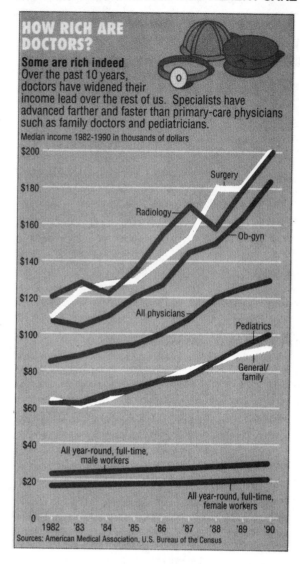

HOW RICH ARE DOCTORS?

Some are rich indeed
Over the past 10 years, doctors have widened their income lead over the rest of us. Specialists have advanced farther and faster than primary-care physicians such as family doctors and pediatricians.

Median income 1982-1990 in thousands of dollars

Surgery
Radiology
Ob-gyn
All physicians
Pediatrics
General/family
All year-round, full-time, male workers
All year-round, full-time, female workers

1982 '83 '84 '85 '86 '87 '88 '89 '90

Sources: American Medical Association, U.S. Bureau of the Census

Canada, 3.7; and in France, Japan, and the United Kingdom, 2.4.

Historically, the highest fees have gone to doctors who perform concrete procedures, such as surgery, endoscopy, or diagnostic imaging. So-called evaluation and management services—in which doctors may examine and question the patient and prescribe a treatment, but don't actually do a specific procedure—haven't paid nearly as well.

In 1990, for instance, internists charged a median of $110 for a comprehensive office visit for a patient they hadn't seen before, according to a survey by Medical Economics magazine. Such a visit involves taking a medical history, doing a physical examination, and talking with the patient about his or her current condition. It can take up 45 minutes of the doctor's time. By contrast, the same survey found internists charged a median fee of $126 for spending 10 minutes to examine the bowel with a flexible fiberoptic device called a sigmoidoscope.

While individual physicians have great leeway in deciding what they will charge for a given procedure, insurance companies have established computerized databanks that help them determine whether or not the fee is "usual and customary" for that procedure. By this standard, a doctor whose fees are at the very top of the local scale may not receive full reimbursement. But there's no track record of cost for new procedures. With the help of medical specialty societies and the AMA, physicians have secured very high rates of reimbursement for new treatments.

"When something is in development, it's new, it's experimental, only a few physicians use it, there's some risk involved, and the price gets set accordingly," explains Joel Cantor, a program officer at the Robert Wood Johnson Foundation. "Then the technology diffuses and gets easier to use. More physicians get good at it. But the price never goes down."

The classic example is the extraction of cataracts and implantation of artificial lenses in the eye. This undeniably useful technology was introduced in the early 1980s and became a standard procedure by the end of the decade. During that time, however, many ophthalmologists became wealthy by charging $2000 or more for a cataract extraction that could be done in about an hour.

Primary-care physicians, such as general internists, family practitioners, and pediatricians, don't do pro-

cedures like that. Instead, they spend their days in office visits, which have long-established, and thus lower, "usual and customary" fee profiles.

As a result, their incomes are much lower than those of specialists. In 1990, the median income for general family practitioners was $93,000, and for pediatricians, $100,000, according to the American Medical Association's annual survey. Median income for surgeons and radiologists, on the other hand, was $200,000. Senior specialists can earn much, much more. Cardiovascular surgeons in group practice averaged about $500,000 in 1990, according to a study by the Medical Group Management Association.

Medical-school students, who must pick a residency program in their senior year, are painfully aware of these economic distinctions. In addition, they're trained in an academic environment that has long rewarded specialists with prestige and research grants. Young physicians, who leave medical school with a huge debt load, are increasingly turning to specialization. Overall, about one-third of U.S. physicians are in primary care. But among 1987 medical school graduates who have now completed their internships and residencies, only one-fourth have gone into primary care, according to data from the Association of American Medical Colleges.

A fed-up Ohio family doctor, responding to a survey by his professional society, the American Academy of Family Physicians, summarized his feelings this way: "Why bother with 60- to 70-hour work weeks, constant phone calls, all night emergency room visits, poor reimbursements, demanding patients, the need for instant exact decisions . . . concerning a million possible diseases, when you can 'specialize' in one organ, get paid $500 for a 15-minute procedure, only need to know a dozen drugs and side effects, and work part time?"

Do we really need our luxurious quantities of cardiologists, dermatologists, neurosurgeons, and urologists? Other countries get along fine with about a 50-50 ratio between primary-care doctors and specialists. The evidence is that we could, too.

A team from the New England Medical Center recently looked at patients who got their usual care from primary-care physicians (internists or family doctors) or from specialists (cardiologists and endocrinologists). The groups were not

than nine competitors within a 15-mile radius. In a smaller-scale study of 747 hospitals, they found that those in competitive areas allowed patients to stay in the hospital longer after surgery—something that tends to please both patients and doctors, but with a high cost and no clear medical benefit.

More specialists, high costs

Just as American hospitals lead the world in high-priced technology, American physicians are heavy purveyors of expensive treatments and diagnostic tests—and reap great personal rewards for using them. Doctors in the U.S. earn much higher incomes relative to their fellow citizens than do doctors in other countries. According to figures from the Organization for Economic Cooperation and Development, in 1987 U.S. doctors earned 5.4 times more than the average worker. In Germany, the multiple was 4.2; in

identical; the specialists tended to have older patients with more medical problems. But even after that difference was factored in, the specialists ran up higher bills, on average, than the primary-care doctors. They put more patients in the hospital, prescribed more drugs, and performed more tests. Yet an analysis still in progress appears to show that the two groups of patients had similar health outcomes.

The medical profession itself acknowledges the imbalance. The principal professional journal for internists, the Annals of Internal Medicine, said in a 1991 editorial: "Given the number of subspecialists already in practice, there are not enough highly specialized cases to go around. . . . We cannot continue to practice this way when cost containment is the dominant health policy issue of our times."

This year, Medicare began an effort to even out the economic imbalance between primary care and specialty physicians. The new program, known as the Resource-Based Relative Value Scale (RBRVS), is essentially a standard, national fee schedule, adjusted for geographic variations in the cost of practice. It increases the reimbursement for evaluation and management services, and greatly reduces the reimbursement for procedures. Physicians, however, may find a way around this constraint, as they have around others. For one thing, doctors can always simply raise their fees for privately insured, non-Medicare patients—although some private insurance companies may eventually adopt a version of the RBRVS fee schedule.

Since the mid-1980s, doctors have also manipulated the reimbursement system by "unbundling" services—that is, charging for two or more separate procedures instead of one. For instance, instead of billing $1200 for a hysterectomy, a doctor can collect $7000 by billing separately for various components of the operation. Commercial services conduct seminars to teach doctors how to maximize reimbursement in this way. But unbundling can cross the line into outright, prosecutable fraud, according to the General Accounting Office's health-care fraud report.

Supplier-side economics

Just as the providers of care have profited hugely over the years, so have those who supply the providers—the pharmaceutical companies and the makers of medical equipment and devices. They can charge top prices for their products, secure in the knowledge that the system will reimburse them. The pharmaceutical industry has been one of the nation's most profitable industrial sectors; it operates with an average profit margin of 15 percent and has given an average annual return to investors of 25 percent over the last decade.

Companies that latch on to new medical technologies can also earn huge profits. In spite of the current hand-wringing over health-care reform, health-care stocks as a group increased in value by fully 50 percent in 1991.

"A lot of people in health care are making a lot of money," says Stephen Zuckerman, a senior research associate at the Urban Institute in Washington, D.C. "They're not unhappy with the current system."

Curiously, the debate over health-care costs in the U.S. tends to assume that the cost of drugs and medical technology is immutably fixed. But international comparisons demonstrate that this needn't be so. In Japan, for example, the national fee schedule pays $177 for a magnetic resonance imaging (MRI) exam, compared with an average charge of about $1000 in the U.S. Pharmaceutical prices, which vary widely from country to country, are also significantly higher in the U.S. than anywhere else.

Nothing for something

As costly as it is, our health-care system might be worth its price if it somehow ended up making us healthier than people in other countries. But it doesn't.

Of the 24 industrialized nations making up the Organization for Economic Cooperation and Development (OECD), the U.S. spends more than twice as much on health per capita as the average. And it devotes a far greater percentage of its gross national product to health care than any other country. Yet the other OECD countries—with the exception of Turkey and Greece, by far the poorest of the group—all have roughly as many doctors and hospitals per capita as we do.

As for health status, of the 24 OECD countries, the U.S. ranks:

◼ 21st in infant mortality.
◼ 17th in male life expectancy.
◼ 16th in female life expectancy.

Dr. Barbara Starfield of the Johns Hopkins School of Public Health compared the U.S. with nine industrialized European nations in three areas: the availability of high-quality primary care, public-health indicators such as infant mortality and life expectancy, and overall public satisfaction with the value of health care. In all three areas, the U.S. ranked at or near the bottom.

The problem, simply put, is that the system is geared to providing the services that can earn physicians and hospitals the most money—not the ones that will do the public the most good. The U.S. has four times as many $1.5-million magnetic resonance imaging devices per capita as Germany does. But at the same

The uninsured aren't welcome From a hospital marketing consultant's brochure: "To promote cardiology services, savvy marketers select all those at higher risk for heart disease, who are between the ages of 35 and 65, privately insured . . . it's target marketing at its best."

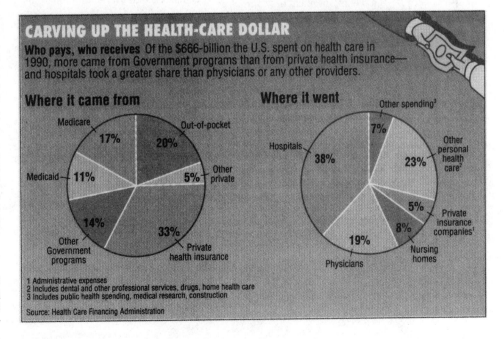

CARVING UP THE HEALTH-CARE DOLLAR

Who pays, who receives Of the $666-billion the U.S. spent on health care in 1990, more came from Government programs than from private health insurance—and hospitals took a greater share than physicians or any other providers.

Where it came from
- Medicare 17%
- Out-of-pocket 20%
- Other private 5%
- Private health insurance 33%
- Other Government programs 14%
- Medicaid 11%

Where it went
- Other spending³ 7%
- Hospitals 38%
- Other personal health care² 23%
- Private insurance companies¹ 5%
- Nursing homes 8%
- Physicians 19%

1 Administrative expenses
2 Includes dental and other professional services, drugs, home health care
3 Includes public health spending, medical research, construction

Source: Health Care Financing Administration

HIGH-TECH COMPETITION

THE CARDIAC MONEY MACHINE

People with heart and circulatory diseases, the leading causes of death in the U.S., have benefited enormously from medical and surgical advances over the past two decades. Until the late 1960s, doctors couldn't do much more than give them a little nitroglycerin or digitalis in the hope of extending their lives moderately. Then came coronary bypass surgery, the first great treatment advance, in which blood vessels from elsewhere in the body are used to bypass diseased coronary vessels and restore more blood to the heart muscle. Next, in the 1980s, came balloon angioplasty, in which a balloon attached to a catheter is passed into the narrowed coronary vessel and inflated to crush the blockage against the wall of the coronary artery.

The last decade has also brought new drugs to dissolve blood clots, to right irregular heartbeats, and to treat heart failure and high blood pressure; new imaging techniques; implantable electronic devices; and, as a last resort, new methods of heart transplantation.

All this, together with changes in diet and exercise habits, has had a dramatic effect. The death rate from heart disease in the U.S. has dropped roughly by half since 1950.

But the improvement has come at a very high cost. New technologies are expensive technologies, and the cardiac field is no exception. Coronary bypass surgery, for example, can easily run $30,000 or more for a single operation.

"It is just well-paid by everybody; even Medicare pays handsomely for it," says Ann Lennarson Greer, a medical sociologist at the University of Wisconsin. "The hospitals are crazy about bypass. Even if they're six blocks from a major heart center, they think they can't afford not to be in on it. People who get coronary problems, namely middle-aged men, tend to be among the best-insured people in our society."

(Uninsured patients may simply not get these costly procedures. One national survey found they were 39 percent less likely than the insured to get coronary angiograms—X-rays to evaluate the heart's blood supply—and 29 percent less likely to have bypass surgery.)

A growing profit center

Just how lucrative the cardiovascular field is was revealed in a 1990 report prepared by the Advisory Board Company, a Washington-based consulting firm, for its hospital clients. The report concludes that nearly one-quarter of all hospital revenues come from cardiology-related business, and of that, more than 80 percent comes from just four procedures—cardiac catheterization, angioplasty, bypass surgery, and heart-valve surgery. Not surprisingly, cardiovascular surgeons bring in the most revenue per inpatient hospital admission of any specialty—$10,942 in 1989, more than twice the average doctor's rate—according to an annual survey by Jackson and Coker, an Atlanta-based physician-recruiting firm.

The profit margins are as impressive as the revenues, according to the Advisory Board report: 70 percent for catheterization, 37 percent for angioplasty, and 40 percent for bypass, compared with overall profit margins for hospitals of less than 4 percent. And, to top it all off, the number of cardiac diagnostic and treatment procedures performed in the U.S. has been growing at an average annual rate of 12.7 percent.

The Advisory Board report uses a real, though unidentified, hospital to illustrate the profit potential. Wanting to increase its cardiology market share, the hospital invested $3-million in state-of-the-art equipment for catheterization and open-heart surgery. The improved equipment (and additional support staff) attracted 25 new cardiologists to the hospital, who brought in hundreds of new patients for catheterization, angioplasty, and bypass. Within two years, the extra business had repaid the entire upfront investment and was adding $1.8-million a year in profits to the hospital's bottom line.

This sort of return on investment has caused hospitals to look increasingly to cardiovascular care to fill their empty beds. In 1980, according to the Advisory Board report, there were 382,000 cardiac catheterizations performed in the U.S. and 340,000 treatment procedures, including bypass, angioplasty, valve surgery, and pacemaker implantations. By 1988, the volume of catheterizations had grown to 965,000 and the volume of procedures to 930,000.

Were all those procedures really necessary?

Doctors' dilemmas

The treatment of heart disease is a classic example of the way in which medical uncertainty produces variable, unnecessary care. Treatments for heart disease are advancing so rapidly that there's often little consensus on what to do or when to do it. What symptoms require a coronary angiography exam? Should a person with mildly uncomfortable angina and blockages in one or two vessels stick with drug treatment, or undergo angioplasty? If angioplasty has failed once, should it be repeated or should the patient get a bypass operation?

Medical journals are filled with debates on those questions. In the meantime, physicians must make daily treatment decisions with little guidance on which course is preferable—but knowing that they will be financially rewarded for ordering the maximum intervention.

Writing in the Journal of the American Medical Association, Dr. Thomas N. James of the University of Texas, Galveston, put it this way: "The same physician who decides whether a diagnostic or therapeutic procedure is to be done is too often also the one who does the procedure, interprets the findings (and decides whether additional procedures are indicated), and is paid for each step of the way.

This is not to say that such physicians are unskillful or that their decisions are necessarily made on the basis of personal gain, but the temptation is inescapably there."

Under those circumstances, it would be surprising if unnecessary procedures were not being done. The evidence is that they are:

■ A study of pacemaker implantations in Philadelphia hospitals found that 20 percent were unnecessary and another 36 percent were problematic.

■ A San Diego team found that, among patients who'd been hospitalized with mild heart attacks, 40 percent of those who got angiograms didn't need them. In addition to running up a bill ranging from $2000 to $3500, these patients were put at a slight risk of complications from the procedure itself.

■ A team from Brigham and Women's Hospital in Boston examined the need for bypass surgery among 88 patients for whom it had been recommended. They advised against surgery for 74 of the 88. Among those 74, 60 accepted the second opinion and didn't have the operation. Over a follow-up period of more than two years, there were only two subsequent heart attacks, neither of them fatal, among this group—an outcome comparable to that of people who receive angioplasty or coronary bypass surgery.

Risky medicine

Despite findings like these, competitive and financial pressures conspire to encourage hospitals to build even more cardiac-care units. Consider the case of Manchester, N.H. Until 1985, Manchester residents who needed open-heart surgery had to travel to Boston or to Hanover, N.H., to get it. That year, a Manchester hospital, Catholic Hospital Medical Center, opened the first local open-heart surgery service. Within one year, the rate of heart surgery among residents of Manchester more than doubled.

What could explain the immediate jump in volume? An analysis by the Codman Research Group, a private health-care consulting firm, found that before the local program started, 90 percent of bypasses done on Manchester residents involved the transplantation of three or more arteries—a sign of serious and extensive disease. By 1988, however, over half the operations were single or double bypasses.

"They were clearly operating on less severely ill patients," says Dr. Philip Caper, Codman's chairman and a professor at Dartmouth Medical School. "The hooker is, nobody really knows whether they were better off. Some doctors think most single bypasses should almost never be done, because the risk is more than the benefit."

While coronary bypass can be life-saving, it is an extremely traumatic procedure involving stopping and cooling the heart, hooking the patient up to a heart-lung machine, then restarting the heart. Handling an operation of this complexity requires a skilled and coordinated surgical team. That's why studies have repeatedly demonstrated that hospitals performing fewer than 150 open-heart procedures a year have higher death rates than those that perform more. In addition to driving up health-care costs, hospitals joining the cardiac gold rush may actually be putting their patients at serious risk.

That was the case in Phoenix in 1985, when the state of Arizona, in the spirit of deregulation, decided to abdicate its authority to control the introduction of new open-heart surgery programs. At that time, four Phoenix hospitals provided open-heart surgery. Almost immediately, seven more began programs. A computer-aided study of Medicare records performed by the Phoenix Gazette and the University of Arizona found that in the first year of deregulation, the local death rate from heart surgery increased by 35 percent. The average cost of the procedure, meanwhile, rose 50 percent.

time, the U.S. system short-changes the basic, low-tech care that has, over the years, proven effective at preventing disease.

The poor and uninsured are most likely to suffer from the imbalance. During the 1980s, while American hospitals were falling all over themselves to add costly, high-tech neonatal intensive-care units, the number of mothers unable to get basic prenatal care climbed, as did the incidence of premature births.

In most states, Medicaid now pays nowhere near the actual cost of delivering care; hospitals lose money on their Medicaid admissions. As a result, many doctors and some for-profit hospitals refuse even to accept Medicaid patients.

People with no insurance at all fare even worse. A group from the University of California, San Francisco, for example, looked at the hospital care given to sick newborn babies in the state's hospitals in 1987. Even though the uninsured babies were, on the average, the sickest group, they left the hospital sooner than insured babies and received fewer services while they were there. The Rand group has also shown that when California cut back on Medicaid coverage a decade ago, the health of people who lost their coverage declined dramatically.

"We've been sucked into believing that if we have a national health program, we're going to have rationing," says Dr. Philip Caper of Dartmouth. "The answer is, we have rationing already. Ask somebody who lost their health insurance, or can't get a bone-marrow transplant because they're on Medicaid. If that isn't rationing, what is?"

Hospitals that serve the poor and uninsured are suffering as well. The success of private hospitals in attracting well-insured patients has put an increasing burden on the public and not-for-profit hospitals still willing (or required) to accept all comers. A 1990 survey of 277 public and teaching hospitals found that 38 percent sometimes held patients overnight in the emergency room because no regular beds were available; 40 percent had turned away ambulances because of overcrowding.

Hospitals in California have even shut down their trauma centers as a way of barring the door against uninsured patients. "Hospitals find themselves jockeying for geography," says Bettina Kurowski, a vice president of St. Joseph Medical Center in Burbank, which closed its

Costs exposed, prices cut After a state government survey revealed it was charging $14,000 more for heart bypass than a local competitor, St. Vincent Health Center in Erie, Pa., dropped its bypass price by $10,000—the first rate reduction in its 116-year history. Estimated annual savings: $5-million.

trauma center when its annual losses hit $1.5-million and threatened the financial survival of the hospital as a whole. "If you can be promised service areas that include freeways, and therefore get trauma cases covered by auto insurance, you can break even. If you don't include freeways, mostly you get penetrating [gunshot and stab wound] trauma, and those patients by and large don't have insurance."

Dissatisfied Americans Pollsters asked citizens of 10 developed nations to rate their health-care systems. U.S. respondents were the unhappiest of the lot. Fully 60 percent said our system is in need of "fundamental changes."

Red tape and red ink

Ultimately, our cumbersome, inequitable system of reimbursement raises the costs for all of us—insured and uninsured alike—and causes problems for physicians as well. "In order to preserve the mirage of a private system, we've created the most bureaucratic, regulated system of any in the world," says David Mechanic, director of the Institute on Health Care Policy at Rutgers University.

A key characteristic of the U.S. system is its obsession with making sure that patients get only what their insurance entitles them to, and nothing more. That means, for instance, that hospitals must keep meticulous track of everything used by a particular patient, down to individual gauze sponges or aspirin tablets—all adding to administrative costs. More important, the burden of dealing with multiple forms from a huge number of insurance companies requires a lot of clerical manpower.

Increasingly, too, doctors and hospitals have to answer to Government and private review panels that evaluate many aspects of the care they offer. Government reviewers work to ensure that Medicare and Medicaid patients are not being undertreated, while private insurers want to make sure that their patients are not being overtreated.

Hospitals in the U.S. spend fully 20 percent of their budgets, on average, on billing administration—compared to only 9 percent for Canadian hospitals. To run a health plan covering 25 million people, Canada employs fewer administrators than Massachusetts Blue Cross, which covers 2.7 million.

Our nation's more than 1200 private health-insurance companies add to the red tape by the necessary maintenance of their underwriting, marketing, and administrative staffs. This overhead consumed an average 14 cents out of every premium dollar in 1990, according to the Health Care Financing Administration.

Private physicians, too, have been forced to hire extra office help to cope with the ever-enlarging demands of third-party review, regulations, and paperwork. Drs. David Himmelstein and Steffie Woolhandler, internists at Harvard Medical School who are prominent critics of the U.S. health-care system, have calculated that the average office-based U.S. physician employs twice as many clerical and managerial workers as the average Canadian doctor. Dealing with the bureaucracy has become so intrusive that doctors have developed a name for it: the "hassle factor."

Dishonest physicians have also taken advantage of the system to bilk insurance companies. According to the General Accounting Office report: "This complex system itself becomes an impediment to detecting fraud and abuse. . . . a physician who bills for more office visits than can reasonably be performed in a day, for example, may not be detected if the billing is split among several payers."

Drs. Woolhandler and Himmelstein, who favor a Canadian-style system, have calculated that about 20 percent of U.S. health-care spending goes for administrative costs: insurance overhead, hospital and nursing administration, and physicians' overhead and billing expenses. Not surprisingly, the private health-insurance industry says this estimate is too high. However, industry representatives decline to offer their own figure.

Universal coverage and uniform fee schedules enable other countries to avoid most of the administrative expense of the U.S. system. The single-payer Canadian system, where all health-care costs are ultimately paid by the Government, devotes about 10 percent of expenditures to administration. The General Accounting Office calculates that if the U.S. were to adopt a single-payer Canadian-style system, we would save about $70-billion a year in insurance overhead and the administrative costs to doctors and hospitals.

Enough for all

No matter what corner of the health-care system is examined—hospital costs, clinical procedures, administrative expenses—at least 20 percent seems to represent waste or inefficiency. If the system could be redesigned to get rid of this excess, it could, in effect, provide 20 percent more necessary service without costing any more than it does now.

Granted, devising a totally efficient system would be difficult, if not impossible, to accomplish. However, there is easily more than enough excess spending in our current system to take care of the roughly 14 percent of the population who are not currently under any public or private insurance plan.

In [the August and September 1992] issues of CONSUMER REPORTS, we'll examine the different options for health-care reform. But it's already clear that the ideal health-care system for American consumers, whatever it turns out to be, will have to be radically different from the wasteful, patchwork system that governs our health care today.

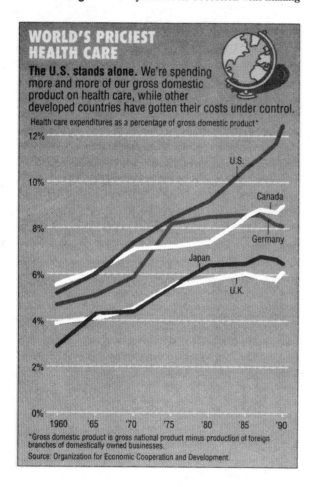

WORLD'S PRICIEST HEALTH CARE

The U.S. stands alone. We're spending more and more of our gross domestic product on health care, while other developed countries have gotten their costs under control.

Health care expenditures as a percentage of gross domestic product*

12%
10%
8%
6%
4%
2%
0%

U.S.
Canada
Germany
Japan
U.K.

1960 '65 '70 '75 '80 '85 '90

*Gross domestic product is gross national product minus production of foreign branches of domestically owned businesses.
Source: Organization for Economic Cooperation and Development.

THE CLINTON CURE

WHAT THE PRESIDENT SAID—AND DIDN'T SAY—ABOUT HIS TRILLION-DOLLAR PLAN TO REVOLUTIONIZE THE SYSTEM

REINVENTING HEALTH CARE

Tom Morganthau and Mary Hager

Barnstormin' Bill Clinton went on the road last week and, in a nationally televised town-hall meeting from Tampa, Fla., displayed remarkable mastery of the arcane details of his plan for health-care reform. The setting was congenial—Ted Koppel as moderator, a large and respectful crowd—and the president was at his best. He seemed at ease and in command. He listened well and gave crisp, clear answers. Insurance coverage for AIDS patients? In-home care for the elderly and disabled? Mental-health benefits? Clinton knew the answers in detail—and time after time the cameras caught questioners nodding as he explained how the plan would affect them. This was vintage Clinton, and it was superb salesmanship. The event, and others like it in the coming weeks, will give Clinton and his cabinet the chance to follow up on his eloquent speech to Congress. It will also help frame the national debate on health reform in terms that are favorable to him.

That's good tactics. But Clinton has not answered (and, in fact, never raised) the two biggest questions before Congress and the voters: how his reform plan would really work, and why he thinks his approach is better than the possible alternatives. This omission was surely intentional. There will be plenty of time in the months ahead for the president to argue the case for his bold (and, some would say, visionary) attempt to overhaul the nation's health-care system. Further, the administration clearly believes that the most important goal for its current marketing blitz is to reassure the country that reform won't hurt, or at least not very much. That is exactly what Clinton said in his speech to a joint session of Congress: "The vast majority of the Americans watching this tonight will pay the same or less for health-care coverage that will be the same or better than the coverage they have tonight. That is the central reality."

But there are many realities in a proposal as revolutionary as Clinton's. He and his advisers want nothing less than a top-to-bottom restructuring of an industry that comprises 14 percent of the U.S. economy—a vast, sprawling and grotesquely ill-managed behemoth that sooner or later touches every single American in profoundly personal ways. Clinton has been candid in saying that health care can never be free, and that reform will cost some Americans more. He has acknowledged that there are large differences of opinion about the right way to fix the system, and he has been candid, up to a point, in describing his hope of attaining more efficiency from doctors and hospitals through "a combination of private-market forces and sound public policy." But he has not told us—not yet, anyway—just how difficult and risky his strategy for reform must inevitably be.

NEWSWEEK's latest polling suggests the public is ready to take risks. An overwhelming majority—79 percent—say the U.S. health-care system needs fundamental changes or needs to be "completely rebuilt." Fifty-one percent approve of the way Clinton is handling the health-care issue, and 56 percent approve of his decision to name Hillary Rodham Clinton to head the administration's task force on reform. Equally important, there is relatively little evidence that the voters have exaggerated expectations for reform. Fifty percent of the NEWSWEEK sample expect to wait longer for health-care services, 49 percent expect to lose the power to choose their doctor and 57 percent expect to pay more for health care. Seventy-three percent think reform will mean higher taxes and, in what may be a warning to Congress and the president, support for higher taxes to finance health care has dropped from 65 percent to 48 percent since February. Still—and this is the good news for reformers—57 percent think Americans will become "more responsible" about using health care and 55 percent think Clinton's proposals would be good for the country.

The Clinton plan is essentially based on two gigantic gambles, and it is only fair to say the administration has been coy about both of them. The first gamble is that there is enough waste and misspending in the system to pay for universal health-insurance coverage for the poor and the uninsured without raising taxes (except, of course, for the proposed new tax on tobacco). Many experts, including analysts for the Congressional Budget Office, are skeptical that the amount of wasteful spending is really as high as Clinton claims. Last week he cited C. Everett Koop, the former U.S. surgeon general, in support of his estimate that we could save $200 billion a year without compromising the high quality of American medicine. Still, Clinton and his advisers have repeatedly avoided specifics of how much waste there is—a crucial issue. "We subjected the numbers in our proposal to the scrutiny not only of all the major agencies in government . . . [but also] to actuaries from major accounting firms and major Fortune 500 companies," Clinton said.

"So I believe our numbers are good and achievable." He didn't say what the numbers *were*—and he didn't say how much it would cost to provide health insurance to the estimated 37 million Americans who don't have it, or how much it would cost to improve benefits for the estimated 22 million Americans who are regarded as underinsured. He also didn't say how much money the administration expects to save by making the health-care system more efficient. What he said, in effect, is "Trust me"—and never mind that if he and his advisers are wrong, the costs of extending health care to the uninsured would ultimately require new taxes.

percent in 1992. That money comes out of workers' paychecks, and it has cost the average American plenty—at least half the increase in real income throughout the 1980s. But the income loss is invisible and the concept of health costs as a percentage of GNP is only an abstraction. And in truth, there is little agreement about which percentage, exactly, is "right" for America. It could be 17.3 percent, which is Clinton's goal for the year 2000, or it could be more: it's our choice.

There can be no dispute that the effort to constrain the nation's health spending must ultimately cost somebody something. That "somebody" could well be the health-insurance industry, which under the Clinton plan will probably suffer a major shakeout at the cost of thousands of jobs. It could be the nation's 630,000 doctors: the Clinton plan almost certainly means that doctors will lose some income, and it probably means that many physicians will see their professional lives changed in dramatic and unsettling ways. It could be hospitals: Michael Bromberg, executive director of the Federation of American Health Systems, predicts that many hospitals will be forced to close. And it could be patients. If government sets limits on health spending nationwide, as Clinton wants to do,

A GUIDE TO HEALTHSPEAK

CAPITATION: Not as painful as it sounds. A way of paying for group care in which doctors get a fixed amount per patient, then hope to spend less on average.

CO-PAYMENT: A small sum HMO patients contribute to their bill for every doctor visit.

CORE BENEFITS: What you'll get in the end, at the minimum; a set of guaranteed medical services.

FEE FOR SERVICE: The old-fashioned way—you pay the full bill (or split it with your insurer) each time you get sick.

GATEKEEPER: Primary-care doctor as traffic cop: he or she OK's all visits to higher-billing specialists.

HEALTH ALLIANCE: Replaces

the more accurate but less catchy "health-insurance purchasing cooperatives" (HIPCs). In short: you and your neighbors, organized by region, buy health services at bulk rates to save money.

HMO: Health-maintenance organization. These managed-care mavens offer all types of care, often under one roof, at a fixed monthly price.

MANAGED CARE: Medicine practiced with an eye to cost. Enthusiasts extol "efficiency"; critics see auditors denying needed care.

MANAGED COMPETITION: The reigning reform theory. The trick is to structure the medical market so doctors and hospitals compete for patients.

MEDICAID: Insurer to the poor has a diminished mission under Clinton plan, as those now eligible would join alliances. Would continue to provide emergency treatment for undocumented residents.

MEDICARE: Insurer of the largest U.S. interest group—the elderly—and Clinton's political football. He'd give new drug and long-term-care benefits in return for higher premiums and $124 billion in cuts over five years.

SELF-INSURED: Some large employers run their own plans. They still could do so, but might be taxed to help fund the alliance system.

SINGLE PAYER: The system used in Canada. The government pays all bills with your taxes. Prices for care are set by the single payer.

ILLUSTRATIONS BY BOB GALE

Clinton's second big gamble is that Congress actually *wants* to limit U.S. health-care spending. Nobody disagrees that health-care costs are out of control. But cutting back on health spending—even the future growth of health spending—can be politically risky. The nation's health budget has soared from 5.9 percent of GDP in 1965 to 14

there must be some reduction in the levels of care and probably restrictions on the style of care that we have come to expect.

The blunt word for this is rationing—and it is arguably true that Clinton's plan implies at least some kind of health-care rationing for all of us. This "rationing" will probably be marginal—delays of service and care that won't particularly affect our health or our lives. And it is a powerfully pertinent fact that America rations health care now, and does it cruelly. Those who can't afford insurance and those who can't get insurance because of "pre-existing conditions" are routinely denied necessary care by the current system. This is morally wrong and economically counterproductive: it is the great failure of the American health-care system. But the issue for all of us—House and Senate members, doctors and hospital administrators and, ultimately, we voters—is whether we are willing to tolerate slightly less medicine in return for a lot more fairness while still controlling costs. That's the trade-off—and it will surely be the primary point of contention when Clinton's plan reaches Congress next month. Do we want to control health spending or not? And if we do, how should we try to do it?

The Clinton plan proposes a double dose of cost containment—the new and largely untested notion of "managed competition," and a backup system of very tough government regulation. These two proposals are designed to work together, with the regulatory system reinforcing the attempt to create competition in the health-care industry. Clinton and his advisers hope competition will slow the growth of health spending without any need for using the regulatory weapons they propose. But no one knows whether managed competition will work on a nationwide scale, and no other nation has tried anything like it. It might work in some areas of the country. Administration officials cite Minneapolis-St. Paul, where spending has dropped sharply, as an example of successful reform. But it may not work, or work well enough, if and when it goes nationwide. And if it doesn't, the regulatory provisions will, as policy wonks say, "kick in."

So what does managed competition really mean, and how does it work? Basically, it is an attempt to promote price competition in the national health-care "market." Like any other market, the health-care industry consists of buyers (patients) and sellers (doctors and hospitals). But as economists see it, medicine differs from other markets because both the buyer and the seller are usually able to ignore the cost of the services that are sold and consumed. The reason is that most Americans do not pay for health care with their own money: doctors' fees and hospital bills are paid by insurance companies from premiums paid mostly by employers. In most cases, these "third parties" do not make the decision to seek care: the patient does that. They also do not make the decision to provide treatment: the doctor does that.

This means the health-care market is broadly dysfunctional when it comes to controlling costs. Consumers rarely know what a specific medical service should cost and almost never price-shop: for obvious reasons, sick people seek the best treatment, not the cheapest. Consumers usually don't know which insurance policies offer the best value. The market is a buyer's nightmare of different premiums, deductibles, co-payments and restricted coverages. Even employers, who pay most of the premiums for working Americans and their families, have trouble sorting out the options. Some insurance companies shape their policies to discourage high-risk patients and attract younger, healthier people. This helps keep losses down and

profits up. But it also undermines the stability of U.S. health-insurance markets by sending disproportionate numbers of high-risk patients to companies like Blue Cross and Blue Shield that are required by law to insure all comers.

All of this would change under Clinton's plan. Insurance companies would be barred by law from refusing coverage to people with pre-existing conditions and from charging discriminatory rates to small companies and high-risk patients. The federal government would define a "core-benefit package" as a benchmark for employers, insurance companies and consumers alike. The creation of this standard package does not mean government will subsidize all health insurance, nor is it primarily intended to establish a certain level of health benefits as an American right (although it would obviously have that effect).

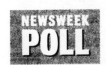

Will President Clinton's proposed health-care plan mean:

61% More security that health care will be available, whatever a person's medical or financial problem
26% Less security

42% More simplicity for doctors and patients
45% More bureaucracy and paperwork

36% Real savings on nation's health-care costs
47% No real health-cost savings

44% Enough choice for patients among various doctors and health plans
39% Not enough choice

55% The same or better-quality health care
37% Lower-quality care

Will the mixture of cost savings, employer-employee payments and new taxes cover the cost of Clinton's plan, or will it require more taxes than he has proposed?
73% More taxes   17% Cover costs

FOR THIS NEWSWEEK POLL, PRINCETON SURVEY RESEARCH ASSOCIATES INTERVIEWED A NATIONAL SAMPLE OF 751 ADULTS BY TELEPHONE SEPT. 23-24. THE MARGIN OF ERROR IS +/- 4 PERCENTAGE POINTS. SOME DON'T KNOW AND OTHER RESPONSES NOT SHOWN. THE NEWSWEEK POLL © 1993 BY NEWSWEEK INC.

The real purpose is to establish an easily understood, fully comparable product for the health-insurance industry. That would make it possible for consumers, employers and the alliances to comparison-shop.

This benchmark benefit package is the beginning of Clinton's attempt to bring competition to the health-care industry. The plan also calls for the creation of wholly new institutions known as health alliances. The health alliances would be quasi-governmental bodies created by the states—large organizations that would represent consumers in a given region, like metropolitan Detroit. They would collect premiums paid by employers, individuals and the federal government, and use those premiums to purchase health-insurance coverage for all their enrollees. (Companies with more than 5,000 employees would be allowed to buy their own insurance or to self-insure.) The health alliances would provide more bargaining power and more expertise in selecting health-care coverage for smaller companies, self-employed workers and the unemployed.

The intent is to "level the playing field" for a more competitive game. The other team consists of health-care providers organized as "plans." As the Clintonites see it, plans could be

---

CLINTON'S CORE BENEFITS

The Clinton plan would guarantee Americans a broad range of care:

PROFESSIONAL SERVICES: Doctors' office visits, emergency-room care, laboratory and ambulance fees.

HOSPITALIZATION: Semiprivate room, unless a private room is medically necessary.

PREVENTIVE CARE: Immunizations, prenatal and infant checkups, cholesterol screening, physicals with increasing frequency as patient ages. Mammograms for women older than 50.

LONG-TERM CARE: Nursing homes and rehabilitation centers are covered as an alternative to extended hospital stays. Maximum of 100 days in a calendar year.

HOME CARE: Also as an alternative to hospital stays. Need for further care would be assessed every 60 days.

EYE AND EAR: Routine eye and ear exams; children's eyeglasses.

OUTPATIENT THERAPY: Occupational, physical or speech therapy to restore functions lost because of illness or injury. Need reassessed every 60 days.

DENTAL CARE: Preventive care for children; adult care would be phased in starting in 2000.

PRESCRIPTION DRUGS: $5 per prescription or a $250 yearly maximum depending on the plan you choose.

HOSPICE: For terminally ill patients as an alternative to a hospital stay.

MENTAL HEALTH: Initially, 30 days of inpatient care per episode of illness, up to 60 days in a year. Thirty outpatient visits to a psychotherapist. By the year 1998, 90 inpatient days; no limit on outpatient visits.

SUBSTANCE ABUSE: Similar to mental health.

MEDICAL EQUIPMENT: Prostheses and braces that improve function or prevent deterioration.

---

formed by doctors, hospitals, insurance companies or any combination of the three. The plans would bargain every year with the health alliances to provide the health services defined in the core-benefit package to the alliance enrollees. These negotiations would include guarantees of quality and service, but they would almost certainly focus on price. The bargaining would force the plans to bid on the basis of a fixed annual payment—about $1,800 for each individual and $4,200 for a family, if the administration's estimates are right.

The result, beyond any doubt, would be a fundamental change in the way physicians, hospitals and health insurers do business. The plans would operate financially much as health-maintenance organizations do now. HMOs sell health care at a fixed, pre-negotiated price, which eliminates the incentive in fee-for-service medicine to run up the bills by ordering more tests and treatments. The Clintonites say fee-for-service medicine would continue to exist, but this is somewhat disingenuous: under the president's plan, fee-for-service doctors would operate under price schedules established by the alliances. Further, many experts think even this regulated version of fee-for-service medicine will gradually be destroyed by the changing economics of the industry. Most doctors would be forced to take salaried jobs as health-plan employees. This change in the structure of the medical profession is well advanced in California, where HMOs and other forms of managed care dominate the market. If the trend goes nationwide—and it already is, owing to pressure from employers to control costs—it would mean the end of medicine as a cottage industry of self-employed professionals.

But the theory many not work. Aside from the vast problems of creating such a system, with all that it entails for the health industry and for government, managed competition may fail to control costs as well as its designers hope. The history of state and federal efforts to contain costs is replete with failure. Time and again, through the Carter and Reagan years, government tried to limit medical spending—and time and again, doctors and hospitals "gamed the system" to frustrate those efforts. When the Feds limited fees, doctors responded by ordering more treatment. When the Feds tried to limit the spread of high-tech, high-cost facilities like cardiac-care units, hospitals and doctors ganged up to beat the regulators. And although managed competition attacks the cost problem at a deeper level, it is perfectly possible the industry will get even. It could do so by forming provider plans so big—as big as General Motors, say—that the bargaining power of the health alliances would be neutralized.

Then what? Regulation. The Clinton plan contains regulatory weapons that would allow the Feds to penalize state government for noncompliance. It would also allow the Feds to intervene in the bargaining between any alliance and any health plan. The primary control mechanism is budgeting—a so-called global budget set every year by a National Health Board, which would then be translated into state-by-state budgets and budgets for each alliance. Computing these budgets is not as difficult as it may seem: it's similar to what HMOs and health-insurance companies do now. And it is therefore highly unlikely that a budget shortfall would leave anyone without health care.

Still, government budgeting would put the whole health-care industry under gradually tightening cost controls. There is a formula in the Clinton plan that sets national spending limits for the first five years of the reform era. It allows health spending to rise by a percentage that is equal to the predicted rise in the cost of living, plus the predicted growth of the U.S. population, plus a three-year fudge factor to ease the pain of transition. It would allow spending to rise from $1.2 trillion in 1996 to $1.5 trillion in 2000. By the administration's estimates, the nation would save about $700 billion through the year 2000. That's paltry, considering the seven-year total ($10 trillion): Clinton clearly hopes to bring soaring U.S. health costs down to a soft landing.

His advisers say this form of cost control differs from all previous regulatory plans because it does not set prices or "micromanage" the industry. They say they are not trying to cut U.S. health-care spending, but merely limit its growth by establishing annual "caps" on premiums. They are probably right on all counts. If budgeting works, it will force doctors, hospitals and health insurers to decide how to control their own costs—there will be no government bureaucrats telling anyone what to do. Crucially, in the Clintonites' view, the annual budgets will stiffen the spines of those who run the alliances in their negotiations with provider plans. Alliance managers can say there is only so much money in the bank—no chance to bid the total up. And if a provider plan fails to control its costs—if it runs over the price it negotiated the year before—it eats the loss. To Ira Magaziner, Clinton's health-care guru, this simply means doctors and hospitals will be forced to operate like all other businesses: bad judgment means less income and possibly even bankruptcy.

Critics—and we will hear all their arguments in the months to come—raise many objections to this part of the Clinton plan. One contention is that the administration wants to limit spending too abruptly and that its five-year budget formula is too severe. Magaziner doesn't buy it: like Clinton, he believes the health industry is full of wasteful spending and unnecessary care. During a recent White House briefing, he said that the budget could be more generous "if we were starting from a system that was already a trim system." But the system, Magaziner said, is "completely bloated" and the administration's proposed budgets are designed to eliminate the fat. "I get frustrated . . . [with] the attitude which says you can never get cost savings," he said. "For the period that we're projecting, from now to the year 2000, we think there's going to be tremendous one-time savings." Maybe. But economist Henry Aaron of the Brookings Institution says that estimating the potential savings from reform is "analytically impossible"—there are just too many unknowns.

And there is real dispute about the whole idea of trying to control costs. Health economist Dr. Rashi Fein of Harvard Medical School, who is skeptical that managed competition will produce real savings, says budget limits are "sensible and necessary." Norman Daniels, the author of a book on health-care policy, says no nation "has kept costs down without some type of budget cap." But the American Medical Association, though officially neutral on the Clinton plan, opposes the very notion of limiting health-care costs through government regulation. The AMA and the American Hospital Association say they are willing to consider flexible spending "targets," but they don't like the hard budgeting in the Clinton plan. Michael Bromberg of the Federation of Health Systems, another hospital group, says that Clinton's attempt to control private-sector spending is unconstitutional—it is, he says, like telling parents how much they can spend on their children's education.

The coming congressional debate is also likely to revolve around the issue of cost controls—according to Magaziner, that is the standard by which any competing plan should be judged. There are bills for a "single payer" system that would turn government into the national health insurer; Washington would control prices the way the Canadian government does, through annual fee negotiations with medical associations. Conservative Democrats and the Republican leadership in the House, on the other hand, want to try managed competition without the global budgeting, which would leave the restructured health-care market to determine national spending levels without limits set by government. Some conservatives want to try tax-deductible "medical savings accounts," which would avoid both managed competition and cost controls. The Clinton plan, with its combination of market reform and government budgeting, lies near the middle of this spectrum. But given the huge stakes for Congress, the health industry and the public, no one can say whether the middle is the right place to be.

But let's assume the Clinton plan passes, and that some day soon—perhaps as early as 1995—we Americans are getting our care from a radically transformed health system. What will happen to us as patients and consumers? Despite the president's attempts to be reassuring about the changes that will ensue, there is a very good chance that our relationship with our current doctor will be disrupted—the physician may leave medicine altogether or join a health plan we do not choose to join. OK, switching doctors isn't the end of the world, at least for the vast majority of Americans who are healthy. But it can be very threatening for those with serious medical conditions, and it can undermine the quality of care. And what about the quality of care? Clinton's staff promises that health alliances will issue annual reports on quality and that we all will know what to expect from the health plans we join. But it isn't that simple—nobody in medicine knows how to measure quality. There is another risk, too—that quality will be eroded when doctors make medical decisions on a cost-conscious basis. It isn't supposed to happen, but it does. "People with the best of intentions, including the Clintons, may create a system that imposes cost constraints," says Dr. Robert Brook of the University of California, Los Angeles, and the Rand Corp. "The thing that slips out is quality."

Brook's research shows that the attempt to eliminate unnecessary care cuts about as much muscle as it does fat—which brings us back to rationing. Rationing—the dreaded R word—is easily exaggerated, and it is very unlikely that we Americans will see doctors or bureaucrats make life-or-death decisions for cost reasons. But that's not the whole story. "What we've found in other countries when the lid has gone on [are] longer waiting lists, deterioration of facilities and a marked slowdown in the adoption of new [medical] technologies," says Dr. James Todd of the AMA. "It's an economic model that does not deal with the real world of the doctor-patient relationship." Todd is wrong: the world is real enough in Germany, Britain and, up to a point, Canada. And the question we Americans face is whether we still want a health-care system that offers care without compromise—or whether we believe it is costing us too much.

With ANDREW MURR *in Los Angeles,* BOB COHN *in Tampa and* DEBRA ROSENBERG *in Boston*

HEALTHTOWN, U.S.A.

The landscape of health care is about to change. Under the Clinton proposal every American will choose one of three basic kinds of health plan—HMO, fee-for-service or a combination. The big questions are how much you will pay and how you will choose your doctors. Lost already? Here's a tour of Healthtown, U.S.A.

HEALTH ALLIANCE

The nerve center of the Clinton plan, though you'll probably never lay eyes on one. Each state will set up alliances with as many as 1 million members. The alliances will then compile the lists of health-care plans from which their members choose. Unless you work for a big company, you're automatically a member.

SELF-EMPLOYED WORKER

The self-employed will pay for their own health premiums—$1,800 for individuals, $4,200 for a family—but could deduct the entire amount from taxes.

RETIREE

Under 65: government will subsidize premium payments, if necessary. Over 65: Medicare pays the bills, plus prescriptions and in-home health care.

FEE-FOR-SERVICE PLAN

Traditional pay-as-you-go doctors. This is the most expensive health plan: after reaching a $400 deductible, the typical family would pay about 20 percent of medical bills up to an annual $3,000 out-of-pocket maximum.

PSYCHOTHERAPIST

The plan calls for comprehensive mental-health care by the year 2000. Until then, limited psychotherapy sessions, in-patient care and psychiatry would be covered.

HMO

You get: all your medical care, either under one roof or from an approved network of doctors, for $10-$15 per visit. You lose: the privilege of choosing your own doctors.

PHARMACY

Trips to the drugstore would become less painful. Under some plans, prescription drugs would cost as little as $5; for others, coverage would kick in after a $250 deductible.

UNEMPLOYED

Clinton wants everyone to pay something toward health care, even people out of work. If your income is 150 percent below the poverty line, the government will help pay the premiums.

MEDICAID

Poor people would join health alliances just like everyone else and pick the health plan of their choice. Federal and state governments would pay the premiums, but only for plans priced at or below the average of all those offered.

WRITTEN BY PATRICK ROGERS. ILLUSTRATED BY JARED SCHNEIDMAN AND GUILBERT GATES

MIDSIZE COMPANY

At companies with more than 50 but fewer than 5,000 workers, the employer would pay 80 percent of an employee's insurance premiums. The worker would be responsible for the rest.

CORPORATION

Businesses with more than 5,000 employees can set up their own private health alliances, offering the same three basic health plans as their government-run counterparts. Big businesses pay 80 percent of their employees' insurance; the workers themselves pick up the remaining 20 percent.

HOSPITAL

From the patient's viewpoint, hospitals will look pretty much the same. But don't expect a private room unless you really need it—or are ready to pay big bucks.

COMBINATION PLAN

Choose a doctor from the plan's network and you pay only a small co-payment—$10-$25. Choose an outside doctor—the old family pediatrician, say—and you pay extra.

HARDWARE

SMALL BUSINESS

The owner pays 80 percent of employees' insurance premiums, the workers pay 20 percent. But for companies with fewer than 50 workers, government subsidies keep health-care costs at 3.5 percent of payroll for all workers making less than $24,000.

DENTIST

For now, only children are covered, and then only for preventive care. Adult dentistry would be added later.

NURSING HOME

Nursing homes and residential treatment are covered when they can be justified as an alternative to hospitalization. A hundred-day yearly maximum.

UNDOCUMENTED WORKER

You can't join a health alliance unless you have working papers. Still, emergency care would not be denied.

COLLEGE STUDENT

If college is far from home, students would join a local health alliance. Otherwise, family policies would cover their health costs.

UNCLOGGING THE
drug pipeline

WHAT THE NEW FDA POLICY MEANS TO YOU

Jon Hamilton

Jon Hamilton covers health care for The Commercial Appeal *in Memphis, Tenn.*

YOU'VE PROBABLY HEARD THE COMPLAINTS:

► There's a backlog of unreviewed drugs at the Food and Drug Administration (FDA).

► Many drugs are sold for years in other countries before they're available here.

► A drug's journey from the test tube to the drugstore shelf typically takes 12 years and costs a pharmaceutical company more than $200 million—costs that are passed on to the consumer when the drug finally becomes available.

► The FDA's stringent requirements deprive people with potentially fatal illnesses of drugs that could save their lives.

The complaints all have a basis in fact, but it appears that the FDA is increasingly determined to do something about this drug "lag." That was underscored last March, when in light of two new studies an FDA advisory committee unanimously recommended approval of tacrine— the first drug to offer hope against Alzheimer's disease—after twice turning thumbs down in 1991. Even more surprising, the FDA reportedly backs the panel and will soon allow the drug's sale—after rejecting appeals for tacrine's approval for years and publicly attacking the doctor who developed it.

"Tacrine received unusual guidance and remarkably swift action from the FDA, despite the agency's initial negative reaction," says Dr. David Knopman, director of the Alzheimer's Disease Clinic at the University of Minnesota.

The agency postponed some required safety tests in animals, which would have delayed human trials by several months. And even before advisory committee approval, thousands of patients were allowed to receive tacrine under a new program that makes unapproved drugs available to desperately ill patients. Finally, FDA officials worked quickly to assemble an advisory committee meeting just two months after the tacrine studies finally showed the drug offered some benefit.

"The FDA stuck by its principles, but it did bend the rules, and it acted quickly," says Knopman. "It did a good job."

Critics of the agency say tacrine illustrates a new era at an organization whose unwritten motto has long been "Better safe than sorry."

"It's a conservative agency," says Dr. Joseph DiMasi, an economist and senior research fellow at the Tufts University Center for the Study of Drug Development, an independent office funded in part by grants from pharmaceutical companies. "There are bureaucratic incentives to be very risk averse, and they're not going to go away." To a large extent, those incentives are side effects of a notorious drug called thalidomide.

The FDA was established in 1906 to protect the public from untested food additives and drugs. It had little power until 1938, when Congress gave it the authority to require that manufacturers prove their drugs safe before marketing, through testing on animals and people. Then came thalidomide, a sedative that was given to thousands of pregnant women in Europe during the 1950s and around 1960 was found to cause severe birth defects. The U.S. narrowly escaped the horrors of thalidomide, because one FDA employee, Dr. Frances Kelsey, questioned the safety data submitted by the drug's manufacturer and held up its approval. (Kelsey, 79, is still at the agency today.)

In the 30 years since, fear of another thalidomide has ensured that drugs are approved only after exhaustive review. That fear has been intensified on infrequent occasions when unsafe drugs have breached the agency's defenses or when drugs have been approved through fraud (see "The Comeback of Generic Drugs").

Nevertheless, the FDA's rigid approach to drug approval has clearly shifted. When drugs for invariably fatal illnesses with no other treatment op-

From *American Health*, October 1993, pp. 78-80, 103, 105, 107. © 1993 by Jon Hamilton. Reprinted by permission.

tions are at stake, the agency is willing to risk making them available even if they might ultimately prove ineffective or even unsafe. This change is a victory for advocacy groups that have pressed for faster drug approval.

One of the most aggressive of these groups is ACT UP (AIDS Coalition To Unleash Power). In October of 1988, in a protest organized by ACT UP members to demand faster approval of AIDS drugs, 1,000 demonstrators blocked traffic entering the FDA's Rockville, Md., headquarters, smashed police barriers, plastered the agency's windows with stickers and scuffled with police. Nearly 200 people were arrested in the demonstration, which received extensive publicity and helped spur the agency's efforts to make drugs available for life-threatening illnesses before they're approved.

Other, less vocal activists have also attracted the FDA's attention. They represent patients with amyotrophic lateral sclerosis (Lou Gehrig's disease), breast cancer, Alzheimer's disease and epilepsy. George Rehnquist, for example, is a retired Knoxville, Tenn., engineer who led the fight for tacrine's approval. His wife, Lucille,

was the first Alzheimer's patient in the U.S. to start taking the drug experimentally in its oral form, in 1984. Rehnquist has testified before congressional committees, helped organize nation-wide letter-writing campaigns, given talks across the country and formed a foundation in Knoxville called Families for Alzheimer's Rights.

Fellow tacrine advocate Woodrow Wirsig, a former magazine editor, wrote a book about his battle with the FDA to obtain the drug for his dying wife; he makes frequent speeches and once attempted to sue the FDA for withholding tacrine. Both Rehnquist and Wirsig have met with FDA Commissioner David Kessler. "I don't think tacrine would have gotten approved without us pushing for it," Rehnquist says.

Drug companies eager to market potentially lucrative products have taken up the drumbeat of the activists. They're joined by allies in Congress who contend that the FDA's slowness in approving drugs is hurting a key industry. Pressure from all these camps has had a considerable effect.

"There have been a number of changes over the past four or five years

that have resulted in very significant improvements in the way we evaluate drugs," says Gerald Meyer, deputy director of the FDA's Center for Drug Evaluation and Research.

One of the most dramatic changes is the agreement reached last year between the FDA and the pharmaceutical industry letting the agency charge "user fees" for reviewing drug applications. Under the agreement, firms pay the FDA $100,000 or more for each new drug application, in addition to fees for drugs already on the market and for manufacturing facilities. The fees—expected to total $325 million by 1997—will allow the FDA to hire 600 new drug reviewers, expanding the review staff 50%. Calling user fees the biggest change at the FDA in 30 years, Commissioner Kessler has said that the added personnel will cut review times for AIDS drugs and other critically important drugs to just six months, compared with the 2½ years it now generally takes to review and approve a new drug.

Those in the pharmaceutical industry are not as optimistic but do expect a somewhat faster review for all drugs. "We believe this is only a partial solution to a slow process," says Thomas Copmann, assistant vice president for biotechnology and biologics at the Pharmaceutical Manufacturers Association. "But it is clear that the FDA is approaching the problem vigorously."

To further speed review, drug companies can now submit their applications on computer discs—a major improvement over the reams of documents that have often overwhelmed FDA offices. Computerization means data can be retrieved and reviewed faster, and it allows several reviewers to check an application simultaneously.

Perhaps most important, the FDA has taken several recent initiatives to speed approval of crucial drugs and make them available to patients before they're given final approval. The Alzheimer's drug tacrine, the AIDS drug didanosine (DDI) and about 40 other experimental drugs have been offered to patients under the FDA's treatment IND (investigational new drug) program. This program makes promising experimental drugs available to desperately ill patients while the drugs are still under review.

Once a sponsor (typically the drug's maker) receives a treatment IND approval, "basically any doctor in the

In Search of Unapproved Drugs

What can Americans do when they want a drug not approved by the FDA? Some of them travel to foreign countries, which typically approve drugs long before the U.S. does and often put fewer restraints on their sale.

Thousands of Americans, for example, have gone to Mexico for Retin-A, a cream said to have antiwrinkle properties; it's available over the counter in Mexico but approved in the U.S. only as a prescription acne remedy. Patients with far more serious problems, such as AIDS and Alzheimer's disease, have also sought out drugs in foreign countries.

The FDA allows Americans with serious illnesses to bring into this country drugs that are sold abroad but are not approved in the U.S. But permission is limited to drugs for personal use and amounts for treatment generally lasting three months or less.

Unapproved drugs can also be obtained through underground sources, including "buyer's clubs." These clubs, formed by patients with AIDS and other diseases, distribute (usually at cost) a wide variety of unapproved drugs, including drugs that come from foreign suppliers or are manufactured illegally in the U.S., as well as herbs and nutritional supplements.

Although the sale of unapproved drugs is illegal, the clubs contend that their activities are protected by the FDA's personal-use policy. For its part, the FDA has decided to monitor the clubs for the time being rather than prosecute them.

Last May the agency sent guidelines to a dozen AIDS buyer's clubs to help ensure that patients won't be harmed by their products. The guidelines ask the clubs to keep written statements from customers to the effect that the drugs they obtain are strictly for personal use. Each statement should also give the name and address of the U.S. doctor supervising the buyer's use of the drug. In addition, the guidelines prohibit clubs from promoting or commercializing their wares and from selling drugs that "represent an unreasonable risk."

Clubs that don't follow the guidelines risk FDA enforcement action, according to Dr. Randolph Wykoff, director of the agency's Office of AIDS Coordination. "We can be aggressive if the situation warrants," he says.

Buyer's clubs say they support the FDA's efforts to prevent profiteering and ensure that underground drugs don't harm patients. "There are justifiable public health concerns," says Sally Cooper, executive director of the People With AIDS Health Group, a New York City–based buyer's club that serves about 5,000 people a year. To minimize risk, she says, her group tests all drugs it distributes and includes physicians on its board.

Nevertheless, Wykoff urges that buyers beware. He points to an increase in reports linking serious side effects to underground AIDS drugs that were impure or contained the wrong dosage. "If you buy something through the underground, there is no guarantee you are getting what you think you are," he says.

country with a patient who might benefit from the drug can apply for it," says Dr. Eileen M. Leonard, special assistant for drug evaluation policy in the FDA's Center for Drug Evaluation and Research. "If their patient qualifies, they can get the drug, and then report back on the patient's progress."

While treatment IND approvals are intended mainly to make drugs accessible, "they also give us a lot of information on adverse reactions that can be very useful when trying to get a new drug to market that hasn't been studied extensively," says Leonard. Even if a drug doesn't have a treatment IND approval, physicians may still be able to obtain it for a patient by requesting approval for what's known as an emergency IND (previously referred to as a "compassionate use" permit).

Along with developing programs to make experimental drugs accessible, the FDA is making efforts to speed up its review and approval.

The agency's accelerated-approval program, announced last year, hastens review of breakthrough drugs for serious illnesses when the drugs promise significant benefits over existing therapies. Such drugs are approved provisionally quite early in development, before their clinical effectiveness is confirmed. So far, several important new drugs have come through this "fast-track" approval program: Approved last year were the AIDS drug dideoxycytidine (DDC) and taxol, the anticancer compound derived from the bark of the Pacific yew tree to treat ovarian cancer. Interferon beta-1b, the first drug ever marketed for treating multiple sclerosis (MS), was approved last July.

Accelerated approval relies solely or partly on so-called surrogate end points—physical signs or laboratory measurements of a drug's effectiveness, instead of more conclusive clinical demonstrations. These shortcut indicators can slash months or years off the time needed to test a drug.

For example, testing of interferon beta-1b relied partly on magnetic resonance imaging (MRI) scans of the brain. MRI scans showed that MS patients treated with a placebo had a greater increase in brain lesions after two years than did patients treated with the drug. It would have taken much longer to win approval if the FDA had insisted on clinically conclusive evidence that the drug slows MS.

Surrogate end points are not foolproof; sometimes a drug may alter an

The Comeback of Generic Drugs

In 1989 several generic drug firms were found to have falsified test results to gain approval for their products—a discovery that severely jolted the Food and Drug Administration (FDA).

The generic drug scandal sparked a federal probe that has led to the recall of dozens of generic drugs and convictions of eight companies and more than 40 people. Fortunately, none of the illegally marketed generics are known to have caused any harm, and other generics were thoroughly tested and judged safe and effective.

Generic drugs are copies of brand-name drugs whose patents have expired. The generics generally cost about half as much as their counterparts and have been hailed for contributing to lower health-care costs.

A generic's active ingredient must be chemically identical to the brand-name version's. Its maker must also prove to the FDA that it's bioequivalent—absorbed into the bloodstream at the same rate and as completely as the original. But two firms cheated on the bioequivalence tests by substituting brand-name capsules for their own generic versions, and other companies falsified drug applications in different ways.

The scandal prompted Congress to pass the Generic Drug Enforcement Act of 1992, which bars generic drug executives from continuing to work in the industry—in some cases permanently—if they've been convicted of a crime involving drug products. In addition, the FDA has beefed up its investigative branch and adopted stricter internal review procedures for all drugs, including generics. Such changes have made it "quite unlikely" that similar problems with generics could occur again, according to Dr. Sidney Wolfe, head of the Public Citizen's Health Research Group in Washington.

Generic approvals plummeted at the peak of the scandal, but are now on the upswing. Major approvals this year include clotrimazole cream, 1% (similar to Gyne-Lotrimin, for vaginal yeast infections), and gemfibrozil capsules (equivalent to Lopid, which reduces serum cholesterol).

---

end point while having no effect on the disease itself. That's why makers of drugs receiving accelerated approval must agree to do follow-up studies to evaluate their drugs' clinical benefits.

Another innovation that could dramatically reduce the drug lag is "harmonization," through which the U.S. works with other countries to standardize requirements for drug studies. A harmonization committee with members from the U.S., Japan and European Community countries has been meeting for two years to find ways to coordinate approvals. A drug approved in another country wouldn't automatically be approved here, FDA officials say, but harmonization could help companies avoid having to repeat costly and lengthy studies merely to satisfy trivially different standards.

Not all these efforts to speed up drug approval have met with applause. Dr. Sidney Wolfe, a consumer advocate and head of the Public Citizen's Health Research Group in Washington, says he's unhappy about efforts to bring the U.S. in line with other nations.

"What's troubling is that some of these other countries differ vastly from the U.S. in their standards for safety and efficacy," Wolfe says. "There should be no change unless it means bringing those other countries up to our standards."

Wolfe also worries that the urge to approve drugs quickly could lead to cursory reviews that jeopardize safety. "Given that many lifesaving drugs are potentially harmful," Wolfe says, "one has to be careful not to do more harm

than good when these drugs are made available to the public."

Early release of promising experimental drugs could actually make it impossible to learn whether they're beneficial, some experts contend. In an editorial this year in the *Annals of Internal Medicine*, for example, Dr. Paul Stolley of the University of Maryland School of Medicine wrote that the wide availability of experimental AIDS drugs has hobbled efforts to recruit patients for clinical trials needed to evaluate the drugs. Once a drug has implicit FDA backing, he argued, patients won't take the risk of receiving a less effective comparison drug. "We have the methods to answer the important questions about new therapies for AIDS," he wrote, "but, because of misguided compassion, we may fail to use them."

Other doctors worry that pressures to be compassionate will bring drugs to market whose modest benefits fail to outweigh their toxicity. Dr. John Growdon, a neurologist and Alzheimer's specialist at Massachusetts General Hospital in Boston, has called tacrine's effect on Alzheimer's patients "very modest"; he notes that the drug caused liver damage among 42% of them. "I haven't used tacrine," he says, "and I don't intend to use it in my practice."

Nevertheless, FDA officials insist that the agency's new willingness to approve drugs faster and make them available sooner doesn't mean the watchdog has muzzled itself. "We've had to adjust to societal pressures," says the FDA's Meyer. "But I strongly believe that nothing the FDA has done has lowered its standards."

Keeping Score

The new trend toward evaluating medical care

David Zinman

David Zinman, a former medical reporter for Newsday, *wrote* The Day Huey Long Was Shot.

Planning to buy a washing machine? You've probably done your homework, perhaps by consulting a consumer magazine to see how the various models compare. But how would you pick the best hospital or surgeon if you needed an operation?

Ironically, we're forced to make crucial medical decisions far less methodically than we go about choosing Maytag over General Electric. Advice from friends or referrals from doctors can help, but what we really need is objective information about quality of care. A revolutionary research technique called outcomes accountability now offers such knowledge.

Once confined to academic research, outcomes accountability is moving into real-world use, assessing health care by focusing on medicine's ultimate bottom line: the impact of treatment. It gathers "hard data" such as treatment costs and whether patients lived or died, plus crucial feedback such as how patients' quality of life was affected.

Applied to states and communities, outcomes accountability holds health care providers publicly responsible for their results by highlighting hospitals and doctors both good and bad. On a larger scale it could revolutionize the practice of medicine by showing which among several competing treatments offers the best results at the most reasonable cost.

"Outcomes accountability is crucial to the success of President Clinton's health plan," says Dr. Paul Ellwood, an outcomes expert and head of Inter-Study, a nonprofit Jackson, Wyo.-based research group. "The Clinton plan emphasizes managed competition—health care providers competing with each other on price and quality—and quality will be measured in terms of outcomes."

The outcomes movement is fueled by the need to rein in health care costs and the knowledge that much of the money spent is frittered away on treatments that don't work and on hospitals and doctors that don't measure up.

"Why shouldn't a patient know which hospital is doing the best job?"

"Our studies indicate that at least one-third of what goes on in the practice of medicine produces little or no health benefit for our patients," says Dr. Robert Brook, a professor of medicine at UCLA and head of the health sciences program at the Rand Corporation in Santa Monica, Calif.

Explains Dr. David Nash, director of health policy and clinical outcomes at Thomas Jefferson University in Philadelphia: "We've finally come to grips with the fact that there is great and un-explained variation in the health care system, and nobody is going to continue paying for it—nobody." As the nation tries to improve medical care while controlling spiraling costs, says Nash, "outcomes management is going to expand and tackle more and more areas. It's the wave of the future, and there's no way to stop it."

Two states, New York and Pennsylvania, are leading the way.

New York's outcomes program has focused on bypass surgery. Since 1989, the state has published yearly mortality rates for hospitals where the surgery is performed—and the program has clearly had an impact.

New York's first report, for 1989, listed Winthrop-University Hospital in Mineola, N.Y., in 26th place among the 30 New York hospitals doing by-pass surgery. Stung by its low ranking, Winthrop took action.

"Our cardiac surgery service is totally different from the way it was two years ago," says Dr. William Scott, chairman of thoracic and cardiovascular surgery at Winthrop, who was hired in early 1990 specifically to turn things around at the hospital.

Scott withdrew operating privileges from two surgeons who, the state data indicated, did too few bypass operations to maintain their skills. He also intensified the monitoring of patients and changed the support personnel in the operating room.

The result: In the report covering 1991, Winthrop soared to second place in statewide rankings, and its mortality rate from heart surgery—"risk-adjusted" to take the severity of illness of its patients into account—plummeted from 9.58% in 1989 to 1.77% in 1991. "We now have a well-organized, well-run service," says Scott, who gives New York's outcomes program much of the credit for his department's transformation.

Winthrop's new ranking impressed Fred Hoschander, an angina patient who underwent a quintuple bypass at Winthrop last December. "My first thought was to go to a larger, better-known medical center," says Hoschander, a 60-year-old retired family physician. "Then I saw the ratings published in *Newsday* [a Long Island, N.Y., newspaper] and Winthrop was second, so I decided to have the operation there."

Six weeks after surgery, Hoschander's chest pain was gone, he felt fine and he strongly supported the state's rating system: "Why shouldn't a patient know which hospital is doing the best job?"

Winthrop wasn't the only New York hospital to shake things up in the wake of the outcomes disclosures. Statewide, the average risk-adjusted mortality rate from bypass surgery dropped from 4.25% in the report covering 1989 to 2.72% for 1991—a decline of 36%.

"That great an improvement in coronary artery bypass surgery hasn't been demonstrated elsewhere in the country," boasts Dr. Mark Chassin, New York's state health commissioner.

Based on this success, New York plans to extend its outcomes research to include annual results from balloon angioplasty (a nonsurgical method of treating coronary arteries narrowed by heart disease). The angioplasty study will look at both mortality and rates of complications, including reclogging of arteries following the procedure. Also afoot in New York are plans to link outcomes to the state's payments to hospitals, with the highest reimbursements going to centers giving the best care.

Since 1988, Pennsylvania has rated its hospitals on a total of 59 treatments and surgical procedures, and included how much they cost, which varies widely. The price of bypass surgery in Pennsylvania, for example, ranges from $21,000 to $84,000—a fourfold difference.

"High cost and quality don't necessarily correlate," says Joseph Martin, a spokesman for Pennsylvania's Health Care Cost Containment Council, which conducts the outcomes program. For example, Philadelphia's Graduate Hospital charged $84,000 for bypass surgery and had a higher-than-expected mortality rate, while the city's Episcopal Hospital charged only $44,000 and had a death rate in the range expected.

Pennsylvania companies are taking advantage of the data. Last January Hershey Foods gave 6,500 of its employees the option of switching to a managed-care health plan that allows them to choose from among 10 hospitals shown to provide excellent care at low cost.

New York and Pennsylvania have now gone beyond hospital data to disclose mortality outcomes for individual physicians. In both states the data involve bypass surgeons. New York was first, releasing names in 1991 in response to a court order. (Until then, physician-specific data were kept confidential and were given only to the hospitals where the surgeons worked.) The information included the names of the 140 New York surgeons doing bypass surgery from 1989 through 1990, mortality rates among their patients for that period, and how many operations they did. The clear message: The busier surgeons—those doing more than 50 operations a year—did significantly better (an average risk-adjusted mortality rate of 3.2%) than surgeons doing fewer (average rate, 7.2%).

Pennsylvania followed in 1992 with a patient-mortality ranking of 170 bypass surgeons. The report named 14 surgeons with more deaths than expected for the operation, two who had fewer than expected, 33 who had performed fewer than 30 operations at any one hospital (the minimum deemed necessary for meaningful assessment) and 121 who fell within the expected patient-mortality range.

Critics contend that outcomes programs such as New York's and Pennsylvania's unfairly penalize the hospitals and doctors treating the sickest patients. Fear of a low score, they say, will motivate doctors to shun high-risk patients in favor of those more likely to survive.

"The programs may make a hell of a contribution one day," says Dr. Frank Spencer, chairman of surgery at New York University Medical Center in New York City, "but right now, any statistician would blow it out of the water."

Defenders contend that the rankings have correctly taken patients' health status into account. They point out that the New York mortality data are adjusted using 21 risk factors selected by a panel of cardiac surgeons that include the patient's age, the severity of the disease and any history of previous heart operations. Pennsylvania's program takes seven factors into account.

"There is no advantage to taking low-risk patients, since their condition is taken into consideration when a doctor's mortality rate is risk-adjusted," says Dr. Sidney Wolfe of Ralph Nader's Public Citizen Health Research Group in Washington.

Despite the debate, outcomes research is spreading. Iowa, Colorado and Florida are now collecting outcomes data on hospitals and physicians. And in at least 14 states, regional employers have banded together to collect outcomes data for hospitals as a way of choosing health care providers.

The most extensive such effort is under way in Cleveland, where 31 hospitals, 2,500 doctors, 50 corporations and 8,000 small businesses have voluntarily collaborated to improve the quality of care in area hospitals. The Cleveland hospital study will collect information on the mortality and length of stay for patients treated in four departments: intensive care, surgery, ob/gyn and general medicine. The scores for each hospital will be compared with the outcome expected based on the risk factors affecting its patients.

The Cleveland study also asks patients to fill out surveys rating hospitals on 11 factors including quality of care, food service, admitting and discharge procedures and billing. A "global satisfaction rating" summarizes patients' responses to three questions: Would you brag about this hospital? Would you come back? Would you send a family member there? The study results will be made public and should help hospitals focus on areas that need improvement.

"Prices have kept going up, but corporations have had no clear basis on which to choose health care other than cost," says Dr. Dwain Harper, executive director of the Quality Information Management Corporation, which runs the Cleveland program. "If hospitals can give corporations a clear understanding about which services are better, then businesses can use that information to choose the most efficient hospitals. Ideally, the better hospitals will be rewarded with more patients."

Certain surgical procedures are done much more often in some parts of the country than in others, with major differences even from one town to the next. For example:

▶ The chance that a man in Iowa with an enlarged prostate will undergo surgery for the problem varies from 15% to 60% depending on the hospital treating him.

▶ The chance that a woman in Maine will eventually have a hysterectomy ranges from 20% to 70% depending on where she lives.

Why the differences? Local preferences, rather than any scientific justification. Determining which treatments are demonstrably superior could improve health care while reducing expenditures on those that are worthless. In 1989 Congress created an agency to provide that kind of information.

The Agency for Health Care Policy and Research (part of the U.S. Department of Health and Human Services) spends a third of its annual $125 million budget on outcomes research. So-called Patient Outcomes Research Teams at universities across the country analyze outcomes data involving thousands of patients. The aim: Identify the most effective treatments for a host of disorders and publish the data in medical journals. The agency also uses these findings in preparing "clinical practice guidelines" to help doctors choose the most appropriate treatments.

So far the agency has published guidelines for urinary incontinence, acute pain, bedsores and cataracts, and has also issued a patient guide for each. (The practice guidelines and patient guides are free and can be ordered by calling **800-358-9295.)** Guidelines are under development for more maladies, including low-back problems, middle-ear infection in children, depression and congestive heart failure.

"The response from the medical profession has been very positive, and the public has expressed extraordinary interest in what we're doing," says Dr. J. Jarrett Clinton, the agency administrator. He says his group has already sent out 3 million pieces of literature in response to requests.

The agency's guidelines are not mandatory, but some congressmen believe they should be. Rep. Duncan Hunter (R.-Calif.) has introduced a bill calling for treatment protocols that would have to be followed when patients are cared for under Medicare. "We need uniform treatments backed up by hard science to insure quality of care and to cut health costs," Hunter says.

The aim: Identify the most effective treatments for a host of disorders.

Some medical specialty groups, including urologists, orthopedists, radiologists and radiation oncologists, are developing treatment guidelines through their own outcomes research. The American Urological Association (AUA), for example, recently spent $1 million on a pilot study on the long-term outcomes of surgical and nonsurgical treatment for an enlarged prostate, which can cause difficulty urinating.

Prostate enlargement is often treated surgically—about 400,000 operations last year at a total cost of about $3.5 billion—but surgery can cause complications, including incontinence and impotence. The AUA study, involving 100 patients, compared surgery with three nonsurgical options (drug therapy, balloon dilation and "watchful waiting").

"It's pretty embarrassing to have to tell patients that we don't know the long-term outcomes of these treatments," says Dr. John McConnell, an associate professor of urology at the University of Texas Southwestern Medical Center in Dallas and one of the urologists involved in the AUA study. With surgery, for example, "we can tell patients their chances of symptom relief are between 75% and 96%, and their chance of impotence ranges from 3% to 35%. But we can't be more precise than that, because not enough patients have been followed yet." Outcomes research, says McConnell, "will

give us the data we need for advising patients about which treatment will relieve their symptoms while interfering minimally with their quality of life."

Some experts are calling for a national outcomes database—an ongoing effort "that would track the conditions, treatments and outcomes of millions of patients in a standard way," says InterStudy's Ellwood. Using office computers, doctors would create the database by entering outcomes data on their own patients; then they'd use the pooled data to help them with their individual treatment decisions. Ellwood predicts such a database will be created within the next four to five years.

Consumer advocates generally favor outcomes research, but some wonder if the information will actually have an impact on medical care. "You can do outcomes research and find out the likelihood of someone's doing well or poorly with certain treatments," says the Health Research Group's Wolfe. "But the question is, will the findings be incorporated in how patients are treated? The public will soon become cynical if outcomes research doesn't affect the way medicine is being practiced."

Other proponents worry that the movement may be stymied by hospitals and physician groups that may not want to share their data or insist that it be kept from the public. "Hospitals and doctors may try to co-opt the process by saying the public will not understand the information," says Arthur Levin, director of the Center for Medical Consumers in New York City. "We may yet see a revival of the old fight on the part of health care providers to see to it that nobody looks over their shoulder."

In general, however, consumer advocates have hailed the outcomes movement. "Outcomes research is a great victory for health consumers," says Blair Horner of the New York Public Interest Research Group in New York City. "Patients deserve to have as much information as they can when they make life-and-death decisions."

The Mainstreaming of
Alternative Medicine

Douglas S. Barasch

Douglas S. Barasch is a freelance writer in New York specializing in medical issues.

There was little more that doctors could do for Catherine Bettez. Afflicted for nearly 10 years with lymphocytic hypophysitis, a rare, incurable disease of the endocrine system that depresses immunity, the 43-year-old woman had become increasingly debilitated by pain and depression, conditions that persisted despite medication. Acknowledging their limitations, her endocrinologist and her psychiatrist referred her to another kind of healer—a practitioner whose treatments were meditation and yoga.

"It seemed off-the-wall," says Bettez, a former proof-reader in Westminster, Mass. "I'm going to sit around and meditate and that's going to make me feel better?"

Because the healer her physicians recommended was not some robed mystic but a professor of medicine at the University of Massachusetts in Worcester, she decided to enroll in his program last spring. Since completing it, Bettez reports, she has been able to cut down on Naprosyn, an anti-inflammatory medication that helps alleviate her pain, and stop taking Ativan for her depression. "This has been a godsend."

In recent years, unconventional therapies such as meditation, acupuncture and homeopathy have begun to gain a foothold in American medicine. Catherine Bettez is one of millions of patients who have been treated with such methods, and her physicians are among the thousands of doctors who either refer patients to practitioners of alternative medicine or use elements of it themselves.

This year, the National Institutes of Health established an Office for the Study of Unconventional Medical Practices to investigate a wide range of treatments, including herbal medicine and massage therapy. Next year, Harvard Medical School plans to offer a course on unorthodox medicine. Similar courses and lectures are already available to medical students at Georgetown University, the University of Louisville, the University of Arizona and the University of Massachusetts in Worcester. Dr. David M. Eisenberg, an instructor of medicine who persuaded Harvard to offer the course after having studied acupuncture in China, says his purpose was not only to introduce students to the theory and practice of alternative treatments but also "to train students to think rigorously about them."

Acupuncture, a mainstay of Chinese medicine for thousands of years, came to Westerners' attention about 20 years ago, when China opened its doors to the modern world. American doctors were intrigued by the use of acupuncture as a surgical anesthetic, and researchers found that it works by inducing nerve cells to produce endorphins, the body's natural painkillers. Scientists have also found evidence to support the view, held by many cultures, that illness can be brought on not only by external forces, like viruses, but by one's state of mind. Stress seems to weaken the immune system and happiness to strengthen it. Personality traits such as impatience increase the risk of heart disease. Studies show that meditation and other "mind-body" therapies confer various benefits, including reduced pain and, for infertile women, a higher conception rate.

Many physicians now speak of a transition from the narrow biomedical model of Western medicine to a "biopsychosocial" one. With this approach, doctors would continue to marshal the tools of Western medicine to do what it does best: save the life of a patient who is acutely ill or in critical condition, by pumping him full of antibiotics when he has pneumonia, for example, or mending his skull after it has been shattered in a car accident. Doctors would also draw on holistic techniques to help prevent killer illnesses such as heart disease, diabetes and cancer, and to treat chronic conditions such as pain, hypertension and anxiety—problems that often do not yield to high-tech medicine. Patients would then have the healer's touch and, if necessary, the MRI.

Under the direction of Jon Kabat-Zinn, a professor of medicine, the Stress Reduction Clinic at the University of Massachusetts Medical Center in Worcester has taught Buddhist meditation and yoga to thousands of patients, most of whom have been referred by physicians. At one recent class there were 30 patients whose ailments included AIDS, muscular dystrophy, hypertension, chronic back pain, anxiety disorder, gastrointestinal distress, coronary artery disease and cancer.

Outcomes studies show that most patients who go through Kabat-Zinn's eight-week program feel much better than they did before, regardless of their illnesses. "They're taking people that the system is not helping. They're taking the toughest patients and having significant outcomes," says Dr. John K. Zawacki, a gastroenterologist at the University of Massachusetts Medical Center.

About 40 miles east, at Deaconess Hospital in Boston, is the Harvard-affiliated Mind/Body Medical Institute, founded in 1988 by Dr. Herbert Benson, a cardiologist at Harvard Medical School. The institute uses meditation, repetitive exercise and yoga to achieve what Dr. Benson calls the relaxation response, a physiological state characterized by lowered blood pressure, heart rate, respiration and metabolism that was the subject of his best-selling book of the same name.

The institute offers programs for cardiac risk reduction and rehabilitation, infertility, insomnia, chronic pain, AIDS and cancer. Cures are not promised. Patients can, however, hope for a reduction in symptoms, or at least a greater ability to cope with serious medical conditions as well as with treatments (such as chemotherapy) that can be both psychologically and physically debilitating.

Dr. Benson has demonstrated the success of his methods in several clinical studies. One published last year in the journal Fertility and Sterility showed that women receiving medical treatment for infertility who also went through his infertility program had about a 35 percent conception rate, compared with a roughly 17 percent rate among women who got only medical treatment. A study last year in The Clinical Journal of Pain found that after going through Dr. Benson's chronic pain program, people didn't feel the need to go to the doctor as often—the number of visits was reduced by an average of 38 percent. And a study published in the Journal of Cardiopulmonary Rehabilitation found that patients who had completed his hypertension program showed reductions in blood pressure, anxiety and depression.

Relaxation techniques as well as other alternative therapies such as biofeedback are now routinely taught to patients at medical centers and doctors' offices around the country. More than 2,000

MILESTONES

1971
The opening of China to the modern world and a New York Times article by James Reston about his experience with acupuncture stimulated interest in Chinese medicine among American physicians and the general public.

1974
"Type A Behavior and Your Heart," a best seller by two cardiologists, Drs. Meyer Friedman and Ray H. Rosenman, suggested that personality traits such as impatience and irritability increase a person's risk of heart disease.

1975
"The Relaxation Response," by Dr. Herbert Benson, a Harvard cardiologist, showed that meditation can lower blood pressure and heart rate.

1979
Norman Cousins, long-time editor of The Saturday Review, wrote that taking vitamin C and watching comedies led to his recovery from an "incurable" disease. Jon Kabat-Zinn, a professor of medicine, established the Stress Reduction Clinic at the University of Massachusetts Medical Center in Worcester, the first hospital-based program to use meditation and yoga therapeutically.

1981
Robert Ader, a professor of psychosocial medicine at the University of Rochester, published "Psychoneuroimmunology," a textbook on the interaction of the mind and the immune system.

1988
Dr. Benson established the Mind/Body Medical Institute at the Dea-conness Hospital in Boston, which uses his relaxation technique to help treat conditions such as chronic pain and cancer.

1989
A study in The Lancet by Dr. David Spiegel, a psychiatrist at Stanford University, showed that women with metastatic breast cancer who get medical care as well as "psychosocial treatment"—including support group meetings and self-hypnosis—live twice as long as patients who receive only medical care.

1990
Another Lancet study, by Dr. Dean Ornish, director of the Preventive Medicine Research Center in Sausalito, Calif., demonstrated that techniques like yoga can help reverse coronary heart disease.

Alternative Medicine Lexicon

Acupuncture—An ancient Chinese practice that involves inserting thin needles into the body at various points and manipulating them to relieve pain or treat illness.

Biofeedback—A technique for teaching people to become aware of their heart rate, blood pressure, temperature and other involuntary body functions in order to control them by a conscious mental effort.

Herbal medicine—The use of balms and medications prepared from flowers, leaves and other parts of plants.

Homeopathy—A medical system based on the idea of treating disease by using minute, highly diluted doses of the very substances that, in large doses, can cause it.

Hypnotherapy—A method of inducing a trancelike state characterized by extreme suggestibility in order to help patients relax, control pain and overcome addictions such as smoking.

Naturopathy—An approach to treating illness with diet, exercise and other "natural" means, rather than drugs or surgery.

Guided imagery—The use of mental imagery to facilitate the healing process.

physicians use acupuncture in conjunction with conventional medicine, according to the American Academy of Medical Acupuncture, and 5,000 use hypnotherapy, according to the American Society of Clinical Hypnosis. Dana Ullman, a board member of the National Center for Homeopathy, estimates that more than 1,000 doctors practice homeopathy.

Alternative therapies have a reputation for being less expensive than conventional medicine, since practitioners prescribe fewer drugs and recommend fewer diagnostic tests and other costly interventions, and because they typically spend more time with patients than regular doctors do. But the fees charged by practitioners of unconventional medicine can be high. An initial consultation with a physician, a nurse or some other certified practitioner of homeopathy costs $60 to $300, depending on the location, although the visit lasts about an hour and a half, says Dr. William Shevin, president of the National Center for Homeopathy. Subsequent half-hour visits range from $45 to $80. Acupuncturists charge $50 to $100, says Dr. Joseph M. Helms, president of the American Academy of Medical Acupuncture. Jon Kabat-Zinn's stress-reduction program runs $565 for nine sessions, and Dr. Benson's programs cost an average of $1,000 for 10 classes.

Insurance reimbursement for unconventional medicine varies by the policy, the therapy, the practitioner and the geographical region. Catherine Bettez's insurance policy covered most of the fee for Kabat-Zinn's relaxation program, and another patient, Ken Hokanson, says his policy covered all of it. Six states—California, Florida, Montana, Nevada, New Mexico and Oregon—require insurers to reimburse patients who see licensed acupuncturists for pain relief. And in Alaska, the services of licensed naturopaths, practitioners who treat disease with nonmedical approaches such as diet and exercise rather than drugs and surgery, must be covered.

Some insurance companies impose their own standards. The American Western Life Insurance Company in California, a $60 million insurer with 300,000 clients, recently launched a "wellness and preventative care health plan," which reimburses patients for alternative therapies such as homeopathy, herbal medicine, shiatsu massage, acupressure, acupuncture, guided imagery, hypnotherapy and biofeedback.

But American Western is clearly the exception. Many major companies, including the Prudential Insurance Company of America and the John Hancock Mutual Life Insurance Company, two multibillion-dollar insurers, cover alternative therapies only if a medical doctor or a licensed practitioner performs them. A therapy must also be deemed medically necessary by the insurance company's own doctors. "It has to be documented to be an effective and safe intervention, not just prescribed by a doctor or provided by a physician," says Dr. I. Steven Udvarhelyi, vice president of medical services at Prudential, which covers meditation, biofeedback, acupuncture and shiatsu massage, but not hypnotherapy. "We base our coverage decisions on a careful and extensive review of the medical literature. We also consider the consensus opinion within the medical community."

The medical community's willingness to accept some alternative therapies has been strengthened by a few ground-breaking studies. In 1990, Dr. Dean Ornish, director of the Preventive Medicine Research Institute in Sausalito, Calif., published a study in The Lancet showing that techniques such as yoga and meditation, when used in conjunction with a low-fat diet, can reverse coronary heart disease, actually reducing the amount of plaque in the arteries. A year earlier, also in The Lancet, Dr. David Spiegel, a psychiatrist at Stanford University School of Medicine, demonstrated that women with metastatic breast cancer who got medical care as well as "psychosocial treatment"—including support groups and self-hypnosis—survived twice as long as patients who received only medical care. These studies "added significantly to the cumulative evidence that emotions and behaviors can influence physical health," says Dr. Halsted R. Holman, a professor of medicine at Stanford.

Scores of other studies have suggested a link between emotions or attitudes and physical health. For example, a report last year in the New England Journal of Medicine found that stress increases a person's chances of catching a cold. Other research has shown that particular alternative therapies are effective against certain ailments. Homeopathic remedies can relieve headaches, colds, flu and allergies, according to several European studies. And a recent article in The Lancet concluded that a traditional Chinese herbal therapy reduces the symptoms of dermatitis.

A s the scientific evidence supporting various unconventional treatments accumulates, some physicians predict nothing less than the transformation of American medicine, from a biomedical model to a biopsychosocial one. Dr. Joel Elkes, professor emeritus of psychiatry at the University of Louisville, believes that within 25 years mind-body techniques will permeate medical practice, from primary care to the treatment of such illnesses as cancer and heart disease. The integration of approaches such as meditation, yoga, acupuncture and biofeedback with drugs and surgery, he says, "will be as important to medicine as the discovery of antibiotics."

"I think that's possible," says Dr. Arnold S. Relman, former editor of The New England Journal of Medicine who now teaches at Harvard Medical School and is writing a book on the health care system. "But it all depends on whether we can get more scientific evidence."

Like Dr. Relman, other gatekeepers of American medicine remain skeptical about much of the research on alternative treatments. Dr. Marcia Angell, executive editor of The New England Journal of Medicine, thinks many of the studies have been poorly designed and "characterized by exuberant interpretation."

Some scientists studying the interaction between the mind and the body are themselves skeptics, who say their work is often erroneously used by practitioners—including many physicians—as justification for alternative therapies.

"I resent being cited as the scientific basis for protocols and approaches that have never been tested scientifically," says Dr. David L. Felten, a leading researcher in the new field of psychoneuroimmunology, the study of the connection between the mind and the body's susceptibility to disease. Dr. Felten, a professor of neurobiology and anatomy at the University of Rochester School of Medicine and Dentistry, who received a MacArthur fellowship in 1983, has been working out the "hard wiring" of mind-body communication. His research has helped uncover a fascinating network of communication pathways between the body's endocrine, immune and nervous systems—a sort of physiological Rosetta stone. This network reveals that neurotransmitters, immune cells and hormones act as messengers between our thoughts and emotions and our immune defenses.

W hat everyone wants to know is which alternative therapies really work. Many medical practices that are widely accepted today met stiff opposition from the medical establishment when they were first introduced. Doctors initially doubted the need to wash their hands before performing surgery to prevent infection, for example, as well as the benefits of anesthesia. More recently, the value of acupuncture has been questioned. "People thought acupuncture was way out, spooky, flimflam, a few generations ago," Dr. Relman says. "But there appears to be convincing evidence that it can relieve or prevent pain, and now it's more respected."

Some of the resistance to alternative therapies is giving way as more scientists study them. "The champions of alternative medicine shouldn't expect to be believed unless they meet rigorous standards," he adds. "But on the other side, the traditional biomedical establishment ought not to prejudge. All biases and prejudices ought to fall before the evidence."

Contemporary Health Hazards

Our level of wellness is influenced by many factors, both external (exogenous) and internal (endogenous). While most diseases result from a combination of internal and external factors, a clear understanding of the differences between these two is crucial to the development of prevention and treatment strategies.

The dynamic interaction between humans and their environment is a constant source of both joy and sorrow. Humans more than any other living species have the ability to shape the environment to their needs and correspondingly must assume responsibility for the quality of the environment. Our tremendous scientific advances over the last 10 years have made us increasingly aware of the impact our behavior can have on both the physical environment and other living things. Because our understanding of nature is incomplete, we are not always able to accurately predict the environmental impact of new technologies and products. We must, therefore, proceed with caution and be prepared to rectify any problems that arise.

During the past few years we have been inundated with health warnings about toxic substances in our air, water, and even the food we eat. Unfortunately, the American public has come to believe that these reports are simply warnings and need not be taken too seriously. Reports of poisonous chemicals polluting our waters, seeping from the earth, and spewing into our skies are indeed overwhelming. Although awareness of the problems has increased, we have yet to make significant strides in our move to clean up our environment. Clearly, the major obstacles to such an effort are the complex economic aspects involved. If we as a people demanded that all offenders stop polluting our environment today, all of us would have to permanently park our cars, risk having our heat turned off, and face losing our jobs. The results would probably be more detrimental to our health than the toxins themselves. Certainly this is not the answer to our environmental problems. The scenario just described, while unrealistic, does demonstrate the relationship between the pollution problem and economics. Cleaning up the environment will be costly, and we must all be willing to shoulder some of the responsibility if we are to be successful in our efforts.

While some improvement has been observed in the areas of air and water pollution, much remains to be done, and new areas of concern continue to surface. Of all the environmental health issues, atmospheric pollution by chlorofluorocarbon compounds (CFCs) and carbon dioxide seems to have generated the most concern worldwide. CFCs are synthetic products that have achieved worldwide acceptance as components of refrigerants, propellants, and solvents. Unfortunately these compounds, when released into the atmosphere, destroy the ozone layer that shields the earth from ultraviolet (UV) radiation. This protective layer is under-going a rapid depletion; consequently, there has been a steady rise in the amount of UV radiation to which we are exposed. Most experts agree that we will witness significant increases in the incidence of skin cancer because of this. To protect ourselves against the damaging effects of this form of radiation, medical authorities have encouraged us to apply liberal amounts of sunscreen to our skin. According to some researchers, adherence to this advice may prove to be deadly. While sunscreens appear to be effective in blocking the UVB rays that cause sunburns, they provide little protection against UVA radiation, which constitutes 95 percent of the UV radiation and is associated with malignant melanoma, the most deadly form of skin cancer. Opponents of sunscreens argue that they disable our bodies' natural alarm system (sunburn response) and expose us to very high doses of the more dangerous UVA radiation. Michael Castleman's article "Beach Bummer" discusses the controversy concerning the use of sunscreens and the prevention of cancer.

Despite the numerous safety precautions taken by the food industry there may be as many as 81 million cases of "food poisoning" annually in the United States. According to the Centers for Disease Control (CDC), food poisoning attributable to botulism and trichinosis is declining, but food-borne illnesses such as salmonella have increased over 200 percent in the last 25 years. Growing concern over salmonella surfaced in January 1992 when New Jersey adopted a statewide regulation that prevented restaurants from serving raw or runny eggs to the public. Another food-borne pathogen, campylobacter, may be even more common than salmonella. Recent studies have confirmed the threat that these pathogens pose by finding evidence of their presence in over 65 percent of all raw meat and poultry sold in this country for human consumption. Because contamination is so widespread, the CDC recommends that consumers view every product of animal origin as if it were contaminated and treat it accordingly. "Gut Reactions" by Jonathan Edlow examines specific types of food poisoning, including symptoms, food sources, and preventative measures.

While AIDS has dominated the press coverage of sexually transmitted diseases, other STDs such as HPV and genital herpes infect hundreds of thousands of individuals each year. HPV, also known as genital warts, is a viral disease for which there is no vaccination or cure. Its symptoms can range from cauliflower-like warts that appear on the genitals to cancer of the genitals, especially cancer of the cervix. Experts estimate that as many as 750,000 people a year are infected with this disease. The article "Dangerous Liaison" presents a frank discussion of the HPV problem and suggests that it may well be the venereal disease of the 1990s. Geoffrey Cowley and Mary Hager's article "Sleeping with the Enemy" provides a short discussion of the eight most common STDs, including information regarding their incidence, symptomatology, and medical complications.

Hepatitis, another infectious illness, infects over 500,000 Americans each year and claims the life of about 16,000 annually. Each of the five different forms of hepatitis—hepatitis A, hepatitis B, hepatitis C, hepatitis D, and hepatitis E—is caused by a different virus. Hepatitis B, the most prevalent form, may be spread by sexual contact. Its virus is extremely contagious and is able to remain contagious outside the body for a week or longer. Of the 300,000 who contract hepatitis B, 150,000 will become acutely ill, and about 300 will die. Six to 10 percent of hepatitis B victims will never completely shake the infection and will become hepatitis B carriers, with about 33 percent developing chronic active hepatitis. Yearly deaths attributable to this condition total approximately 5,000. There is currently no reliable cure for any form of hepatitis. The good news is that there is an effective vaccine for hepatitis B, but as with all vaccines, it must be taken before one is infected if it is to provide immunity. Rob Stein's article "The ABC's of Hepatitis" discusses the five different forms of hepatitis and provides information regarding mode of transmission, preventative measures, prognosis, and methods of treatment.

Another health hazard is rape, an act of violence against another human being. Date rape or acquaintance rape has recently emerged as a major security issue at numerous colleges and universities throughout this country. It is difficult to determine whether this form of sexual violence is relatively new, or if it has been going on for years, undetected, like wife beating or sexual harassment. We do know that date rape is widespread, with the number of reported cases growing rapidly. In 1989 it was estimated that between 13 and 25 percent of all coeds attending American universities were victims of date rape. Statistics also indicated that in most cases the victims knew their assailants. Sexual violence has become so common on college campuses that it frequently surpasses theft as the foremost security issue. Lauren David Pedin's article "What Every Woman Needs to Know About Personal Safety" discusses the safety measures women can take to reduce their risk of becoming victims of rape or some other violent crime.

While this unit focuses on exogenous factors that influence health, it is important to remember that health is a dynamic state representing the degree of harmony or balance between internal and external factors. This concept of balance applies to the environment as well. Because of the intimate relationship between people and their environment, it is impossible to promote the concept of wellness without also safeguarding the quality of the environment. Perhaps the greatest environmental challenge yet to be faced is the blending and balancing of technological change with environmental evolution.

Looking Ahead: Challenge Questions

What do you consider to be our greatest environmental health hazard today?

Are you concerned about the damaging effect of UV radiation on your skin? What steps are you taking to prevent such damage?

What steps can an individual take to reduce the risk of contracting food poisoning?

What could the government do to help cut the spread of STDs? What are you personally doing to reduce your risk of contracting them?

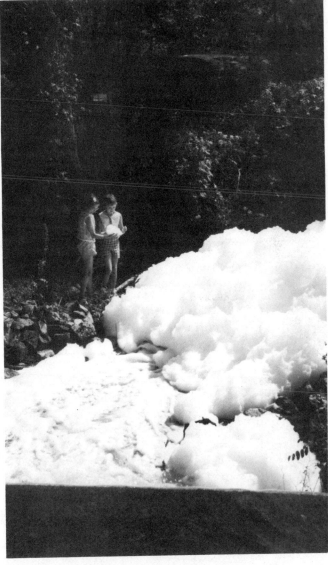

Beach bummer

New evidence suggests that sunscreens don't prevent skin cancer and may even promote some forms of it. The manufacturers know it. Some researchers know it. Why don't consumers?

Michael Castleman

Medical journalist Michael Castleman writes for national magazines and has authored six books, most recently An Aspirin A Day *(Hyperion). Kerry Lauerman of* Mother Jones *contributed additional reporting to this story.*

Anyone who's ever heard a smoke alarm go off knows how horrid its whine can be. Why keep it around? Because a little unpleasantness can prevent injury or death in a fire. But in the last few decades, millions of people who cherish smoke detectors may have disabled one of nature's equally protective, if annoying, alarms. They've rubbed on sunscreen, never thinking that sunburns, like smoke alarms, might prevent a greater harm.

As experts persuaded more and more Americans to use sunscreens, melanoma became an epidemic, with new diagnoses roughly paralleling sunscreen sales.

Ironically, sunscreen devotees have turned off their dermatological smoke detectors in the name of preventive medicine. Sunburn, experts say, is a key risk factor for malignant melanoma, the potentially fatal skin cancer that's become a headline-grabbing epidemic since 1980. Forget what used to be called a "healthy tan." Today, experts insist, we're paying for decades of naïve, post–World War II, beach-blanket sun worship with an unprecedented melanoma rate. But there's hope, they tell us. If you can't avoid the midday sun, pour on the sunscreen.

Unfortunately, the public health authorities who urge routine, liberal use of sunscreen (especially on children) fail to mention that *sunscreens have never been shown to prevent melanoma.* The medical research community knows this. The Food and Drug Administration knows it. And sunscreen makers know it. Yet, as a result of scientific myopia, bureaucratic inertia, and the almighty bottom line, they've essentially told us to use sunscreen and not to worry.

But two San Diego epidemiologists, Cedric and Frank Garland, *are* worried. Best known for their work linking sunshine with the prevention of breast and colon cancer, the Garland brothers (with research associate Edward Gorham) have compiled a body of evidence suggesting that sunscreens dupe the public into believing they're covered by state-of-the-art melanoma protection, when, in fact, they may be highly vulnerable to the disease. Even worse, the Garlands' research suggests that sunscreen use just might *promote* melanoma.

Unfortunately for the public health, the Garlands refuse to discuss their theory for fear of professional ostracism. After they presented their case against sunscreens at a 1990 epidemiological meeting in Los Angeles, both the *New York Times* and the *Washington Post* ran articles explaining their theory. Epidemiologists accused the Garlands of grandstanding for speaking to the press before publishing their analysis in a scientific journal. Stung by this criticism (which could threaten funding of their other work), the brothers have since avoided journalists. But anyone who examines the Garlands' claims might feel, well, burned by sunscreens.

Meanwhile, most dermatologists, epidemiologists, and sunscreen makers continue to suggest that sunscreens prevent melanoma. With a $380 million market at stake, the sunscreen industry in particular has an interest in keeping the Garlands' argument out of the public eye. Perhaps, as the industry claims, sunscreens prevent melanoma; perhaps they promote it. No one knows for certain, but worse, almost no one is trying to find out. So before you rub on another drop of sunscreen, consider the evidence. Because sunscreen makers are watching out for everything except your health.

Malignant melanoma's dark, mole-derived tumors are the fastest-rising cancer under the sun. From 1975 to 1992, the number of melanoma cases reported annually in the U.S. tripled, increasing more than any other cancer. Since the 1950s, melanoma rates have also risen dramatically among fair-skinned Australians, Brits, Canadians, and Scandinavians (it is extremely unusual for dark-skinned people to get skin cancer).

Melanoma now strikes thirty-two thousand Americans each year and kills sixty-eight hundred. But before 1950 it was quite rare. Two other skin cancers, basal and squamous cell skin tumors, were dermatologists' major concern. These slow-spreading cancers usually occur in white men over forty-five who work outdoors or live near the equator. They are by far the nation's most prevalent cancers, with 600,000 new diagnoses each year, but they rarely prove fatal, with successful treatment in 99 percent of cases.

Around the turn of the century, doctors linked risk of basal and squamous cell tumors with lifetime sun exposure—the more sun, the more risk. They also discovered a far rarer—and more fatal—skin cancer, later dubbed malignant melanoma, which they believed had nothing to do with sunlight because it usually appeared in people who spent little time in the sun. Victims of the fatal cancer had only two things in common—fair skin and red or blonde hair. Doctors concluded that the cancer was a consequence of being fair-skinned and light-haired.

But by the late 1960s, numerous studies showed a connection between melanoma and the ultraviolet radiation in sunlight, demonstrating, for example, that whites who live near the equator have higher melanoma rates than those in temperate climes.

The fact that outdoor workers rarely develop melanoma was apparently explained when researchers shifted their attention from sun*light* to sun*burn*. They hypothesized that deeply tanned skin protects against melanoma, even though it increases the risk of basal and squamous cell cancers. Indoor office workers have brief, intense exposures to the sun—the kind that cause sunburn, which in turn could lead to melanoma.

During the 1970s, scientists used the sunburn theory to explain the dramatic rise in the melanoma rate in the second half of this century. After World War II, they argued, record numbers of Americans became white-collar workers, which limited their sun exposure and, as a result, increased their risk of weekend sunburns. In addition, sunbathing became a national pastime, and women's swimsuits became more revealing.

Because melanoma has been associated with teenage sunburns, but the median age for diagnosis is in the forties, researchers concluded that melanoma, like many cancers, takes decades to develop. Estimating a twenty-five- to thirty-year lag time, proponents of the sunburn theory claim that postwar sunbathing resulted in the melanoma epidemic of the 1980s.

There is no animal model for melanoma (as there is for squamous cell skin cancer, which mice can contract), so it is impossible to conduct laboratory experiments to discover exactly what causes the disease. And, although the

New kid on the (sun)block

When the Garland brothers took aim at sunscreens that protect skin only from UVB rays, many sunscreen makers referred media calls to the Academy of American Dermatology, which issued a rebuttal stating, "No studies have suggested direct relationships between melanoma and ultraviolet A."

Less than three years later, the AAD is recommending UVA protection and it is the major focus of sunscreen marketing efforts. Part of the reason is the FDA's approval of the UVA-screening chemical Parsol 1789 (until recently available only in Herbert Laboratories' Photoplex). Although previous sunscreens had claimed to block UVA, they blocked only about one-third of the UVA spectrum. In fact, in 1990 the FDA warned Schering-Plough, makers of Coppertone, that adopting its own proposed UVA rating system would constitute "false and misleading" labeling.

If the Garlands are right about the dangers of sunscreen, then UVA-blockers might go a long way toward solving the problem. Of course, that's what everyone thought twenty years ago about blocking UVB. . . . So before you rush out to buy Photoplex or any other broad-spectrum sunscreen, remember: scientists still don't know what causes or prevents melanoma. Assertions that UVA blockage protects against melanoma are purely speculative.

Hot tip

"Sun Protection Factor" (SPF) numbers may not be as useful as you think. A sunscreen's protection depends not only on the SPF, but also on the thickness and uniformity of the application and the product's chemical stability. The SPF standard assumes liberal application. A thin coat might provide only half the SPF on the product label.

—M. C.

sunburn theory is an advance over the "fate of the fair-skinned" theory, it fails to explain a few things.

For instance, sunburn was a common medical problem long before people started wearing bikinis. Turn-of-the-century medical texts dealt with it as a fact of life, and folk medicine abounds with remedies. Yet melanoma was extremely rare before 1950.

Many of the social changes sunburn-theory supporters attribute to the 1950s actually occurred about thirty years earlier. Sunbathing first became popular during the 1920s, thanks to fashion designer Coco Chanel, who launched a tanning chic after returning from a yachting vacation with a golden tan. Assuming a lag time of twenty-five to thirty years, the melanoma rate should have risen considerably starting in the mid-1940s. It didn't.

Furthermore, several studies suggest that melanoma actually may have a short lag time. Sunspots, which cause complex effects in the upper atmosphere, appear cyclically on the sun's surface about every eleven years. A study of sunspot activity between 1935 and 1975 showed that every sunspot cycle was followed a few years later by a small but significant increase in the melanoma rate.

A Scottish study corroborated the idea of a short lag time by finding a "highly significant" correlation between melanoma diagnoses and severe sunburns occurring just five years earlier. Melanoma diagnoses in fifteen- to twenty-four-year-olds have increased noticeably since 1973. And studies in Sweden, Hawaii, and the continental U.S. have shown consistent seasonal patterns in melanoma diagnoses, another hallmark of biological events with short lag times.

But if melanoma has a lag time of only a few years, then the explosive increases of the 1960s, 1970s, and 1980s can't be blamed on changes in beach attire of the 1920s *or* the 1940s. The factor that accounts for these changes must have appeared in the middle or late 1950s and become gradually more significant as time has progressed.

No one knows what this factor is. But Cedric and Frank Garland are afraid that it may be sunscreen use.

Most sunscreens block about 5 percent of ultraviolet radiation—the UVB rays that cause burning. The other 95 percent of the UV spectrum, UVA, has long been thought to play a minor role in sunburn, so sunscreens block only a small portion of it (see box on preceding page). But studies have shown that UVA may play an important role in skin cancer. UVA radiation penetrates more deeply into the skin than UVB, down to the melanocytes, the cells that turn cancerous in melanoma.

Scientists have yet to identify exactly what corrupts healthy melanocytes, largely because there is no animal model for melanoma. But mice develop *non*melanoma skin cancers under UV light.

The sunscreen-melanoma link might also explain why professionals are at greater risk than clerical workers.

Proponents of the sunburn theory are quick to point to a Danish study in which sunscreen was shown to delay (but not completely prevent) the development of squamous cell tumors in mice exposed to artificial sunlight. The higher the sunscreen's sun protection factor, the longer it took the mice to develop tumors. To date, this is the closest scientists have come to establishing the preventive value of sunscreens.

However, another study at the same lab should give sunscreen advocates pause. In this experiment, mice exposed to artificial sunlight developed a small number of squamous cell tumors. But ones exposed to artificial sunlight followed by additional UVA developed more than twice as many tumors.

Not only does this study suggest that UVA may play a role in skin cancer, it also points to the particular danger of sunlight

What about the ozone?

The melanoma epidemic became a major news story six years ago when the ozone "hole" (thinning is a more accurate description) opened up over Antarctica. However, what's been happening over the bottom of the world has nothing to do with the melanoma rate in the U.S.

In a 1991 report, the Environmental Protection Agency estimated a 5 percent ozone loss over the U.S. during the last decade. But the amount of UV radiation striking the country actually decreased a bit, according to the National Cancer Institute, because of another UV filter—air pollution. If ozone loss on the order of Antarctica's happens over the U.S., our melanoma rate might well soar in the future. But melanoma epidemiologists agree that, to date, Antarctic ozone loss has played no role in our Melanoma epidemic.

—M.C.

followed by UVA alone—a cycle similar to that which occurs when people use sunscreen. They hit the beach, playground, or ballfield and remove some clothing, exposing themselves to full-spectrum sunlight. Then they apply sunscreen, blocking UVB, but continuing their exposure to UVA. As the sunscreen wears off, they're again exposed to full sun. After reapplying sunscreen, they get additional UVA—and possibly cancer.

Of course, mice are not human beings, and squamous cell cancers are not melanoma, so either study (or both) may mean nothing. But melanoma experts trumpet the implications of the first study, that sunscreens help prevent skin cancer, while ignoring those of the second, that sunscreen use fosters a cancer-promoting pattern of UV exposure.

The Garlands have more disturbing news about sunscreen: by impairing the body's production of vitamin D, it may also remove a defense against cancer. According to studies, vitamin D has a hormone-like effect that interferes with the growth of several tumors, including those associated with melanoma and colon and breast cancers. Although we get small amounts of the vitamin from milk and cold-water fish, most of our bodies' supply is produced when skin is exposed to UVB. By blocking UVB, sunscreens interfere with vitamin D synthesis. A recent study shows that habitual sunscreen users have unusually low vitamin D levels—sometimes low enough that researchers call them "deficient."

A sunscreen-melanoma link might also illuminate a peculiar fact unexplained by the sunburn theory: melanoma risk rises with income. Although both professionals and clerical workers work indoors, the former have a significantly higher melanoma rate. Because health consciousness is generally an upper-income phenomenon, sunscreens presumably appeal to the more affluent.

Even if sunscreen is one day shown to protect against melanoma, the Garlands worry that it may give users a dangerously false sense of security. No one knows how large doses of

UVA might affect the body. Historically, whites would have been dangerously sunburned long before they received the levels of UVA radiation that they may now get in one sunscreen-wearing day at the beach. Whatever UVA's role in causing melanoma, the Garlands strongly recommend that you not make yourself a guinea pig.

Remember those old Coppertone ads with the puppy pulling down the little girl's bathing suit? Suntan lotions, introduced in the mid-1950s for cosmetic purposes, were the first commercial use of sunscreens. As sales increased throughout the 1950s and 1960s, so did the melanoma rate.

During the 1970s and 1980s, suntan lotions were repositioned as sunscreens, which, experts said, prevented skin cancer by preventing sunburn. Sales in 1991 were $380 million, more than twice as much as a decade earlier. But as experts persuaded more and more Americans to use sunscreens, melanoma became an epidemic, with new diagnoses roughly paralleling sunscreen sales.

This epidemic has been a godsend for sunscreen makers. According to the journal *Drug and Cosmetic Industry,* "Every indicator that skin cancer is on the rise, every utterance by a dermatologist . . . seems to reinforce the need for consumers to use more of these products. The missionary work required to double the market [by 1995] has already been done, and not just by the industry."

Sunscreen makers frankly admit that their products have never been shown to prevent human skin cancers. "The studies show that sunscreens prevent squamous cell cancers in animals," says Patricia Agin, sunscreen product manager for Schering-Plough, whose brands, including Coppertone, account for one-third of the market. "I think they do the same in humans. But . . . we don't know for certain. Because there's no animal model for [melanoma], we don't know if sunscreens prevent it. I see no reason to think that they wouldn't, but we have no proof that they do."

Jack Surrette, marketing vice-president of Tanning Research Laboratories (makers of Hawaiian Tropic sunscreens), goes further. "To some extent, when you protect only for UVB, it would seem to run a risk for potential skin cancer," he says. "UVA is a more damaging ray. We may be hurting ourselves by protecting ourselves too well on the UVB side."

Unfortunately, sunscreen labels do not reflect Agin or Surrette's understanding of the research. They echo the claims of dermatologists and cancer-education organizations: "Regular use may prevent skin cancer." Of course, when a label says "skin cancer," sunscreen makers insist that it means nonfatal squamous cell skin cancer. But if the label doesn't distinguish between melanoma and other skin cancers, then how can consumers be expected to?

Further confusing consumers, most sunscreens carry a seal of approval from the nonprofit Skin Cancer Foundation, which claims to alert people to safe products. More than 130 different suncare products have earned the right to display this seal—for a price. In addition to submitting their products for testing and review, corporations also dole out ten thousand dollars to use

What you can do

To prevent malignant melanoma, start by using common sense instead of just sunscreens. First, assess your risk. Risk factors include: fair skin; blonde, red, or light brown hair; blue or green eyes; a family history of melanoma; an indoor occupation; outdoor leisure activities; numerous moles; freckling on the upper back; a tendency to sunburn easily and tan poorly; and actinic keratoses, rough, red, sun-induced bumps which sometimes develop on fair skin. The more risk factors you have, the more concerned you need to be. Anyone, even a black person, can develop melanoma, but for those without risk factors the danger is slight.

Dermatologists, the Skin Cancer Foundation, and the American Cancer Society all agree that the best way to prevent harm from sunlight—burning, wrinkling, and all forms of skin cancer—is to avoid direct sun between 10 a.m. and 3 p.m. Just take reasonable precautions: Don't sunbathe. If you love the beach, invest in an umbrella. Don't patronize tanning salons. In summer, adjust your schedule to engage in outdoor activities in the early morning or late afternoon. When out on summer days, wear a hat, sunglasses, and lightweight, long-limbed clothing. In winter, particularly if skiing, cover up with clothing.

There's no such thing as a "healthy tan," so don't go looking for one. Even if you take all the precautions listed above, you'll still acquire some color in the summer without significantly raising your melanoma risk.

How to spot it

Few people understand how life-saving early melanoma detection can be. Seventy percent of melanoma tumors develop from pre-existing moles. So examine your moles regularly—or have someone else do it—and know the ABCD's of melanoma detection:

- Asymmetry. Most normal moles are round and symmetrical. Melanomas are oddly shaped and asymmetrical.
- Border. Most normal moles have smooth edges. Melanomas often have notched or scalloped edges.
- Color. Most normal moles are a single shade of brown. Melanomas are black, blue, pink, and multicolored.
- Diameter. Most normal moles are less than one-quarter inch in diameter. Early melanomas grow outward and become larger.

Even before melanoma moles undergo visual changes, they often itch. If one of your moles starts to itch, or if you become nervous about a mole for any reason, ask you doctor for a referral to a dermatologist. If you have significant melanoma risk factors, see a dermatologist annually.

—M. C.

the seal. John Epstein, who sits on the Skin Cancer Foundation's four-member seal review committee, says he can't recall anyone ever being denied the seal, but companies that file inadequate paperwork must resubmit their requests. (A foundation spokesperson claimed that some companies have withdrawn rather than resubmit their applications.)

The foundation, which boasts celebrity backers such as Tom Selleck, Lauren Bacall, Dick Cavett, Paul Newman, and Joanne Woodward, earns about one-fourth of its $1.7 million budget from corporate donations. Recently the foundation sent sixty thousand elementary schools posters that urge students: "Always use sunscreen when you go outdoors, no matter the season or the color of your skin."

The Skin Cancer Foundation isn't the only case of corporate funding blurring the boundary between public health and the bottom line. The Skin Phototrauma Foundation (acronym: SPF) was founded by Ortho Pharmaceuticals (whose parent company, Johnson & Johnson, makes Sundown sunscreens), Procter & Gamble (Bain de Soleil), and Mary Kay Cosmetics (Sun Essentials). Even the Academy of American Dermatology, a medical association that counts 98 percent of dermatologists in the United States and Canada among its members, uses corporate donations to fund its public-education efforts.

So who should consumers turn to for an untainted view of sunscreens? The likely choice would be the Food and Drug Administration. Sometime this year, the FDA plans to release new labeling regulations for the first time since 1978. One proposal would require all sunscreen labels to carry "sun alerts," warning consumers that preventing sunburn may not protect them against wrinkling and skin cancer. But even after new regulations are released, the public and sunscreen makers will have eighteen months to comment before the FDA issues its final regulations, probably in 1995.

When the Garland brothers first presented their case against sunscreens at the 1990 meeting, a few epidemiologists expressed guarded interest. Dr. Leonard Kurland of the Mayo Clinic called their analysis "intriguing and worth exploring further." But most supporters of the sunburn theory considered the brothers' argument ludicrous.

The Garlands openly admit that the case against sunscreens is not airtight. The controversial assertion that melanoma has a brief lag time needs corroboration. The study showing that UVA promotes squamous cell tumors in sun-exposed mice may not be applicable to human beings. And a recent study showed no correlation between vitamin D levels and melanoma risk.

But the best theory is the one that answers the most questions, and the sunburn/long-lag-time theory looks shaky. It ignores the studies showing a brief lag time. It doesn't address why sunburn rarely caused melanoma before the 1950s. It sheds no light on why melanoma risk is linked to income. And it fails to explain why increases in the melanoma rate have so closely paralleled the rise in sunscreen use.

Despite these shortcomings, the sunburn theory continues to be the dominant scientific theory, and it often takes decades to overturn a dominant theory. It took almost twenty years for researchers to accept a connection between sunburn and melanoma, and no one was out there saying, "Get burned. It's good for you." Today leading scientists *are* saying, "Use sunscreens. They're good for you." If sunscreens provide a false sense of security, or worse, promote melanoma, convincing the scientific establishment could take well into the next century.

GUT reactions

Don't let food poisoning turn a pleasant meal into a nightmare

Jonathan Edlow, M.D.

Jonathan Edlow, M.D., is a physician and writer in the Boston area.

It might have been the pizza, or maybe it was the frozen yogurt that threw 25-year-old Becky Gilbert into a tailspin. "I couldn't even leave the bathroom for 12 hours," recalls the Philadelphia medical student. "The cramps were incredible. And I became so dehydrated, I had to get IV fluids in the emergency room. It was two or three weeks before I felt normal again. I never realized food poisoning could make you feel so sick."

Unfortunately, Gilbert's miserable experience was not just a freak occurrence. "Food poisoning," a phrase that refers to a variety of illnesses caused by eating food that's contaminated by bacteria, viruses, parasites or toxins, affects some 6 1/2 million Americans every year, according to Dr. Mitchell Cohen, director of bacterial and mycotic diseases at the Centers for Disease Control (CDC). Other experts in the field indicate that there may be as many as 81 million cases of food poising in the U.S. annually.

The incidence of food poisoning is difficult to track because most infections are never reported. But while some types, including botulism (caused by potentially deadly bacteria most often found in improperly canned goods) and trichinosis (caused by a parasite in pork), are on the decline, others appear to be on the rise. Reported cases of salmonella, a food-borne illness caused by bacteria in poultry, eggs, beef and unpasteurized dairy products, increased from 18,649 in 1963 to 43,776 in 1988, according to the most recent data from the CDC. Last January, growing concern about salmonella led New Jersey officials to pass a statewide regulation preventing restaurants from serving raw or runny eggs (the ruling is now being modified because of public outcry). And another food-borne pathogen called campylobac-

ter, found in poultry, unpasteurized dairy products and ground water, may now be more common than salmonella, say some experts.

Studies have shown that salmonella and campylobacter are in about 65% of raw meat and poultry.

In this age of modern medicine, why is food poisoning still a health threat? The CDC offers several reasons: Food animals are now raised in close quarters, which promotes the spread of diseases such as salmonella; as food processing becomes more centralized, a single contaminated ingredient may show up in several different products; every year, we import more foods from developing countries where food hygiene is not as advanced as it is in the U.S.; and an increasing number of Americans lack a basic knowledge of proper food handling.

While most people recover from food poisoning in a few days, others, like Becky Gilbert, feel rotten for longer. And for some people, food poisoning can be far more serious: According to Cohen, food-borne illness kills about 9,000 Americans each year. Those at greatest risk include infants, the elderly and people with weakened immune systems, such as those infected with HIV. Patients with severe liver disease, cancer and sickle cell anemia are also at increased risk. Pregnant women should be especially careful too.

Symptoms vary depending on the type and amount of the contaminant. The most common types of food poisoning—salmonella, campylobacter and staphylococcus—lead to vomiting and diarrhea, among other symptoms. Other illnesses, such as botulism, trichinosis, scombroid

poisoning and food-borne viruses such as hepatitis A, produce a wide range of symptoms, including hives and neurological problems. (For a complete description of the causes and symptoms of different types of food poisoning, see "The Facts About Food Poisoning.") The time it takes for symptoms to appear also varies: Scombroid poisoning, caused by improperly chilled fleshy fish including tuna and mackerel, may produce symptoms such as hives and a burning sensation in the throat in just five minutes, whereas salmonella symptoms may take six to 48 hours to appear.

Fortunately, there are measures we can all take to greatly reduce our chances of getting sick. First, know the enemy: Meat, poultry, eggs, milk, cheese and fish are most often implicated in outbreaks of food poisoning. Studies have shown that salmonella and campylobacter are in about 65% of raw meat and poultry intended for human consumption. (The U.S. Department of Agriculture [USDA] is experimenting with a chicken feed that significantly reduces salmonella, but chickens raised on it probably won't be in the supermarkets until 1993 or early 1994.) Cohen's advise: "Assume that every product of animal origin is contaminated, and handle it accordingly."

A few foods should be avoided entirely: unpasteurized milk and cheese made from unpasteurized milk (some brie, as well as feta and blue cheese, may be made from unpasteurized milk—check the label or ask a store clerk to find out), as well as raw or undercooked eggs. This means no caesar salad dressing, hollandaise sauce or eggnog made with raw eggs, and no raw cookie dough. (Pasteurized liquid whole eggs, available in some supermarkets, can be substituted in recipes calling for raw eggs.) The USDA says eggs should be cooked until the white and yolk are solid, since even soft-boiled, soft-scrambled and sunny-side up eggs pose some risk. Honey should not

THE FACTS ABOUT FOOD POISONING

TYPE	OCCURRENCE	SYMPTOMS	ONSET AFTER EATING
Campylo-bacter	Common	Muscle pain, nausea, vomiting, fever and cramps; occasionally bloody diarrhea	2 to 10 days
Clostridium perfringens	Common	Diarrhea and cramps	9 to 15 hours
Hepatitis A	Common	Fever, nausea, abdominal pain and loss of appetite; after 3 to 10 days, dark urine and jaundice	15 to 50 days
Norwalk virus	Common	Nausea, vomiting, diarrhea and headache	1 to 2 days
Salmonella	Common	Nausea, vomiting, diarrhea, cramps, fever and headache	6 to 48 hours
Staphylo-coccus	Common	Vomiting and diarrhea; occasionally weakness and dizziness	30 minutes to 8 hours
Scombroid poisoning	Uncommon	Facial flushing, headache, dizziness, burning sensation in the throat, hives, nausea, vomiting and abdominal pain	5 minutes to 1 hour
Botulism	Rare	Double vision; difficulty speaking, breathing and swallowing; nausea, vomiting, abdominal pain and diarrhea	12 to 48 hours, sometimes as long as 8 days later
Listeria	Rare	Flu-like symptoms, including fever and chills; can cause spontaneous abortions and stillbirths, as well as severe illness in newborns and immune-suppressed people	2 to 4 weeks
Trichinosis	Rare	Fever, edema (swelling) of the eyelids and muscle pain	1 to 2 days

be given to babies, since it can lead to infant botulism.

February's *Consumer Reports* magazine reported widespread fish contamination; it urged pregnant women, women who expect to become pregnant within a few years and children under six to avoid salmon, swordfish, lake whitefish and tuna because they may contain polychlorinated biphenyls (PCB's) or mercury. But the Food and Drug Administration (FDA) believes all cooked fish is safe for the general population as long as consumers are careful when buying, preparing and cooking it. Some reasonable precautions people can take: Eat a variety of fish, not just one type; shop in large commercial markets, where fish is likely to be fresh and of good quality; and don't eat fish caught in heavily polluted areas. Many health authorities, including the FDA, believe raw fish (such as sashimi and sushi) and raw shellfish pose a health hazard. Some experts advise everyone—especially those in high-risk groups—to avoid raw shellfish altogether; the FDA says people should limit their consumption to cold-weather months, when shellfish tends to be less contaminated.

But most foods simply need to be handled and cooked properly. When shopping, get the groceries home within two hours (if the outside temperature is more than 85°, get them home in an hour). Keep meat and poultry separate in your shopping cart, to prevent meat fluids that might contain bacteria from dripping on other foods. Pass up foods in damaged containers, and if a product has a "use by" or "sell by" date, make sure it hasn't expired. Also, avoid foods that don't look fresh. This advice is particularly important when buying fish, since scombroid toxins cannot be destroyed by cooking. Whole fish should have clear eyes, red gills and firm, unmarred flesh; fillets and steaks should appear bright and shiny. Fresh fish should not have a strong, unpleasant odor. Don't buy fish that's stored above 33°—it should be on ice or in a refrigerated case with a thermometer—and don't buy precooked fish that's displayed with potentially contaminated raw fish. Shellfish should be kept damp and properly ventilated at a temperature under 40°; mollusk shells should be closed (or they should close quickly when you tap them).

Once you get home, store perishables

in the refrigerator or freezer immediately. Leave eggs in their carton: Jostling them in egg trays on the refrigerator door may cause tiny cracks. Use eggs within three weeks. Keep ground meats and stew meats in the refrigerator for no more than two days and in the freezer for no more than four months; other fresh meats keep for three to five days in the fridge and six to 12 months in the freezer. Poultry stays fresh in the refrigerator for a day or two and in the freezer for up to nine months. Fresh fish should be buried in a shallow pan of ice in the refrigerator and eaten the same day it's purchased. (For information on storage times for other foods, and answers to any other questions about food poisoning, call the **USDA's meat and poultry hotline at 800-535-4555.**)

It's also a good idea to check your refrigerator and freezer temperatures: The maximum safe temperatures are 40° for the refrigerator and 0° for the freezer. Thaw meat and poultry in the fridge or the microwave, not at room temperature. (You should also marinate food in the refrigerator.)

FOODS FOUND IN	PREVENTIVE MEASURES
Meat, poultry, eggs, unpasteurized dairy products, fish, shellfish and untreated water	Cook meat, poultry and eggs thoroughly; wash hands and work surfaces before and after contact with raw animal products; don't drink unpasteurized milk or untreated water
Meat and poultry	Keep cooked foods above 140° while serving; cook, cool and reheat foods thoroughly
Raw shellfish, untreated water and any food handled by contaminated people	Wash hands thoroughly and frequently; avoid raw shellfish
Raw shellfish and any food handled by contaminated people	Wash hands thoroughly and frequently; avoid raw shellfish
Meat, poultry, eggs and unpasteurized dairy products	Cook meat, poultry and eggs thoroughly; wash hands and work surfaces before and after contact with raw animal products; don't let foods sit at room temperature for more than 2 hours; don't drink unpasteurized milk
Cooked meat and poultry; meat, poultry, potato and egg salads; cream-filled pastries	Cooking does *not* inactivate the staph toxin; wash hands and utensils before preparing food; don't let food sit at room temperature for more than 2 hours
Mackerel, tuna and bonito	Make sure fish is fresh; if it has a peppery taste, stop eating it
Improperly canned goods and honey (for infants)	Follow established guidelines for home canning; don't buy damaged canned goods; cook and reheat foods thoroughly; don't eat cooked foods that have been left at room temperature for more than 2 hours; don't give infants honey
Unpasteurized milk and cheese made from unpasteurized milk; processed meats	Avoid raw or undercooked animal products, especially if you're pregnant or immune-suppressed
Pork	Cook pork thoroughly (to an internal temperature of 160°)

SOURCE: CENTERS FOR DISEASE CONTROL AND THE U.S. DEPARTMENT OF AGRICULTURE

An ounce of prevention counts in food preparation too. After touching raw meat and poultry, wash your hands with soap and hot water for at least 20 seconds. Let's say you cut a fresh chicken into parts and then, without washing your hands, prepare a bottle for the baby: You could contaminate the bottle sufficiently to infect the child. You should also wash the counter top, cutting board and any utensils that come in contact with raw food: People have gotten salmonella from eating foods sliced with contaminated knives. A plastic cutting board is best for meat and poultry, since raw juices can seep into porous wood boards.

Perhaps the most effective weapon against food poisoning is cooking. Thorough cooking will kill parasites (such as the one that causes trichinosis), most bacteria and some viruses and toxins (such as the one that leads to botulism). The USDA recommends that beef, veal, lamb and pork be cooked to an internal temperature of 160° and that poultry be cooked to 180°. If possible, use a meat thermometer to check; if you're cooking only parts, such as a chicken breast, make sure the meat juices run clear and the meat isn't pink inside. The FDA recommends that fish be cooked until it's opaque and flakes easily with a fork.

Be careful with foods cooked in the microwave, since microwaves are notorious for heating unevenly. If your microwave doesn't have a turntable, rotate the food by hand periodically. Correct heating is also very important when doing home canning, since this will prevent botulism. (For the brochure "Principles of Home Canning," send a check for $2.75 to the **Superintendent of Documents, U.S. Government Printing Office, Washington, DC 20402.**)

The last defense against food poisoning is proper serving. Both hot and chilled foods should be served quickly, using clean silverware and dishes—not the ones on which you stored or prepared the food. At buffets, place small amounts of food on the table and restock serving dishes from a refrigerated or heated supply rather than letting food sit for a long time. Cold foods should be kept below 40° and hot foods above 140°. Promptly refrigerate leftovers in small, shallow containers so the food is chilled thoroughly and quickly, and reheat leftovers completely.

If you brown-bag your lunch or pack a lunch box for your child, refrigerate the perishables at work or school if possible. Otherwise, put something cold in the lunch bag, such as a cold drink, a plastic container partially filled with water and frozen, or a freeze pack. Wash plastic lunch containers every night and use a new, clean bag every day.

When eating out, avoid restaurants that don't look clean; if the dining area seems dirty, the kitchen probably is too. If the food isn't served steaming hot, send it back. At salad bars, foods should be kept on beds of ice to ensure they're properly chilled.

If despite all your efforts, you still fall prey to food poisoning, get plenty of rest and drink lots of juice, broth or flat soda. Avoid foods that contain lactose, such as milk, butter, yogurt and cheese, since these may make your diarrhea worse. And wash your hands thoroughly and often to keep food poisoning from making the rounds in your house. If you're in a high-risk group, if you can't keep down liquids or if you have a persistent fever, dizziness, severe pain, bloody stools or any neurological symptoms, consult a doctor.

DANGEROUS LIAISON

A Mysterious, Sexually Transmitted Virus Threatens to Trigger a New Epidemic

Janny Scott

Janny Scott is a Times *medical writer.*

There is something pure and innocent about Patty and Victor Vurpillat. She was 18 and he was 19 when they met in 1988. They fell in love. She moved in. Within 10 months, they were married. Everybody freaked, as Victor tells it; it was like the 1950s.

The newlyweds found a sunny little apartment in Pacific Palisades. She stocked the refrigerator with health food and began training for a marathon. He enrolled at Santa Monica College, bringing home A's and B's. Conversation turned to babies.

But then Patty and Victor came down with a most un-1950s disease—a condition fraught with all the uneasiness of sexual relations in the age of AIDS, caused by a virus with disturbing links to cancer that threatens to become the venereal disease of the 1990s.

It all started with some bumps on Patty's cervix. Genital warts, the nurse-practitioner at the clinic pronounced them. A closer examination turned up an area of abnormal tissue. The clinic recommended a biopsy to check for signs of cancer.

Suddenly Patty was on her back with a microscope perched between her thighs. A nurse peered in and snipped away at her insides. Later, Patty returned to have the warts frozen off. It was creepy: She could feel her cervix defrost.

Victor, too, had to be vetted. There he lay in a women's clinic, surrounded by women. They put his feet up in stirrups; there were little mittens on the stirrups. Two nurses set about removing tiny warts, one by one.

Back at home panic colored Patty's thoughts: She would get cancer; she would have a hysterectomy; there would never be any children. She tried reminding herself that the risk was small. But fear ached in her gut.

"It was just awful—not knowing what's going on with your body and if you're going to be OK or not," she said recently. "There's a certain percent chance you're going to be all right. But then, maybe you're not."

Patty and Victor Vurpillat are infected with a strain of human papilloma virus—HPV—the virus that lurks behind one of the country's fastest-spreading sexually transmitted diseases and is rapidly becoming a prime suspect in the search for the causes of cervical cancer.

As much as 15% of the population may already be carrying the virus—a fact that many health officials view with alarm. It is estimated that 750,000 people become infected every year—most of them teen-agers and young adults who are healthy, sexually active and entering their peak reproductive years.

For most of them, HPV infection will mean nothing more than a frustrating struggle with the virus's most common visible symptom, genital warts—small, cauliflower-like growths that usually can be removed with various disconcerting and less-than-perfect treatments.

But, for a few, HPV may contribute to a profoundly disturbing form of cancer—cancer of the genitals, and in particular, cervical cancer, a condition that threatens the core of one's sexuality, the ability to reproduce and, occasionally, life itself.

The difficulty is, it is impossible to predict who will fall into which group.

As a result, millions of Americans find themselves condemned to a sentence of life beneath the cloud of HPV, carrying in their tissues an incurable and highly infectious virus that may eventually unleash a devastating cancer.

The burden falls especially hard on women. Both sexes can carry and spread the virus, but symptoms are more pronounced in women. Although the virus has been associated with cancers of the penis and anus, the greater risk appears to be cancer of the cervix.

What's more, some people are spreading the virus unknowingly: It is transmitted by contact with warts, and warts often go unnoticed. Some physicians suspect that HPV may even occasionally be spread indirectly—perhaps on a tanning bed, toilet or washcloth.

For that reason, it may not be possible to protect oneself completely. Physicians strongly recommend condoms. But they acknowledge that even condoms are not foolproof; some warts remain exposed, and contact can occur before or after the condom is used.

What are the long-term implications of the spread of such a virus?

Many researchers insist that HPV is unlikely to produce a significant increase in the number of deaths from invasive cervical cancer in the United States, because cervical cancer is highly treatable and, in most cases, even preventable if women are screened regularly.

Nevertheless, some have noticed a worrisome trend—an apparent rise in the incidence of cervical dysplasia, abnormalities in the cells on the surface of the cervix that, although treatable, in some cases turn out to be antecedents of cancer.

Some physicians also have reported an increase in adenocarcinomas, a particularly nasty subset of cervical tumors. Those tumors now seem to strike younger women in particular, researchers say; and they may be especially difficult to detect early and cure.

Both of those trends, which some researchers believe may be linked to HPV, suggest a startling shift in the demographics of cervical cancer: A disease that in the past has afflicted mostly women in their late 40s and beyond is now threatening women in their prime.

"My guess is that the teen-age cervix is phenomenally sensitive, in that there is a tremendous amount of cell division," says Dr. Stephen L. Curry of Tufts University. "If they are exposed to whatever carcinogens there are, there will be a higher incidence of cancer."

Even more troubling is the fact that as many as half of all women in the United States don't undergo annual cervical cancer screening, without which it is impossible to detect and treat the cancer's precursors, staving off more serious disease.

At a large public-health clinic near downtown Los Angeles that serves mostly low-income Latinos, women are turning up with the earliest stages of cervical cancer at twice the national rate, and their average age is just 24.

HPV infection is rampant among her clients, says Catherine Wylie, who oversees the family-planning program at the H. Claude Hudson Comprehensive Health Center at Adams Boulevard and South Grand Avenue. The spread will continue, she says, until the law requires that partners of people who have HPV be tracked down and treated.

"Our women have sex early because they marry at 16 to 18," Wylie said recently. "As long as this disease is not reportable, and there's no partner follow-up and treatment, I think we're going to have an epidemic of cervical cancer."

There is nothing new about warts—on the genitals or elsewhere. They have been around for millennia. As early as the 1st Century AD, physicians described the more ignominious form—warts on the genitals and anus, also known as condylomata.

But it was not known until this century that warts came from viruses—a specific family of viruses called human papilloma viruses. (It is now known that some strains cause common warts on the hands and feet and other strains cause genital warts.)

That discovery led to an intriguing glimpse of HPV's mysterious links to cancer.

In the early 1930s, researchers discovered that a form of papilloma virus caused benign tumors (also known as papillomas) in cottontail rabbits. When exposed to certain chemicals that were otherwise innocuous, those tumors quickly turned malignant.

Even today, those initial animal experiments remain a model for examining the way papilloma virus-induced abnormalities can progress to cancer, researchers say. But the links between HPV and human cancers would remain unrecognized for another 40 years.

In the meantime, it became clear how HPV is spread.

The first report of sexual transmission of HPV came in 1954. Twenty-four women came down with genital warts after their husbands returned from the Far East. All 24 husbands admitted to having had sex overseas, and all had recently had penile warts.

Sex with a partner who has untreated warts is known now to be extremely risky, since the virus is highly concentrated in warts. In studies, most partners of people with warts developed warts themselves within weeks or months. Cuts and abrasions appear to increase one's infection with the virus.

There is at least one other form of transmission: HPV can be spread to an infant during childbirth. In rare cases, the infection produces a life-threatening condition in which warts on the infant's larynx interfere with his or her ability to breathe.

And because physicians have seen instances of HPV spreading in cases in which no sexual contact is believed to have occurred—for instance, among non-intimate members of the same household—some wonder whether HPV is spread in other ways. Those cases, however, are difficult to prove.

By whatever routes, genital warts began proliferating in the 1960s under the influence of increased sexual freedom and declining use of barrier contraceptives. Statistics on visits to U.S. physicians indicate a 12-fold increase in cases in just 20 years.

According to the National Disease and Therapeutic Index, the number of visits for treatment of genital warts leaped from 160,000 in 1966 to 1 million just a decade later. By 1988, that number had reached 1.2 million.

In the meantime, HPV research languished, in part because of an obstacle that has yet to be overcome. Scientists had never managed to grow HPV in the laboratory, making it difficult to study its transmission, its treatment and how the virus affects cells.

Then in the mid-1970s, a pathologist working in a laboratory in Canada began noticing a peculiar pattern under his microscope: He found striking similarities between cells from genital warts and cells from pre-malignant lesions on the cervix.

The pathologist, Alexander Meisels, a professor at Quebec's LaVal University, was intrigued by two features in particular. The cells he was studying seemed to have in common an unusual cavity around the nucleus and an overabundance of a protein called keratin.

Suddenly, it dawned on Meisels: The lesions must have come from the same source as the warts. If HPV caused not just warts but cervical lesions as well, and lesions were known in some cases to develop into cancer, then HPV had a role in the process leading to cervical cancer.

"The cells seem to have to be infected [with HPV] first," says Meisels, who is also head of the department of pathology and cytology at Saint-Sacrement Hospital. "But that is not sufficient. Something else is acting on them."

Cervical cancer has long been thought to be caused at least in part by a sexually transmitted infectious agent. Among the most important risk factors for the disease is simply the number of sexual partners a woman has had and the number of partners her partner has had.

Worldwide, cervical cancer is a top cancer killer. Half a million women come down with it annually. Half of those women will die within 2½ years, mostly in countries with poor access to health care and inadequate cervical cancer screening.

In the United States, the death rate has plummeted since the Papanicolaou smear made it possible to identify and treat the precursors of cervical cancer. This year, there will be about 13,500 new cases of invasive cancer and 6,000 deaths—down nearly 70% since the 1950s.

Even so, some researchers are worried by recent reports of an increase in the especially virulent adenocarcinomas—an apparent rise that some believe may come from a sexually transmitted infectious agent, perhaps HPV.

Twenty years ago, this particularly aggressive type of tumor made up just 5% of all invasive cervical cancers. Now that figure is 30%, says Dr. Alex Ferenczy, a professor of pathology and obstetrics and gynecology at McGill University in Montreal.

Sex with a partner who has untreated warts is risky, since that's where the virus is concentrated.

There are also signs that invasive cancer is striking at a younger age. According to Ferenczy, 22% of all invasive cancers in developed countries are now diagnosed in women aged 35 and younger. That figure is up from less than 10% just 15 years ago.

"That's a heavy-duty increase," Ferenczy says. "This has major clinical implications for whoever screens women for cervical cancers. They have to remember that invasive cancer is no longer and not necessarily a disease for elderly women."

That lesson is not lost on Dr. Louise H. Connolly, medical director of the Manhattan Beach Women's Health Center, a full-service medical clinic operated by Centinela Hospital on a busy South Bay thoroughfare a few miles from the beach.

A graduate of Yale Medical School, Connolly opted for a career in obstetrics and gynecology. What appealed to her was the possibility of practicing preventive medicine—as she puts it, protecting a woman's right to sexuality without harmful consequences.

But these days, harmful consequences walk into the office every day. About one in five of Connolly's patients is infected with HPV. The average age of those women, Connolly figures, is 22. News of the diagnosis, and the risk of cancer, comes as a rude shock.

"When you're 18 to 25, you feel that your health is guaranteed. You feel invulnerable to major disease," Connolly says. "I think initially they're shocked and frightened

that they're 18 or 20 years old and they have something that might lead to cancer.

"Right behind that, they feel they have a sexually transmitted disease and they may feel dirty," she added. "So it's fear and shame together. It cuts them off from asking people for support—from family, boyfriends and friends."

One woman, who asked to be identified simply as Annie, was in her mid-40s when she discovered that she had genital warts. She was divorced at the time, sexually active and in a relationship with a man she has since married.

Annie had no gynecologist, so she told her family doctor. For a year and a half, they fought a losing battle against the warts. Annie would go in for treatment with various ointments, the warts would disappear, and within several months they would be back.

"It's emotionally painful and it's demeaning," Annie says. "You've got a sexually transmitted disease and someone is fooling with your bottom. And to be honest, one of the hardest parts about the whole thing was my husband's lack of understanding.

"He just didn't understand what I was going through emotionally," she says. "It was more like an imposition to him. He'd see me going for another treatment and he'd think, 'She's going to be out of commission for a week.' "

After eight or 10 episodes, even the physician was becoming impatient. So when the next wart arrived, Annie went to see Connolly. "When she examined me, she said, 'This is not a wart,' " Annie recalls. "It's something else, and I want to remove it.' "

Connolly cut off the growth and sent it in for a biopsy. The results came back: Annie had early cancer of the vulva. (Vulval cancer is another genital cancer that has been linked to HPV but is less common than cervical cancer.)

Fortunately, Annie's cancer was at its earliest stage. It was confined to the top layer of the skin and could be cut off easily. Simply removing it and a surrounding margin of normal tissue for a pathologist's scrutiny would probably be sufficient treatment.

But Connolly had Annie return for colposcopy, an extensive internal examination with a binocular microscope that magnifies and illuminates the vagina and cervix. Through the scope, Connolly would be able to detect any warts or more troubling changes.

"It was horrible, just horrible," Annie remembers, referring to her fear of what Connolly might find. "There you are, spread-eagle, for [nearly half] an hour. None of it really hurts. . . . But every time she'd stop and look at something, I'd think, 'Oh God, oh God, oh God.' "

HPV infection contributes to a range of manifestations in women. They fall along a continuum from barely significant to severe. Some people suffer no symptoms, some suffer just one. Others proceed at varying rates of speed from one to the next.

The least serious are warts and so-called subclinical infections—barely perceptible changes in the cells that cover the cervix. A specialist scrutinizing cells scraped off during a Pap smear might detect the virus's distinctive footprint—

clumps of oddly misshapen cells.

More-extensive cell changes create a condition known as dysplasia, or cervical intraepithelial neoplasia (CIN). Those abnormalities can be detected through Pap smears or colposcopy, where they appear as areas of white tissue where it should be smooth and pink.

Dysplasia can range from mild to severe. Many cases will clear up spontaneously, some become worse. A small minority seem to advance to become carcinoma *in situ,* an early and highly treatable form of cancer confined to the top layer of tissue of the affected organ.

Finally, there can be invasive, or malignant, cancer.

Deep in the vastness of Los Angeles County USC Medical Center, Carol Carriere peers through a microscope at a small glass slide. Thousands of cells from a woman's cervix are smeared on the slide, clustered like dense constellations of stars.

Carriere is chief cytotechnologist in the Department of Cytology at County USC. Some 30,000 slides pass through her lab every year. Most are from Pap smears, and many carry the tell-tale signs that HPV has invaded the cells.

Scanning the slide, Carriere looks for subtle changes—say, a cell with an oversized nucleus or cells in abnormal patterns of clumping. A key tip-off to HPV's presence is that enlarged and irregularly shaped nucleus, often surrounded by a widening cavity.

In moderation, she says, those changes suggest subclinical infection or warts. More extensive abnormalities may indicate pre-malignant cells.

Treatment of HPV-related diseases depends upon the symptoms. There are no drugs that can rid the body of the virus, just as there is no vaccine. So physicians such as Connolly treat the manifestations: They freeze or vaporize or slice off the warts and areas with abnormal cells.

The first line of attack is a variety of chemicals, administered either by the patient or physician. For persistent warts and warts on the cervix, many physicians use cryosurgery, freezing the wart and surrounding tissue with a low-temperature probe.

Another option for extensive warts and dysplasia is laser surgery, in which a concentrated beam of light serves as a scalpel. Finally, a so-called cone biopsy is occasionally used to slice a cone-shaped chunk of abnormal tissue from the cervix.

It is not really known why such approaches work, but they seem to. Many people treated for warts and dysplasia never experience a recurrence. By removing a repository of virus, the treatments may be diminishing the load of virus in the body. Or, they may be triggering an immune response.

Nevertheless, there are limitations.

"It's clear that you can't cure a viral infection by burning the skin off," says Dr. Kenneth L. Noller, chairman of the department of obstetrics and gynecology at the University of Massachusetts Medical School. "It would be like trying to cure a cold by burning off the lining of the lungs."

Connolly, for one, also prescribes what she discreetly terms "pelvic rest" until the warts or areas of dysplasia have been treated and have healed. She advises frequent Pap smears—as often as every three to six months—a repeat colposcopy in a year and examination and treatment of any partners.

"Most of them drag their feet," Connolly says. "Some couples break up: She gets angry, they have a fight, he leaves."

Genital warts are common in men as well as women. They can occur on the penis, anus, scrotum and in the urethra. But they are often less visible than on women, noticeable only with close examination. So, many men unknowingly infect their partners.

There may also be certain "high-risk males"—men for whom a succession of partners or wives develop cervical cancer. Some researchers have speculated that such men are

---

There are no drugs that can rid the body of the HPV virus, just as there is no vaccine.

---

transmitting some carcinogen, probably an infectious agent, perhaps a strain of HPV.

Gynecologists say many men's physicians are unfamiliar with HPV infection.

"Some of them will just go to their family practitioner, who just eyeballs them and says, 'No, you don't have it,' " says Dr. Virginia A. Siegfried of Los Angeles. "That may be part of the problem in some of the patients we seem to keep getting back again: They're just re-exposed."

"You need a urologist or dermatologist who will go over the entire penis, urethra, scrotum and peri-anal area carefully," Connolly says. "They should check the opening of the urethra to make sure there isn't one tiny wart sitting in there that's going to infect someone."

Nan Singer (not her real name) discovered in her early 30s that her husband had warts on his anus. When she asked him about them, he conceded that he had had them for seven months. But he had neglected to tell her and had neglected to have them treated.

Even after she confronted him, her husband was reluctant to see a doctor. Then he expected Nan to be responsible for seeing that he used the medication, and even for administering it. Nan felt betrayed and disgusted; their sexual relationship deteriorated. Existing problems in their marriage grew worse.

"The thing that shocked me was that he was so uninformed," says Nan, who believes her husband's response to the disease contributed significantly to their subsequent divorce. "He knew what they were, but he made no effort to understand what it could mean to me."

Nan began having Pap smears every four to six months. One after another, they came back normal, or Class 1. Then, during one four-month period, the results switched suddenly from Class 1 to Class 3, signifying cell changes consistent with dysplasia.

Nan's gynecologist recommended laser surgery, a process Nan likens to "taking napalm to your insides." She describes her recovery as protracted and painful, sloughing off dead tissue for days. The smell seemed so foul, she feared co-workers noticed.

Neither Nan nor Annie has had any further problems. But both are familiar with their gynecologists' waiting rooms. They go in every few months and have tried to make peace with the unsettling knowledge that trouble could surface any time.

Nan has become one of those women Connolly set out to protect: She is now a veteran of HPV, herpes infection, three ectopic pregnancies and pelvic inflammatory disease; but at 34, she remains determined to preserve her ability one day to conceive and bear a child.

"I've lived with a lot of pain and this bad equipment for years," Nan said bitterly one morning recently, in an interview at her home near Los Angeles. "I [am not] about to lose it for venereal warts."

Unfortunately, there are as many questions as there are answers about HPV.

Many more people are infected than come down with any visible symptoms. What percentage will develop symptoms remains unknown. "People are flipping up figures," Ferenczy says. "Probably 5% to 15% will show up with some sort of HPV-related disease."

Of those who do, most will develop warts or dysplasia. In many of those, the conditions might clear spontaneously if left alone. In a small percentage, HPV infection will lead to cancer. What percentage that will be, and who they are, is impossible to say.

"I'm not sure now we know what the true risk is to a woman who has HPV infection," says Dr. John Curtin, a gynecologic oncologist at the USC School of Medicine.

The infection can remain hidden for long periods, surfacing at any time. One 65-year-old woman in Minnesota recently developed genital warts inexplicably, leaving her physician, Dr. Leo B. Twiggs, wondering why her symptoms emerged when they did.

According to Twiggs, director of the Women's Cancer Center at the University of Minnesota Hospital, research suggests that symptoms may surface when a patient's immunity is down. Other factors probably cause the immune suppression, he says; but maybe the virus can, too.

"Once the virus is interlocked into the cells, it's like a small computer program or a mini-computer hooking into a mainframe," Twiggs says. "The question is, where does it sit? Next to what operations systems? What's it doing there?" No one really knows what turns the program on.

Another question is one foreshadowed a half-century ago in the initial experiments with papilloma virus infection in rabbits: What are the so-called co-factors that encourage the progression to cancer? Are there ways women can minimize their risk?

One prime suspected co-factor is cigarette smoking. Opinion is divided on oral contraceptives. Other possible co-factors include additional infectious agents, such as the herpes virus, hormonal influences, genetic background and environmental and dietary factors.

The National Cancer Institute is preparing to try to answer the co-factor and risk questions with the help of a study of 15,000 to 20,000 women. Researchers will track them for several years to determine who among them develops the kinds of abnormalities known to precede cervical cancer.

They will then screen the women for HPV infection and those possible co-factors that might have played a role in their symptoms. Thus, researchers hope to be better able to predict the consequences of HPV infection and what puts people at greatest risk.

"What's certain is if you have an abnormal Pap smear or dysplasia, you are more likely to have the virus detected," says Dr. Mark Schiffman of the National Cancer Institute. "But if you have HPV today but are normal, does that mean you will get an abnormal smear?"

"People assume that women with the virus will go on and get dysplasia," Schiffman says. "Maybe the answer is no. Maybe most women can fight off the virus with their immune system. . . . We are trying to determine for physicians and women the meaning of infection."

It is also possible that, in some women, warts and mild dysplasia will disappear without treatment. For that reason, there is disagreement among physicians about when treatment is warranted and how much difference it makes.

Dr. Jonathan S. Berek, director of gynecologic oncology at the UCLA School of Medicine, believes that some women are being over-treated—at considerable pain and expense and with limited evidence that the therapy really helps.

But other physicians argue that they cannot afford to wait. If even a small minority of patients risk developing cancer, they suggest that it would be irresponsible to not do everything possible to protect those patients.

"Since we don't have the tools to say which will progress . . . you're almost forced to over-treat the others,"

Physicians disagree about when treatment is warranted and how much difference it makes.

Connolly says. Furthermore, many patients are anxious to be rid of their warts.

There is similar controversy about the value of a new form of HPV testing.

There are now some 60 known strains of the virus. (In 1987, they were being identified at a rate of three a month.) Some are found primarily in benign warts; some turn up in connection with dysplasia. A few seem to be linked primarily to invasive cancers.

But the associations are not hard and fast.

Several companies have developed tests capable of identifying the strain with which a person is infected. The first test on the market appeared in the United States early last year and is being offered by some commercial labs.

The manufacturer suggests that the test be used with the Pap smear to alert physicians to the presence of a potentially cancer-causing virus. The company claims that once physicians know the strains involved, they can monitor their patients accordingly.

But some physicians counter that all patients should be closely monitored anyway. They say the association between specific strains and symptoms is not yet sufficiently clear to justify alarming, or reassuring, patients on the basis of the test.

"I'm not sure how to use it, to tell you the truth," says Siegfried of Los Angeles. "It doesn't change how we treat the patients, and I'm concerned that it might cause more anxiety if the patients are told they have the type that is more closely linked to cancer."

In the end, researchers say that panic about HPV is counterproductive.

Most people never will develop cervical cancer, they repeatedly point out. The disease's antecedents are easily detected and treated. And in most cases, the rate of progression is slow enough that a single missed Pap smear will not be crucial.

But with nearly half the women in the United States not undergoing regular screenings, says Berek of UCLA, attention should be focused on encouraging those women to change their lifestyles and get regular checkups.

Berek would like to see more public resources devoted to comprehensive cancer screening of all Americans—an approach he and others point out repeatedly has been proven cost-effective but rarely attracts much political support.

"So I think the broader issue here is not so much that we've identified a virus that causes warts—a small proportion of which are virulent and probably are associated with the development of genital cancers," Berek says. "The issue is who's getting screened and why can't we save those other 6,000 lives?"

But statistics offer little comfort to people such as Patty Vurpillat.

In Patty's case, the warts on her cervix returned within a few months of treatment. When the clinic advised a second biopsy, she balked. She feared the pain of another biopsy and was losing confidence in the clinic where she was being treated.

Unsatisfied and anxious, she sought a second opinion. In December, the new physician suggested waiting three months. Warts sometimes regress. If they don't go away, the physician said, she might try once more freezing them off.

So these days, Patty Vurpillat is waiting.

"I've been worried," she said sadly one recent afternoon. "It's always in the back of your mind: I'm thinking, 'Could something really be messing up my reproductive system?' I'm going to turn 20 this week. And I feel like I'm going to turn 40."

Sleeping With the Enemy

Be careful out there;
there's much more to watch out for than AIDS

Five years ago, stunned by the fact that 25,000 Americans had developed AIDS, health experts warned that the disease could eventually claim more lives than the Korean or Vietnam War. Today the death toll from AIDS stands at about 120,000—more than the two wars combined—and it's still accelerating: more Americans will die of AIDS in the next two years than have died in the past 10. But AIDS isn't the only argument for safer sex. The genital tract can harbor a menagerie of disease-causing organisms, and though none of them is as deadly as HIV, their consequences are often devastating. Gonorrhea and chlamydia are leading causes of infertility. Untreated syphilis can ravage the heart and brain. The sexually transmitted viruses that cause hepatitis and genital warts also foster certain cancers. And many venereal infections can pass from mother to child at birth, leaving the baby blind, brain damaged or dead. All these diseases are preventable, and some are easily cured. Yet many are on the rise. They strike 12 million Americans, including 3 million teenagers, every year.

1 SYPHILIS
Annual incidence: 130,000 cases

Unleashed on the world five centuries ago, apparently after Spanish explorers took it home from the Americas, venereal syphilis spread largely unabated until the 1940s. Penicillin tamed the disease during the '50s, and it was largely forgotten until the mid-1980s, when drug abuse, poverty and declining health care fueled new inner-city outbreaks. Syphilis is still rare compared with other sexually transmitted diseases, but reported cases have doubled since 1984. The rate among black males (157 cases per 100,000) is now more than 54 times the corresponding rate for whites.

The syphilis bacterium (*Treponema pallidum*) often causes genital lesions known as chancres within six weeks of infection. The sores heal readily by themselves, but without treatment the disease advances. Within 12 weeks, most sufferers experience fevers, aches, rashes, hair loss and mouth sores. Only at later stages does syphilis invade the heart, eyes, brain and other organs. The greater risk is that an infected woman will unknowingly pass the disease to her unborn baby. The germ can cross the placenta any time after the fourth month of pregnancy, causing meningitis, deformities or stillbirth. Antibiotics can stop the disease at any stage, but they can't undo its damage. Syphilis testing is a good idea for any sexually active person who develops genital sores or who learns that a partner was infected. Blood tests can detect antibodies to the bacterium, but antibodies may not show up in the blood for six weeks or more. Specialized microscopes can spot the bacterium in tissue taken from a chancre.

2 GONORRHEA
Annual incidence: 1.4 million cases

Gonorrhea declined markedly during the 1980s, suggesting that large segments of the population have gotten the message about safer sex. But the disease is still 10 times as common as syphilis, and the racial disparities are more striking than ever. The rate of new infections, 12 times higher among blacks than whites a decade ago, is now 39 times higher. Like syphilis, the condition is easily treated with antibiotics.

The gonococcus bacterium thrives in moist, warm cavities, including the mouth and throat as well as the rectum, cervix and urinary tract. Genital symptoms such as burning, itching or unusual discharge normally show up two to 10 days after infection. If those symptoms go unnoticed, as often happens in women, the infection can spread into the fallopian tubes, causing such complications as infertility and tubal pregnancy. Doctors can readily detect gonococcal infection by analyzing penile or cervical discharge under a microscope. Testing is recommended for anyone who experiences symptoms or who has unprotected sex with more than one partner. Since the germ can infect a child's eyes at birth, many experts also favor testing for all pregnant women and antibiotic eyedrops for all newborns.

3 CHLAMYDIA
Annual incidence: 4 million cases

The government has never tracked chlamydia as closely as syphilis, gonorrhea or AIDS, but health officials rank it the nation's most common sexually transmitted disease. An estimated 4 million Americans contract this bacterial infection each year. The most common symptom is an inflammation of the urethra that causes painful urination or a discharge of pus or mucus. In addition to painful urination and vaginal discharge, women sometimes experience general pain in the lower abdomen. Like gonorrhea, chlamydia can lead to sterility in women who don't receive treatment.

Unfortunately, the disease is easy to miss until complications set in. One in four infected men, and at least half of all infected women, experience no initial symptoms at all. So experts recommend that anyone with more than one sex partner—especially women still in their childbearing years—be tested annually. Until recently, testing for chlamydia involved culturing genital secretions. The process took several days, and because gonococcal bacteria don't grow readily in culture, the results

 From *Newsweek*, December 9, 1991, pp. 58-59.

were unreliable. Using new diagnostic techniques, doctors can reliably analyze the secretions in the course of a 30-minute office visit. Tetracycline is the usual treatment for chlamydia. The drug can't be taken during pregnancy, but substitutes are available.

4 PID
Cases treated annually: 420,000

Gonorrhea and chlamydia can both lead to pelvic inflammatory disease, or PID, the most frequent complication of sexually transmitted disease in women. The trouble begins when an infection spreads from the cervix into the fallopian tubes (a process that vaginal douching and the use of intrauterine devices may hasten). The tubes become scarred, and the scar tissue impedes passage of fertilized eggs to the uterus. Besides obstructing pregnancy, PID can cause fertilized eggs to lodge in the wall of the fallopian tube, destroying the embryo and endangering the mother's life.

PID seems to be waning along with gonorrhea; a recent study by the Centers for Disease Control showed a sharp drop in incidence between 1982 and 1988. But the disease still afflicts nearly 11 percent of the nation's childbearing-aged women—one in 10 whites and one in six blacks. Some 420,000 sufferers seek treatment every year, at a cost of $2 billion. The warning signs of PID, easily spotted during a routine pelvic exam, include swelling or tenderness in the cervix, uterus or surrounding tissue. A cervical smear can confirm that the lower reproductive tract is infected or inflamed. But diagnosing more widespread PID often requires laparoscopy, an outpatient surgical procedure that involves inserting a scope into the abdomen through a small incision below the navel. Antibiotics can stop the disease. To avoid reinfection, women who develop PID should get their partners tested for the responsible bacteria.

5 GENITAL HERPES
Annual incidence: 500,000 cases

Unlike a bacterial infection, genital herpes can't be cured with antibiotics. Once infected with a herpes simplex virus, you're infected for life. Some 30 million Americans carry these common pathogens (there are two types), and most never suffer any consequences. But an estimated half-million people develop new cases of active genital herpes each year. The number of patients seeking treatment has grown sevenfold since the late 1960s.

In adults, the condition is more an annoyance than a health threat. The virus causes cold-sore-like lesions on the genital area. They normally appear within 10 days of infection and heal within three weeks. But many carriers experience occasional flare-ups, and anyone with an active lesion can pass the virus to a sex partner—even if the lesion is unnoticeable. Women with active herpes can also infect their babies during delivery, causing brain damage or death. Though no drug can root out the infection, daily doses of acyclovir, an antiviral drug, can help control it. And Caesarean delivery can reduce the risk to a newborn.

6 GENITAL WARTS
Annual incidence: 1 million cases

Like herpes sores, genital warts are caused by viruses that medical science has yet to tame. No one knows just how many people carry the culpable strains of human papilloma virus (HPV). Nor is it clear whether symptom-free carriers can spread the infection. But health officials estimate that 1 million Americans develop active warts every year and that two thirds of their sex partners contract the infection. The hard, fleshy bumps typically appear within three months of exposure to the virus, and they can show up well inside the vagina or the cervix, making self-diagnosis difficult for women.

The warts themselves are more unpleasant than dangerous; doctors can usually remove them by freezing, burning, chemical solutions or, when necessary, surgery. But experts worry about possible links between HPV and cancers of the penis, vulva and cervix. Cervical cancer strikes 14,000 American women a year, and kills 6,000. The malignancy is treatable if detected early, so women with a history of genital warts should have annual Pap smears as a precaution.

7 HEPATITIS B
Annual incidence: 300,000 cases

Hepatitis B isn't generally thought of as a sexually transmitted disease, but it should be. The virus infects an estimated 300,000 Americans every year, causing 5,000 deaths, and sex is the leading mode of transmission. Overall incidence hasn't changed much in recent years. But while the rate among gay men plummeted during the '80s—apparently in response to AIDS-inspired precautions—heterosexual transmission surged by 38 percent. Anyone with more than one partner is at risk.

The hepatitis B virus (HBV) attacks the liver, causing a tenacious flulike illness marked by jaundice. There is no cure; most people recover naturally and develop immunity to future infection. But HBV can take root in the body, remaining contagious and leading slowly to cirrhosis or liver cancer. There is a proven hepatitis B vaccine; the government recommends it for all sexually active gay men and for heterosexuals with more than one partner. But while 28 million heterosexuals are at risk, less than 1 percent have taken advantage of it.

8 AIDS
Total U.S. cases: 199,406*

An estimated 1 million Americans are infected with the AIDS virus—many of them unknowingly—and any infected person can pass the virus to sexual partners. Gay men still constitute the largest risk group for AIDS, followed by intravenous drug users. Only 6 percent of all U.S. cases have been traced to heterosexual contact. But heterosexual transmission is the norm throughout much of the world, and experts agree it will become more common here as the epidemic matures.

HIV often causes a brief, flulike illness at the time of infection, but it can remain silent for a decade or more before causing the fatigue, fevers, diarrhea, weight loss and susceptibility to infections that mark the onset of full-blown AIDS. Within a month or two of infection, the body produces antibodies that a blood test can detect. Testing is recommended for anyone with multiple partners or a history of sexually transmitted disease. The antiviral drugs AZT and ddI can slow the progress of HIV disease, and new treatments have made some AIDS-related infections more manageable. But safer sex is still the best medicine. The disease is incurable, and unlike the others, it always kills.

GEOFFREY COWLEY *with* MARY HAGER

*Through October 1991.

The ABC's of HEPATITIS

The viruses that cause liver disease grow ever more insidious

Rob Stein

Rob Stein is a science editor at National Public Radio in Washington.

In November of 1989, Eileen Johnson of Central Islip, N.Y., was hit by overwhelming fatigue. She began vomiting frequently, and her skin took on a yellowish cast. Her worried family rushed her to the hospital, but the 36-year-old woman's condition continued to deteriorate, and she soon lapsed into a coma. Only after 10 days did she regain consciousness, and seven weeks later she was still too weak to walk.

Johnson had been struck by acute hepatitis caused by the hepatitis B virus. Two years after falling ill, she returned to work, but she has yet to fully recover her strength. "I don't know if I'll ever be the same," she says. "I always think I'm going to get sick again. The illness has changed my life forever." That her friends and co-workers dismiss hepatitis as a trivial problem especially bothers her.

"They just don't realize how easily they can become infected with hepatitis," says Johnson. "A lot of them say to me, 'You stay in bed a couple of weeks—what's the big deal?'" The big deal is that the hepatitis viruses—five different varieties designated by the letters A through E—are approaching HIV, the virus that causes AIDS, in their collective contribution to illness and death.

Last year, HIV infected 40,000 Americans, bringing the number of HIV-infected people in the country to about 1 million, with a yearly death toll that now exceeds 31,000. By comparison, more than 500,000 Americans become infected with some form of hepatitis virus each year, and about 16,000 die annually from the complications.

The hepatitis viruses can be transmitted in different ways and vary widely in their health impact. But they all have one feature in common: They infect liver cells and cause inflammation of the liver, the body's largest internal organ and one of its most important. (The table "The Deadly Alphabet" compares the various hepatitis viruses.)

The liver performs a host of vital functions, which include storing energy, ridding the body of toxins and metabolizing drugs and alcohol (long-term alcohol abuse is the major cause of *nonviral* hepatitis). Loss of liver function can eventually be fatal, although deterioration usually takes years or even decades. Johnson's rapid decline was an exception to what is usually an insidiously extended process.

"These viruses generally don't kill you quickly," says Dr. Jay Hoofnagle, a hepatitis expert at the National Institutes of Health (NIH). People typically are infected for years without knowing it, with liver damage proceeding all the while. "These are infections that people acquire when they're young, some through sexual activity, and that kill them in their 50s." Most deaths are from long-term complications that include cirrhosis (scarring of the liver due to chronic inflammation), liver failure and liver cancer.

Our run-through of this dangerous viral alphabet begins with letter A:

▶ **HEPATITIS A:** It's the least malevolent of the hepatitis viruses to which Americans are exposed, for one main reason: It doesn't result in chronic hepatitis or its deadly complications, since the infection eventually clears up.

Hepatitis A is contracted orally, mainly through fecal contamination of food or water. Infections are especially prevalent in developing countries with poor hygiene and sanitation. There, major epidemics are caused by contaminated drinking water or food. In a 1988 outbreak in Shanghai, more than 300,000 people developed acute hepatitis A after eating infected raw clams.

In the U.S., hepatitis A outbreaks result mainly from food handlers with poor personal hygiene; from close contact among household members or in places with inadequate hygiene, such as day care centers; or from eating raw shellfish—which is how Gino Benza believes he got infected.

Benza, a 29-year-old marketing manager from New York City, bought raw oysters from a Manhattan street vendor. Less than a month later, he lost his appetite and noticed that his urine seemed unusually dark. Then his skin and the whites of his eyes took on a yellowish hue. He missed only one day of work, and after a few weeks, his appetite returned. "I was definitely lucky," Benza says. "It could have been a lot worse."

Day care centers are prime locations for hepatitis A outbreaks. "You get a lot of young children fond of mouthing everything," says Dr. David Nalin, director of clinical research for infectious diseases at Merck Research Laboratories in Blue Bell, Pa. "There's a lot of diaper changing, and the virus can easily spread to many children, who take it home to their siblings and parents."

An estimated 71,000 Americans became sick from hepatitis A in 1991. Deaths are rare and mainly involve the elderly and people with underlying liver disease, who die from acute hepatitis and its symptoms, including fever, nausea and vomiting. Most, however, recover within about two weeks.

Hepatitis A infections *can* be prevented, at least temporarily. Before visiting developing countries, for example, travelers can protect themselves by getting an injection of immune globulin containing antibodies against the hepatitis A virus; one shot, available from a physician or health department, may provide protection for three to four months. Similarly, a prompt dose of immune globulin (within two weeks of exposure) can help protect people who have been in close contact with someone recently diagnosed with hepatitis A. And an even better form of prevention may be available soon.

Last year a major study in *The New England Journal of Medicine* showed that a vaccine made from inactivated hepatitis A virus was extremely effective in preventing the infection in a New York community prone to outbreaks. During the nearly four months after 1,037 children got either one shot of the vaccine or a dummy injection, 34 cases occurred in the placebo group, vs. none in the vaccinated group. Some experts are already recommending the vaccine for all children in day care, and it should also prove valuable for travelers and others at risk for infection. It may receive approval from the Food and Drug Administration (FDA) this year.

►**HEPATITIS B:** Perhaps the most prevalent of the hepatitis viruses is hepatitis B, the type that afflicted Eileen Johnson. With 300,000 Americans infected every year, about one in every 20 citizens has now been exposed to it. Most people don't think of hepatitis B as a sexually transmitted disease (a recent Gallup survey found that only 11% of respondents knew it was). But as shown by the chart, more than half of all hepatitis B infections are transmitted that way.

Hepatitis B can also be transmitted from a woman to her infant at birth, when IV drug users share needles and, less commonly, when people receive transfusions. In fact, hepatitis B is transmitted in virtually the same ways as HIV, albeit with some important differences.

While only about 8% of HIV infections are transmitted through heterosexual intercourse in the U.S., 41% of hepatitis B infections are spread this way. And while most HIV infections can be traced to some form of risky behavior—IV drug use or unprotected intercourse, for example—a whopping 26% of hepatitis B cases, including Johnson's, have no known source. The probable reason: Hepatitis B is extremely contagious. The

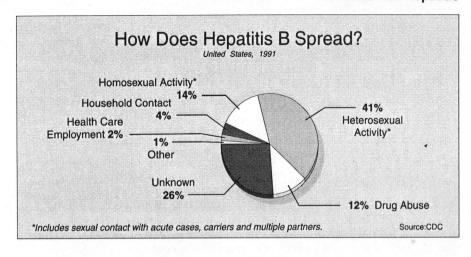

How Does Hepatitis B Spread?
United States, 1991

Homosexual Activity* **14%**
Household Contact **4%**
Health Care Employment **2%**
1% Other
Unknown **26%**
41% Heterosexual Activity*
12% Drug Abuse

Includes sexual contact with acute cases, carriers and multiple partners.

Source: CDC

virus can occur in very high amounts in blood (100 times greater than HIV), so exposure even to a minute amount of blood may result in infection.

Hepatitis B is also much hardier than HIV. Even outside the body—in dried blood, for example—B can remain infectious for a week or longer.

"I think many people whose infections can't be traced are getting it either sexually or through living in a household with a carrier who hasn't been identified," says Dr. Miriam Alter, chief of the epidemiology section of the hepatitis branch of the Centers for Disease Control and Prevention (CDC). "All you need is a minute amount of blood getting into your blood stream, say by brushing your teeth with an infected person's brush or using the same razor." By contrast, those sorts of casual contacts have never been implicated in spreading HIV.

Like Johnson, about half the 300,000 people infected with hepatitis B each year become acutely ill; some 300 die. The other 50% show no symptoms (or minor ones they mistake for a cold) and usually never realize they were infected.

The great majority of newly infected people, whether they become ill or not, manage to lick the infection completely. But from 6% to 10% of infected adults (and between 25% and 90% of infected children under five) can't shake the virus and become hepatitis B carriers.

Carriers have chronic infections that they can potentially transmit to others. While most carriers don't become seriously ill, about one-third go on to develop "chronic active hepatitis"—a progressive, smoldering disease that can lead to cirrhosis, liver failure or liver cancer. Yearly deaths from these hepatitis B complications total about 5,000.

Last year a drug treatment was ap-

proved for people with chronic hepatitis B infection. It's a genetically engineered version of alpha interferon, a naturally occurring hormone that revs up the body's immune response. Hepatitis patients must inject themselves with the drug, sold as Intron A, three times a week for six months, and many suffer flu-like side effects and depression. Alpha interferon appears to produce remissions in about 40% of patients.

Far easier than treating hepatitis B is preventing it—and a safe and effective vaccine against hepatitis B has been available since 1982. But it hasn't been widely used, and yearly cases of acute hepatitis B have actually increased 40% in the past decade (see "Preventing Hepatitis").

►**HEPATITIS C:** For years, 57-year-old Joan Smith (not her real name) of Long Island, N.Y., endured regular episodes of what seemed like the flu: exhaustion, sore throat, aching joints and tender glands. Smith, a working mother, would take a few days off from her secretarial job and return to work when she felt better. But the bouts got progressively worse, and she eventually was tired all the time. One day in 1988 she lay down to rest at work and couldn't get back up. "My doctor said, 'Go home and stay in bed for a couple of weeks,'" Smith says. "I thought, 'Two weeks' rest and I'll be raring to go.' But I'm still home four years later."

Smith has hepatitis C—a recently identified virus that is increasingly recognized as a major health problem. Hepatitis C's best-known victim is country singer and actress Naomi Judd, forced to retire from singing in 1991 due to her illness. About 150,000 Americans became infected with hepatitis C last year. The infection's early symptoms, includ-

Preventing Hepatitis

WITH NO reliable cures for any form of hepatitis, the best of all treatments is prevention. Since sexual intercourse helps transmit hepatitis B and C, condom use can help prevent infection. But vaccines are even better. The best of all preventive measures, experts say, would be for people at risk to receive the hepatitis B vaccine, the only hepatitis vaccine now approved.

The development of a hepatitis B vaccine was a pioneering achievement: the first (and still the only) vaccine for a sexually transmitted disease, and—since liver cancer is so clearly linked to hepatitis B infection—the first and only anticancer vaccine. But the vaccine has failed to fulfill its potential for eliminating hepatitis B as a health threat.

Hepatitis B is most often contracted through sex, and those who could benefit most from vaccination are sexually active adults, both straight and gay, since 75% of cases affect people between the ages of 18 and 39. (To protect that age group, the American Academy of Pediatrics [AAP] recently recommended that all adolescents be routinely immunized against hepatitis B.) Unfortunately, only 1% of Americans aged 18 to 39 have been vaccinated.

Others for whom the hepatitis B vaccine is recommended include: health care workers exposed to blood; dialysis patients and hemophiliacs; people who live with and/or have sex with hepatitis B carriers; IV drug users; and travelers to developing countries.

For the past decade, health officials have aimed their vaccination efforts at these high-risk groups but failed to reach many people who most need the vaccine. So in 1991 the Centers for Disease Control and Prevention (CDC) embarked on a different strategy, recommending that all infants be vaccinated against hepatitis B. The rationale: Infants are more accessible than adults. And the vaccine may protect against exposures to hepatitis B decades later. But the CDC's recommendation, which was endorsed by both the AAP and the American Academy of Family Physicians, has been resisted by doctors and parents.

Parents skittish about yet another vaccination question whether their children will ever need this one. "Parents say, 'My kid isn't going to be a drug abuser or a homosexual,'" says Dr. Edgar Marcuse, a clinical professor of pediatrics and epidemiology at the University of Washington in Seattle, who helped formulate the new recommendations for the AAP. "You then say, 'How can you predict if your kid may one day be the sexual partner of a sexual partner of someone at high risk?' Most parents will accept that."

Many doctors also question the need for the vaccine, as shown by a 1992 survey of North Carolina physicians that found only 37% of pediatricians and 26% of family practitioners felt it was warranted. Some doctors point to uncertainty over how long the vaccination remains effective, noting that a child could conceivably lose protection just when he's most likely to be infected—in adolescence or early adulthood.

But proponents point to evidence that the vaccine provides protection for at least a decade, and they say a single booster shot may be all that's necessary. They also note that when infected, children under five are much more likely than adults to become lifelong hepatitis B carriers.

Both doctors and parents complain about the price—as much as $60 for a series of three shots—although President Clinton's comprehensive childhood vaccine proposal could make it available at little or no cost.

Experts on infectious disease strongly believe that the vaccine's benefits outweigh its costs. "Universal immunization of our children is the only way to ensure protection from hepatitis B and the illnesses and deaths it causes," says Dr. Richard Duma, executive director of the National Foundation for Infectious Diseases in Bethesda, Md.

ing fatigue and loss of appetite, are usually mild, and many cases initially go undiagnosed.

The hepatitis C virus wasn't identified until 1988, and researchers soon realized it was responsible for most cases of what had been known as non-A, non-B hepatitis—including most cases of posttransfusion hepatitis. Its identification led to a blood test in 1990 that has greatly reduced though not eliminated the number of hepatitis C infections among transfusion recipients.

Although transfusions now account for only about 4% of new hepatitis C infections, contaminated blood remains a major route of transmission. About 30% of patients have a history of IV drug use, 2% are health care workers and about 1% are dialysis patients. But many infected people—including Joan Smith—don't fit into any of the high-risk categories, and just how they become infected amounts to a major medical mystery: "I never had a blood transfusion, and I don't have a job that exposes me to blood. I'm not a drug addict. I just have no idea," says Smith.

A study published earlier this year in *The Journal of the American Medical Association* suggests that a significant portion of unexplained infections may result from sexual activity. This study of 170 heterosexual couples identified two cases where a partner appeared to have become infected with hepatitis C through sexual contact. The authors concluded that even though hepatitis C is infrequently transmitted sexually, the large number of carriers means "sexual behavior could nonetheless transmit a significant proportion of new infections in the United States annually."

The more experts learn about hepatitis C, the more dangerous it appears to be. The virus seems to be causing a silent epidemic, with increasing numbers of Americans—now totaling perhaps 2 million—becoming infected, usually without knowing it. (Fully 70% of infections cause no initial symptoms; even when present, the symptoms of hepatitis C are milder than those of hepatitis B.) But according to a recent study, virtually all those infected with hepatitis C may become carriers: infected (and infectious) for life and at high risk for serious complications.

Up to 40% of carriers will eventually develop chronic active hepatitis (a higher percentage than for any of the other hepatitis viruses), and many with the

The Deadly Alphabet

Type	Description, Transmission and Treatment	Risk Groups
HEPATITIS A	Infections are acute, not chronic, so there are no long-term complications. Contracted orally, mainly through fecal contamination of water or food. Cases per year: 70,000; deaths per year: 100.	Children in day care, people who eat raw shellfish, travelers.
HEPATITIS B	The only form of hepatitis for which an effective vaccine has been approved. Half of all infections produce no symptoms. From 6% to 10% of infected adults become chronic carriers, and 30% of carriers develop chronic active hepatitis that can lead to cirrhosis or liver cancer. About 55% of infections occur through sexual intercourse. Cases per year: 300,000; deaths per year: 5,000. Treated with alpha interferon.	Homosexual males, people with multiple sexual partners, IV drug users, children born to infected mothers, health care workers exposed to blood.
HEPATITIS C	About 70% of infected people have no initial symptoms; symptoms typically are mild when present. Virtually all those infected may become carriers, up to 40% of whom develop chronic active hepatitis—making hepatitis C a major cause of chronic liver disease. Spread by exposure to blood (often through IV drug use), but often untraceable. Cases per year: 150,000; deaths per year: 10,000. Treated with alpha interferon.	IV drug users, health care workers exposed to blood, sexual contacts of carriers.
HEPATITIS D	Only affects people also infected with hepatitis B. The most severe form of viral hepatitis, fatal to 20% to 30% of those infected. Spread mainly by contaminated blood. Vaccination against hepatitis B prevents hepatitis D too. Infections per year: unknown, but 70,000 Americans are thought to carry the virus; deaths per year: 1,000.	IV drug users, recipients of contaminated blood products.
HEPATITIS E	Resembles hepatitis A in how it's spread and lack of chronic infections. Affects those Americans exposed in other countries. Cases per year: none in U.S. (there is no current test for detection); deaths per year: none in U.S.	Travelers to developing countries.

Symptoms All hepatitis viruses infect the liver. Sometimes there are no symptoms; at the other extreme, acute life-threatening illness may occur. Hepatitis typically produces flu-like symptoms (weakness, loss of appetite, fever, diarrhea) and jaundice. For all types except A and E, infection may persist and, perhaps decades after initial exposure, lead to life-threatening complications, including cirrhosis and liver failure. *Statistics are for the U.S.*

active form will go on to develop life-threatening illnesses. In fact, hepatitis C appears to be a major cause of chronic liver disease, the ninth leading cause of death in the U.S.

Until recently, experts had assumed most cases of chronic liver disease (primarily cirrhosis) resulted from alcohol abuse. But a study reported last year by the CDC highlights hepatitis C's largely unappreciated role. The study found that the hepatitis viruses—mainly hepatitis C and to a lesser extent hepatitis B—were the underlying cause for up to half of all chronic liver disease deaths, with hepatitis C alone causing 36% of them. About 10,000 Americans die yearly from hepatitis C's complications.

Unfortunately, there is no vaccine for hepatitis C and little chance of developing one soon. That hope was dashed last year, when NIH scientists found in chimpanzee studies that prior exposure to hepatitis C offered no protection against infections that came later.

On the bright side, the first drug for treating hepatitis C was approved in 1991. The drug—alpha interferon (Intron A)—is the same one used against hepatitis B. Intron A is reserved for people with chronic active hepatitis—the kind Smith has, which can progress to cirrhosis. Given as a series of injections over six months, alpha interferon reduces inflammation and liver damage in about half of hepatitis C patients. But half of those who improve relapse when the often unpleasant treatment is discontinued. Smith endured one year of alpha interferon but learned she was among the patients not helped by it. "It's been rough emotionally and physically. It's just been terrible. I just try to make the most of life every day."

Fortunately, a potentially better hepatitis C drug may be available soon. Ribavirin, first developed in 1970, has shown promising results in treating hepatitis C patients in several clinical trials. It can be taken orally, causes few side effects and is expected to receive FDA approval in the near future.

►**HEPATITIS D:** This type infects only people who are already infected with hepatitis B. Hepatitis D causes a "super-infection" that magnifies hepatitis B's severity. Most infections in the U.S. involve IV drug users. Hepatitis D is considered the most severe form of hepatitis, killing one-fifth to one-third of those it infects. Since only people with hepatitis B are susceptible to D, getting the hepatitis B vaccine prevents hepatitis D as well.

►**HEPATITIS E:** This final known member of the hepatitis alphabet—hepatitis E—is similar to hepatitis A in that it's spread mainly through fecal contamination of water and does not progress to chronic hepatitis. So far, hepatitis E outbreaks have occurred mainly in Asia, Mexico and Africa, with sporadic cases affecting American travelers in those areas. For unknown reasons, this virus is often fatal to pregnant women. Efforts to develop a vaccine against hepatitis E are under way.

what every woman needs to know about personal

Safety

Are you scared silly? It's time to get scared *smart*. Trade fear for caution by understanding when and where you're most at risk and how to protect yourself against crime.

Lauren David Peden

Are you afraid to walk down the street alone at night? Let a repairman into your house when your husband isn't home? Accept help from a stranger if your car breaks down on the road? More women than ever answer yes. They're scared, and for good reason. One violent crime is committed every 17 seconds in the United States, with the number of murders and rapes each increasing 9 percent from 1989 to 1990.

And everywhere a woman turns, it seems, she is reminded of the danger. Switch on the television or go to your local movie theater and you're confronted with a slew of "jep" movies—the name that the entertainment industry gives to films in which a woman is in jeopardy of being raped, mugged, beaten, duped or worse. Movies such as *Cape Fear, Sleeping With the Enemy* and *The Hand that Rocks the Cradle* send shivers through female viewers by implying that they could be next. Even everyday life seems more dangerous. Newscasts, top-heavy with stories of crime and tragedy, compound the scare factor with "special reports" on the

perils of everything from eating fresh fruit to shaving your legs.

The result of such menacing messages? Mean World Syndrome, a perception that danger lurks around every corner and that one is perpetually on the verge of being victimized. "Basically we're terrorized by the media," says George Gerbner, professor emeritus of communications at the Annenberg School for Communication in Philadelphia, who coined the term and has studied the phenomenon extensively. "Television shows are full of violence, and news programs dole out risk information without comparison, context, perspective or other relative values. It makes people panicky, particularly women." According to Gerbner, women are afflicted with the syndrome more than men and children primarily because of Hollywood's unnerving depiction of females. "On a typical TV drama, male characters outnumber females by three or four to one, but when there's violence, women are more often portrayed as victims," he explains. "In turn, women perceive the world as fraught with more danger than really exists." And Gerbner's studies have shown that the more hours women log watching TV, the more they suffer from Mean World Syndrome.

But experts are quick to point out that while these fears are exaggerated, they are still very real. It's how women put them in perspective that makes the difference between being reasonably cautious and hyper-afraid. The fact is, a woman *does* have a one in three chance of being raped in her lifetime and a one in 348 chance of being murdered. But when these statistics are stacked up against other odds, they're easier to live with. Overemphasized risks may be inconsequential, and underemphasized ones may deserve more attention. For instance, while you have only an 82 in 100,000 chance of being struck by lightning (an oft-depicted tragedy on reality-based TV shows like *Rescue 911*), your chances of drowning are significantly higher at 4,199 in 100,000.

The key, then, is knowing where your real risks lie and keeping your guard up in those situations but relaxing in others. Statistics show that terrible things happen to good people, but they're not inevitable. In fact, sometimes they're *very* unlikely. We'll discuss the most common dangers you should be concerned about and what you can do to minimize them. So you can learn to look over your shoulder prudently, not constantly, and concentrate on the good things in life.

How to Feel Safe in Your Home

Crime hits hard on the home front, and Americans know it. We spent $3.4 billion on home burglar-alarm systems in 1991. Are such security systems worth the money? Maybe, but before you get out the checkbook, consider this: When criminals were asked what *they* would use to protect their homes, they said dogs, not alarms. Here are the biggest risk factors and some smart measures to keep you safe and sound at home.

• **Fifty-five percent of all burglars enter homes through an unlocked door or window,** says the National Crime Prevention Council. Keep all points of entry locked at all times. And be vigilant about it. Instill the habit in your kids too.

• **In almost all other cases, burglars enter homes through forced entry—** bashing in a window, prying a door away from its frame. Make sure the locks on doors are heavy-duty dead bolts and that the doors themselves are made of metal or solid-core wood that is at least 1 3/4 inches thick. Bolster window safety by installing specially designed pins through the casings to prevent windows from being opened from the outside (contact your local fire department for instructions). In suburban areas, thieves often enter houses by kicking in a basement window. Install bars over cellar windows that thwart break-ins.

• **A criminal may disguise himself to get into your home.** Criminals have been known to masquerade as salespeople, police officers and even victims of car accidents. *Never open your door to strangers.* First look through a peephole or window to see who it is. If you don't know the person, either ignore him until he goes away or ask what he wants through the locked door.

A New Kind of Street Smarts

Even if you don't live in a big city where street smarts are the way of the land, chances are you don't feel completely comfortable walking down the street alone at night (or even during the day in some areas). In fact, according to the National Victim Center, women are so concerned for their safety that 75 percent of them say they limit the places they go by themselves. Over half of all robberies and muggings occur on a street or highway, and driving doesn't afford any additional protection. Carjacking (stealing cars from drivers at gunpoint) is a growing phenomenon, so new that statistics on it aren't yet available. Here are three common crimes that women need to be on guard against.

• **Purse snatching.** The safest way to carry your purse is tucked snugly under your arm like a football with the strap wrapped around it. If the bag has a clasp closure, carry it clutched in your dominant hand, clasp side down. Should someone try to grab it, release the clasp and let the contents spill on the ground. A thief usually won't stop to sift through the mess.

• **Robbery by force or weapon.** Criminals scope out *easy* targets. Appear confident by walking with a strong gait, your hands out of your pockets. If you suspect you're being followed, don't go home. Even if the criminal passes you up, he'll learn where you live. Instead, cross the street, abruptly change direction or head toward an open store, restaurant or well-lit residence and call the police.

• **Carjacking.** According to the FBI, more than 1.6 million cars were stolen in 1990, a jump of over 50 percent since 1981. Increasingly, thieves are stealing cars from their owners right on the road. When you're driving, always keep doors locked and pay attention to other cars and pedestrians around you, particularly at traffic lights and stop signs. If a suspicious person approaches your car, lean on the horn and drive away, even through a red light if necessary. If the person threatens you, relinquish your car to minimize your chances of being hurt.

How to Feel Safe at Work

According to the U.S. Department of Justice, a surprising 13 percent of all violent crimes and 20 percent of all thefts occur on the job. Why the office? It's a contained environment where people spend at least eight hours a day—and it's easy for a criminal to blend in with the crowd or hide in isolated areas, such as rest rooms and stairwells. Here are two concerns to be especially aware of in the workplace.

• **Theft.** The simplest deterrent: Hide all valuables. Keep your purse and other important items in a locked desk or file-cabinet drawer, *not* on the floor under your desk.

• **Physical assault.** In this case, you're most at risk before and after regular hours. Stay alert when coming in early or staying late. Lock your office door while you're working if you're alone or in the company of other employees you don't know well. Keep the phone number for building security taped to your telephone. If your building doesn't have guards at the main entrance, make sure that door is locked too, if possible. And wait to use the bathroom until coworkers arrive or, if you'll be working late, use it before everyone has left for the day.

Stress and Mental Health

Years of medical research have significantly advanced our knowledge and understanding of the human body to a point where not only can organs be transplanted, but machines can be built to replicate their functions. The one organ that still mystifies and baffles the scientific community, however, is the brain. While more has been learned about this organ in the last five years than in all the rest of recorded history, our understanding of this complex organ is still in its infancy. What has been learned, however, has spawned exciting new research and has contributed to the establishment of new disciplines such as psychophysiology and psychoneuroimmunology (PNI).

Traditionally, the medical community has viewed health problems as either physical or mental, treating each type separately. This dichotomy between the psyche (mind) and soma (body) is fading in light of scientific data revealing profound physiological changes associated with mood shifts. The discovery of this complex interaction between mind and body has stimulated intense research regarding the role of stress in health. "How Anger Affects Your Health," "The Mindset of Health," and "Stress" explore the psychophysiology of emotions and its impact on health. "Mind Over Malady" by Peter Jaret discusses the origins of PNI and presents findings that appear to demonstrate a connection between emotional states and the functioning of the immune system.

Hans Selye, the father of stress research, described stress as a nonspecific physiological response to anything that challenges the body. He demonstrated that this response could be elicited by both mental and physical stimuli. Some general characteristics of this response include increases in heart rate, muscle tension, blood pressure, blood sugar, blood fats, and blood coagulability. While these responses are adaptive during times of crisis, Dr. Selye found that the same mechanisms could provoke physiological dysfunction if they persisted for prolonged periods of time. His findings clearly suggest that stress can play a crucial role in the etiology of various diseases.

Mental illness, which is generally regarded as a major dysfunction of normal thought processes, has no identifiable etiology. One may speculate that this is due to the complex nature of the organ system involved. It may also be that many conditions labeled as mental illnesses are not really illnesses at all, but rather behaviors that society has deemed unacceptable. While the latter seems to be true for conditions and behaviors such as homosexuality, drug abuse, child abuse, and sexual dysfunctions, there is mounting evidence to suggest an organic component to the more traditional forms of mental illness such as schizophrenia, chronic depression, and manic-depression. Even as researchers are identifying specific neurochemical disturbances associated with these conditions, experts are locked into a debate as to whether these findings represent the cause or the effect of the mental illness.

The fact that certain mental illnesses tend to occur within families has divided the mental health community into two camps: those who believe there is a genetic factor operating in mental illness, and those who see the family tendency as more of a learned behavior. Regardless of which side is correct, the evidence strongly supports mental illness as yet another example of the weak organ theory.

The reason one person is more susceptible than another to the damaging effects of stress may not be altogether clear, but evidence is mounting that an individual's perception and interpretation of the stressor may be key factors. For some time now psychologists have known that our thoughts create a mind-set or view through which we see our world that colors our perception of it. Given this premise, it would seem reasonable to assume that changing a person's view or mind-set could alter his or her response to a given stressor. "Stress" by Elizabeth Stark examines the issue of perception and concludes that minimizing feelings of isolation, and feeling in control of one's life are central to successful stress management. Ellen Langer, in her article "The Mindset of Health," examines the relationship between mind and perception. She describes how mental states influence health, and how it may be possible for someone to direct his or her own health through a process she terms *mindfulness*.

While the media has alerted the public to the dangers of stress, it has also created the belief that all stress is bad and should be avoided. Avoiding all stress is not only an impossible task, but an undesirable goal as well. Current thinking on this issue has changed the focus from the elimination of stress to an approach that views stress as an essential component of life and a potential source of health. The notion that stress could serve as a positive force in one's life was presented by Dr. Selye in 1974 in his book *Stress Without Distress*. He said that there were three types of stress: negative stress (distress), normal stress, and positive stress (eustress). He maintained that positive stress not only increases a person's self-esteem, but inoculates him or her against the negative effects of distress. The distinction between these three types of stress is a subjective assessment based solely on the perception of the individual. If these assumptions are correct, then the most effective way to change distress into eustress is to work on changing the context or mental state.

Recent studies in the area of occupational stress strengthen the assertion that perception plays a vital role in the stress equation. These studies also challenge the commonly held notion that executive jobs are the most stressful due to their decision-making requirements. Current findings suggest that while executive positions do entail a relatively high level of stress, it is generally of the eustress variety. This is in sharp contrast to the distress experienced by workers at the bottom of the job ladder. Their jobs emphasize performance and provide little latitude for decision-making or control. It is this perceived lack of control that makes these jobs particularly stressful.

According to a recent government document, the incidence of mental illness among adult Americans is approximately 19 percent and growing; this statistic is based on a broad definition of mental illness that includes 230 categories, including tobacco dependence, sexual dysfunction, and developmental defects. Reports such as this, coupled with increasing evidence that mental stress is a contributing factor to many health problems, are prompting researchers to develop therapeutic interventions that will protect individuals from the damaging effects of stress and treat those already experiencing some degree of dysfunction. While tranquilizers have been the traditional treatment of choice, a new branch of medicine, termed *behavioral medicine,* is utilizing techniques such as biofeedback, meditation, self-hypnosis, mental imagery, progressive relaxation, exercise, and nutrition counseling to control stress. In addition to these techniques, many stress management programs include time management training, assertiveness training, and goal setting as stress control strategies. While these techniques may serve a valuable function in a stress management program, none of them is universally effective. "Slow Down, You Breathe Too Fast" by Royce Flippin presents startling new evidence that hyperventilation (a form of overbreathing), once considered a symptom of anxiety and fear, may actually trigger these feelings by lowering blood carbon dioxide levels. These findings validate the usefulness of stress reduction techniques such as meditation and hypnosis, which emphasize the importance of slow deep breathing.

While significant gains have been made in our understanding of the relationship between body and mind, much remains to be learned. What is known suggests that the mind-set of an individual is the key factor in shaping his or her response to stress. In order to be successful in converting distress into eustress, some people may need to make significant alterations in their philosophies of life and thus their mind-sets.

Looking Ahead: Challenge Questions

How have humankind's stressors changed over the last 5,000 years?

How do you manage the stress in your life?

Why do some people respond to stress differently? How do genetics and perception influence one's response to stress?

What is eustress? How can it enhance the wellness of an individual?

What is meant by "mindfulness"? How can this concept be used to promote health?

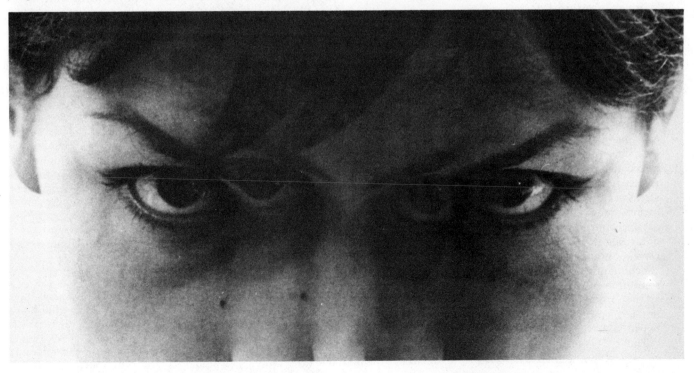

STRESS
It's All Relative . . . and Relatively Easy to Manage

Elizabeth Stark

Elizabeth Stark is a freelance writer specializing in health and behavior.

It's that time of year again: time to send out your holiday cards, buy presents for everyone from your mother to your mail carrier, wrap those gifts, rush from one holiday party to another, travel to see friends and family, and, most likely, eat and drink too much. Is it any wonder that many people consider this the most stressful time of year?

Lest holiday demands turn you into another Ebenezer Scrooge, you should know that you have more control over stress than you may think. And contrary to popular belief, stress often isn't caused so much by external events—such as standing in line for an hour at the post office—as by the way we perceive and cope with them.

Many of us view stress as the unavoidable price of modern life. Nearly nine out of 10 Americans say they experience high levels of it at least once or twice a week, and one in four complains of high levels every day. In the late 1960s, psychiatrists Thomas Holmes and Richard Rahe created a "life stress scale" that listed dozens of events, ranging from things like getting a promotion to the death of a spouse; they assigned each a certain number of points. By checking off those you had experienced in the preceding year and adding up your score, the test implied, you could assign a number to your stress level.

The problem with tidy stress charts is that our reactions to events vary from person to person. What frazzles one may excite or challenge another. Research increasingly shows that it's not the amount of stress that matters, but one's ability to control the situations that engender it.

Understanding stress is further complicated by the fact that the term itself is "one of those words that everyone knows the meaning of but no one can define," says psychiatrist Sanford Cohen, director of the Stress and Clinical Biobehavioral Medicine Center at the University of Miami. For example, many of us refer to upsetting external events as stress, when those are in fact *stressors*. To a psychologist, stress describes the body's reaction to such events. Dr. David Jenkins, a professor of psychiatry at the University of Texas Medical Branch at Galveston, likens stress and an individual to water in a bathtub: "Just as whether the water spills over the top depends in part on the tub's size, people who have a large capacity to deal with challenge may not 'overflow' under stress."

But what happens when your body *does* overflow with stress? First the voluntary nervous system, which responds to sensory input and controls intentional movements, sends messages to your muscles, preparing you—as in prehistoric days—to fight or flee. Then the autonomic nervous system, which regulates involuntary body functions, sends extra blood to your muscles to get you going and slows down other bodily functions such as digestion. In addition, the neuroendocrine system releases adrenaline, the hormone that primes

> Often, external events don't cause stress. How we perceive and cope with them does.

the body for action, and cortisol, another hormone that magnifies and prolongs adrenaline's effect.

This surge of chemicals may have ensured our early ancestors' survival in dangerous situations, but it can wear us down when it results from the unremitting saber-toothed tigers of today: anything from financial woes to that most modern lament, "too much to do, too little time." Bodies exposed to constant, unresolved stress never have a chance to recover. The symptoms that result include headaches, backaches, insomnia, anxiety, depression, arthritis, asthma, gastrointestinal upsets, skin disorders, weight problems and drug and alcohol abuse. In fact, according to the American Institute of Stress (AIS) in Yonkers, N.Y., 75% to 90% of all visits to physicians involve stress-related complaints.

Researchers in the field of psychoneuroimmunology, the study of the relationship between our health and emotions, have even linked stress to specific illnesses. "We now know the mechanisms of many stress-related disorders," says Dr. Paul Rosch, president of the AIS and a professor of medicine and psychiatry at New York Medical College in Valhalla. He believes that chronic, insidious types of stress such as lone-

From *American Health*, December 1992, pp. 41–42, 44–47. © 1993 by Elizabeth Stark. Reprinted by permission.

liness and poverty can affect the immune system; some studies indeed suggest that stress can increase the risk of catching a cold, perhaps even of being struck by cancer or AIDS. Anger, on the other hand, may increase production of hormones such as adrenaline and noradrenalin, which also reduce the body's ability to fight disease and can lead to higher blood pressure and heart attacks as well. Anxiety, another common stress symptom, often affects the gastrointestinal system, contributing to the development of ulcers, colitis and irritable bowel syndrome.

A growing body of evidence indicates that some people are biologically more stress-resistant than others. Genes may play a role. "There seem to be heritable differences in the degree of activity of different body parts," Cohen says. "One family may be susceptible to gastrointestinal reactions, while another gets high blood pressure or headaches."

Research is also focusing on temperament's role in stress reactions. People who seek out challenges that many others would find upsetting fall into a category that Dr. Frank Farley, incoming president of the American Psychological Association and a professor of psychology at the University of Wisconsin in Madison, calls "Type T," for thrill-seeking and risk-taking personality. Partly for physiological reasons, he argues, such people tend to be more creative and extroverted and to take more risks than others, whether positive or negative. A new University of Washington study of high school athletes highlighted a particular dimension of Type T stress resilience: Players who fit Farley's criteria lost less time because of injuries than those with a lower threshold for thrills, probably because they're more tolerant of negative events.

Contradicting a popular prejudice, recent studies by Dr. Redford Williams, a behavioral medicine researcher at Duke University, suggest that having a hurried, impatient Type A personality doesn't necessarily put one at risk for coronary disease. Says Williams: "If you're racing around because you're a go-getter—you're enthusiastic, you're positive—the evidence is that it doesn't

hurt you." So-called hostile Type A's, on the other hand, react to anger with an excessive surge of adrenaline; moreover, the neurological responses that normally counter this reaction are weaker in these people. Compared with others, hostile Type A subjects in Williams' studies were also more overweight, consumed more alcohol, smoked more cigarettes, had worse lipid profiles and consumed more caffeine. "Our findings suggest that the hostile Type A's autonomic nervous system is balanced differently," Williams says. "Since that's a biological characteristic, it does make you think that genetic factors play a more important role in stress than previously thought."

Although biology may lay the foundation for how well we deal with life's stressors, the ways we've learned to defuse them dramatically affect our resilience too. After looking at 1,200 men and women who deal well with stressful situations, Dr. Raymond Flannery, an assistant clinical professor of psychology at Harvard University Medical School, found that they tend to control their lives and look for active solutions to problems; they're committed to meaningful goals; they use little nicotine and caffeine, relax at least 15 minutes a day and get regular aerobic exercise; and they're actively involved with others. "People who live by these principles have better physical and mental health and a greater sense of well-being," Flannery says. When others learn the precepts in his 10-week program, called Project SMART (Stress Management and Relaxation Training), they too report better functioning at home and work and improved health.

While most of us have developed some skills for dealing with stress, says Flannery, we tend to underestimate the importance of social interaction. "Studies show that social contact may lower pulse rate and blood pressure, enhance the immune system and boost the production of endorphins—neurochemicals that make us feel good. When you're in a caring relationship with another person, all these health benefits can accrue."

When your stress load weighs especially heavily, the first step is "to distinguish between things you can do something about and things you

can't," the AIS's Rosch says. "Otherwise, you'll be constantly frustrated." He recommends making a list of your stressors, then separating them into those two categories. As simple as this process sounds, he says, many people don't take the time to think in these concrete terms. Yet, as Flannery says, "none of us can have it all. Life requires each of us to make choices."

Those who learn certain precepts report better health.

One of the major sources of stress is the workplace, where picking and choosing aren't always possible. More than a quarter of the respondents to a 1990 survey from Northwestern National Life, a Minneapolis-based insurance company, said job stress was the single greatest strain in their lives; seven out of 10 said it lowered their productivity and caused frequent ailments. "There are many unhappy, ineffective workers," says Wisconsin's Farley. "I think much of that problem can be laid at the doorstep of an ill-fitting interaction between a person and his environment. People often choose jobs unwisely because they don't know enough about themselves." He cites those ubiquitous lists of the "10 Most Stressful Jobs," which usually include air-traffic controller and police officer. The problem, says Farley, is that some people crave the excitement and danger of being a cop, while others need the familiarity and predictability of, say, an assembly line job. He proposes that "there aren't that many absolute stressors. Stress is an outcome of who you are and what you are doing." That's why, says Rosch, "Type A's thrive in highly demanding jobs as long as they're in control."

Of course, some sense of control is important to *all* workers. Studies have shown that those who feel they have a lot of responsibility and yet have little or no say over decisions that affect them suffer the most stress. Even race-car drivers often say that they feel far more stress sit-

Holiday Stress

Supposedly all-joyous celebration, the holidays are often a time of tremendous tension. Who hasn't experienced that feeling in the pit of the stomach upon realizing it's December 15th and there's still a mountain of gift buying, card sending and cooking ahead?

At this time of year, a big part of the stress load is physical—eating and drinking too much at parties, battling crowds and squeezing just one more event into the day. More insidious is the psychological strain. Merchants and media dictate an impossible holiday ideal. Personal heartaches—about everything from people no longer with us to our unrealized dreams—tend to be magnified at this time. Add in our childhood memories of "perfect" holidays, and how can reality measure up?

Changing demographics have made many traditional holiday expectations unrealistic, says Jo Robinson and Jean Coppock Staeheli, authors of *Unplug the Christmas Machine* (William Morrow, 1991, $8.95). When they examined the causes of holiday stress among thousands of people, they found that in this age of divorce and widely dispersed relatives, the warm, fuzzy image of whole families gathered around groaning boards is long outdated. Considering that both parents in most families work outside the home, lavish feasts and elaborate decorations are also anachronistic.

To bring holiday expectations back down to earth, researchers offer these suggestions:

► BE REALISTIC: Set achievable goals. Don't expect to be happy every minute or for everything to be perfect.

► SET PRIORITIES: Take a hard look at how you've been spending holiday time in the past, and eliminate elements that aren't important to you.

► SIMPLIFY: Do you really need to serve three desserts? Can you scale back on gift giving? Some families draw names from a hat, and have each member buy one terrific gift for the person whose name they pull.

► ENLIST THE HELP OF OTHERS: Mothers often carry an unfair burden of holiday responsibilities. Ask other family members and friends to help.

► TAKE CARE OF YOURSELF: Try not to eat or drink too much. Keep your sleep schedule as regular as possible. Take time out for long walks or hot baths.

► GET SOCIAL SUPPORT: Spend time with those you care about. If you're lonely, seek out people and groups who can make the holidays warmer.

—*E.S.*

ting in the pit while the crew works on the car than when they're barreling around the track.

Still, there will always be people doing jobs for which they're ill-suited and encountering stressful situations that can't be avoided. When you can't change the situation, stress experts recommend that you try to change your outlook. "Most people's problems have to do with faulty perception—perhaps unnecessarily seeing a situation as hopeless—and they have the power to change that," Rosch says. "You can develop certain cognitive skills, such as assertiveness or the ability to manage time better."

If psychological approaches don't appeal to you, you may want to try exercise. Along with providing physical release and mental distraction, it produces natural opiates that elicit calm and euphoria. Experts particularly recommend aerobic activities such as running and swimming. Techniques such as relaxation, biofeedback, visualization, yoga, massage or meditation can also be effective, but you may have to try various approaches to find the one that suits you best. The Type A person,

for example, might have a difficult time meditating, even becoming more stressed in the process.

Before prescribing treatment for her clients, Dr. Suzanne Miller, an associate professor of psychology and medicine at Temple University, determines whether they are "monitors," who want as much information about a stressful situation as possible, or "blunters," who like to distract themselves from it. Because monitors do better with more intellectual, problem-solving approaches, one effective method for them is setting aside a certain period each day as "worry time." When fretful thoughts intrude at other moments, they write them down and go back to the business at hand. The blunter's coping style lends itself much more readily to relaxation and meditation techniques. Although blunters handle stress better in the short term, they often ignore its warning signs, only to find themselves faced with major stress-related ailments later on.

A high-tech way to handle stress, biofeedback allows us to monitor seemingly involuntary body functions. In a biofeedback session, the

patient is hooked up to a machine with painless sensors attached to various parts of the body, such as the hands, arms and face. These sensors measure physiological reactions such as heart rate and muscle

---

Race-car drivers report more stress waiting in the pit than on the track.

---

tension, and produce a flashing light or a beep in response to changes. Using these signals as a guide, the patient learns to control his response, usually by controlling his thoughts. A trainer typically stands by to offer suggestions for improving performance.

If none of these strategies work, a stress-management program may help, particularly one offered by a major medical center or university hospital. Unfortunately, Rosch has found that many "stress-reduction experts"—who aren't licensed—are merely opportunists with little training.

Flannery suggests that if you're considering enrolling in a program, you should ask some questions first: Does the practitioner have a background in counseling or health psychology? Has he demonstrated some mastery in the field? Where was he trained? What does he consider to be reasonable expectations for the program? "A lot of these things are offered as four-hour, quick-fix workshops on a Saturday morning," Flannery says. "But it's going to take a lot longer to enhance your capacity to cope with stress. Look at how long it takes a person to get into physical shape. You'll feel better once you start, but expect to spend anywhere between six months and two years before you enjoy the full benefits." Still, Flannery believes that no one who goes the distance will regret it. "Once people start, they say, 'Why didn't I do this years ago?' And they don't go back to their old ways."

How the Body Responds

Much more than just a feeling of unease, emotional stress triggers a series of bodily responses: The heart races, blood pressure surges, breathing revs up and a rush of adrenaline primes the muscles for action. Embedded in our genes, this so-called fight-or-flight response was intended to protect us from predators. But in a world in which predators often wear pinstriped suits, it's more likely to trigger several physical illnesses.

► HEADACHES. "There's no question that emotional stress has an impact on headaches," says Dr. Ed Blanchard, a professor of psychology at the State University of New York at Albany. Stress, he says, is a major cause of tension headaches—the most common type of headache—and of migraines as well. Stress reduction techniques have been found useful in treating both kinds.

► IRRITABLE BOWEL SYNDROME. Almost everyone experiences gastrointestinal distress occasionally. But frequent problems, including abdominal pain, cramping, bloating, diarrhea and constipation, may be signs of irritable bowel syndrome (IBS), which afflicts 15% to 20% of Americans.

IBS has no known cause or cure, and physical exams usually don't detect it. The majority of those with the problem aren't under exceptional stress and don't even seek medical help. Yet studies have found that IBS patients are more prone than others to the effects of stress, particularly intestinal upheavals. In many cases the symptoms can be soothed by doing relaxation exercises, adding fiber to the diet and avoiding high-fat foods and caffeine. If the problem persists, a doctor may prescribe antidiarrheal or antispasmodic drugs.

► ULCERS. The excess stomach acid triggered by stress has long been considered a major cause of ulcers. But recent research has found stress to be more contributor than cause. The new prime suspect: a type of bacteria present in 70% to 80% of all stomach-ulcer patients and nearly everyone with duodenal (small intestine) ulcers.

"Stress itself won't cause ulcers," says Dr. David Graham, the gastroenterologist at the Veterans Affairs Medical Center in Houston who has been researching the bacterial species, known as *Helicobacter pylori*. "But if you have the bacterium in your system, the increase in gastric acid caused by stress can worsen the ulcer." A two-week antibiotic regimen can eliminate the bacteria.

► HEART DISEASE. Two key risk factors for heart disease—high blood pressure and elevated blood cholesterol levels—can both be exacerbated by stress.

Although elevated blood cholesterol stems mainly from a high-fat diet, a recent study found that people performing mentally stressful tasks experience a temporary rise in cholesterol levels. And earlier research detected a dramatic rise in blood cholesterol levels in income tax accountants every year just before the April 15th deadline.

Men in high-stress jobs are known to be three times more likely than their low-stress counterparts to have high blood pressure. Stress-management techniques such as biofeedback, meditation and yoga can sometimes help lower blood pressure, especially if used over the long term.

Growing evidence is confirming what researchers have long believed: Once people have heart disease, stress increases their chances of dying from it. In studies of heart disease patients, those who were socially isolated or financially strapped died much sooner than more fortunate patients.

Another kind of emotional stress—anger—may also be dangerous to the heart. In a recent study, men with mild heart disease were asked to describe an incident that made them angry. In response to the stress, the pumping efficiency of the men's hearts dropped significantly. The drop meant that the coronary arteries weren't providing the heart muscle with enough blood, perhaps because anger was sending the diseased arteries into spasm.

But many deaths from stress can probably be prevented. A recent study suggests that blood pressure drugs known as beta-blockers can prevent heart malfunctions that occur when cardiac patients are under emotional stress. And minimizing stress can also help: In another recent study, teaching heart attack survivors simple stress reduction techniques lowered their risk of cardiac death by half compared with a control group.

—*Winifred Conkling*

SLOW DOWN, YOU BREATHE TOO FAST

Doctors suspect chronic hyperventilation is behind many "psychological" ailments

Royce Flippin

Royce Flippin is a Senior Editor at AMERICAN HEALTH.

Do you work yourself into a dither about money, relationships or your job? Do situations such as speaking in public or flying turn you into a basket case? Your friends may tell you it's all in your head, and perhaps you agree. But a growing number of scientists say the problem may be you're breathing too fast. Hyperventilation, or "overbreathing," is now a prime suspect in a number of psychological disorders, particularly those involving anxiety and irrational fears.

It's a well-documented fact that people with chronic anxiety are more prone than others to hyperventilation. Until recently, though, hyperventilation has been considered a symptom of anxious feelings (it's still listed that way in the *Diagnostic and Statistical Manual,* the official U.S. handbook of mental disorders). Some researchers are now revising this theory. They believe anxiety is really more a chain of events: It begins when some sort of psychological stress causes a person's trunk, neck and throat muscles to clench. This restricts the lungs and makes the breathing faster and more erratic. It's the erratic breathing pattern—not fear of the stressful situation—that accounts for the uncomfortable sensations of fear and nervousness. Curb this "hyperventilation response," the theory goes, and the apprehensive feelings will evaporate.

"Hyperventilation can magnify any psychological disorder or emotional conflict," says Dr. Herbert Fensterheim, a clinical professor of psychology in psychiatry at Cornell University Medical College in New York City. "The trigger doesn't have to be negative, either. Depending on the person, any emotional stimulation can set off overbreathing."

Fensterheim cites the example of one of his patients, a woman who was having difficulty maintaining relationships with men. It turned out that she would hyperventilate (without being aware of it) whenever she thought about a man she liked. Fensterheim prescribed sessions with a breathing therapist. "Once she learned to breathe properly," he says, "her social problem disappeared."

There's nothing new about a connection between slow, even breathing and a sense of inner peace; it's been a part of various Eastern philosophies, including Taoism, yoga and many martial arts, for millennia. But Western scientists remained largely unconvinced until they learned how to measure carbon dioxide in the blood stream and discovered that the blood's carbon dioxide level drops sharply when a resting person breathes rapidly. This forces the arteries, particularly the large ones going to the brain, to constrict. The result is a reduced blood flow and a shortage of oxygen in the body—regardless of how much is going into the lungs.

Oxygen deprivation has a couple of effects. It switches on the nervous system's "fight or flight" mechanism, creating a physical sensation of nervous arousal. But the biggest influence is on the brain. Besides feeling fearful, overbreathers often complain of poor concentration plus a sense of unreality and detachment. In severe cases they may even experience auditory or visual hallucinations. Dr. Ronald Ley, a professor of psychology and a hyperventilation researcher at the State University of New York in Albany, speculates that oxygen shortages in the brain trigger a subconscious feeling of suffocation that leads to "irrational thoughts and feelings of imminent doom."

Indeed, one of the most insidious effects of overbreathing is that obsessive ideas and apprehensions tend to gain the upper hand more easily. "Fear of death," explains Fensterheim, "is a common symptom among hyperventilators."

Any strong emotion can trigger overbreathing—even thinking about someone you find attractive.

A single, sharp exhalation can reduce your carbon dioxide level by as much as 20% (it will take 30 seconds to return to normal); breathing hard 30 times in a minute will cut your carbon dioxide level nearly in half. According to the hyperventilation theory, such quick drops in carbon dioxide levels—or mini-attacks of hyperventilation—can occur almost imperceptibly in stressful situations, giving rise to anxious feelings.

If anxiety can be a byproduct of faulty breathing, does it follow that anyone who has ever felt anxious has a breathing problem? The more devout hyperventilation theorists stop just short of saying it does.

"To quote Sir Thomas Lewis [a 19th century respiratory specialist], 'hyperventilation is the commonest affliction in civilized society today,' " says Dr. Claude Lum. Now 95, Lum is the retired chief of respiratory physiology at the Papworth Hospital in Cambridge, Great Britain, and is considered the grand old man of breathing study. In the past 30 years, he's treated more than 3,500 patients for hyperventilatory disorders. "At any given time, 10% of the population in Great Britain is clinically hyperventilating," he says.

For all the trouble it causes, chronic overbreathing is hard to detect in all but the most severe cases. The only outward clues are a tendency to gasp or sigh, especially during speaking, and a rising and falling of the upper chest when at rest (in healthy breathers, it's the abdomen that moves). While hyperventilating you're unlikely to feel you're breathing too fast—in fact, because of the brain's "air hunger," you may feel you're not breathing fast enough.

Even doctors can have trouble detecting overbreathing. In his book *The Hyperventilation Syndrome,* Dr. Robert Fried, director of the stress and biofeedback clinic at the Institute for Rational Emotive Therapy in New York City, writes: "It is not infrequent that hyperventilation goes unnoticed in the clinical practice of the psychiatrist, psychologist, social worker, or other mental-health practitioner."

To get a rough idea of your own breathing pattern right now, count your breaths for a minute or two. If you took more than 14 to 16 breaths a minute, you're breathing faster than what's considered appropriate. Now observe the

movement of your chest and abdomen as you breathe. If your chest moves more than your abdomen, chances are you're hyperventilating.

The habit of overbreathing can start early, even before the age of five, according to Fensterheim. "The problem doesn't usually become apparent, however, until the person is confronted by the stresses of adult life," he says. The underlying cause appears to be chronic tension in the muscles of the chest, back, neck and shoulders. This tension interferes with the normal breathing action of the diaphragm muscle. Under stress, a person prone to hyperventilation begins to breathe quickly and shallowly, using

HOW TO CATCH YOUR *Breath*

BREATHING re-education, with muscle and/or breath flow monitoring. This is classic biofeedback training, the type of therapy most likely to be prescribed by a doctor. Learning proper breathing technique takes anywhere from one to six months. Unfortunately, no central directory of breathing therapists exists at this time. To find treatment in your area, contact a local hospital or your state medical association. In the New York City area, contact breathing therapist **Barbara Wiegand at 212-737-0944.**

▶**YOGA BREATHING.** Many YMCA's and YWCA's now offer yoga classes; so do many health clubs. Techniques vary from class to class, but the underlying premise of slow abdominal breathing remains the same. Here are two basic exercises from *The Sivananda Companion to Yoga* (Simon & Schuster, 1983, $12.95):

Abdominal breathing. Sit in a relaxed, upright position, either in a chair or cross-legged on the floor (advanced meditation students can use the lotus posi-

tion). Exhale sharply, pulling in the abdomen, and then inhale slowly, allowing the abdomen to relax. Repeat 20 times. On the last breath, exhale completely, then inhale deeply and hold your breath as long as you can before slowly exhaling.

Alternate nostril breathing. When doing this exercise, known as a "round," count to two for each inhalation, count to eight while holding your breath, and then count to four as you exhale.

Close your right nostril with your right thumb, and breathe in through the left nostril. Hold your breath, closing both nostrils. Breathe out through the right nostril, closing your left nostril (the authors recommend using the ring and little fingers of your right hand). Then reverse the process: Breathe in through your right nostril, close both nostrils, and then breathe out through the left nostril. Begin with three rounds, and gradually work up to 20.

▶**PERCEPTIBLE BREATH.** This therapy was developed by Ilse Middendorf, a German breathing expert who be-

lieves becoming aware of our unconscious breathing patterns is the key to physical and spiritual enlightenment. During an hour-long session, the patient is encouraged to relax completely while the therapist uses gentle body manipulations to guide the movement of breathing. For more information, contact **Marion Mancini, a perceptible-breath practitioner, at 212-769-0925.**

▶**DIRECTED BREATHING.** Developed by Valerie Anne Kirkgaard, a family therapist in Santa Monica, Calif., this therapy's goal is to imagine you are directing your breath into areas of chronic muscle tightness to release long-held physical and emotional tensions.

Kirkgaard's instructions: Pick an area of your body that usually gets constricted under stress (such as the neck). Sitting in a relaxed position, take a deep breath and direct the breathing sensation into the tense area. Hold your breath, concentrating on the feeling of tension. Then think

of the first image that enters your mind. Often this is a memory from childhood. "Within a short period of time, most people get some sort of picture," she says. Exhale, and take another deep, directed breath while keeping that image in your mind. Kirkgaard believes this process, done repeatedly, can uncover buried childhood traumas. For more information, contact **Valerie Anne Kirkgaard at 213-453-8987.**

▶**SKIN CONDUCTANCE BIOFEEDBACK.** This is a do-it-yourself breathing technique developed by Dr. Erik Peper, a behavioral scientist at San Francisco State University and the acting director for the Institute of Holistic Healing Studies. He's developed a program called "Breathing for Health," which is available on cassette tape. It includes a small biofeedback device that fits in your palm and measures the electrical conductivity of the skin on your fingers. As your breathing gets less hurried, skin conductivity decreases. An earphone lets you "hear" your improvement. For more information, contact **Thought Technology at 800-361-3651.**

the upper chest muscles to gulp in small amounts of air at a rapid rate.

"Many people can't help overbreathing because they're chronically tensed up," says Fried. "Over the years, their psychological tensions have turned into habitual muscle contractions."

In breathing therapy, patients learn to do slow, deep "belly breathing" at a rate of six to 10 breaths a minute, allowing the elastic diaphragm muscle to contract down and forward from the rib cage on each inhalation. Therapists also try to teach their patients to control each exhalation instead of cutting it short with a gasping intake of air.

You don't need to visit a specialist, however, to regulate your breathing. Meditation, yoga or any other muscle relaxation technique can help. Breathing through your nose rather than your mouth also tends to keep carbon dioxide levels properly elevated because the smaller opening gives you more control over each inhalation and exhalation. An ancient yoga relaxation device is to obstruct one nostril while breathing slowly in and out of the other.

You can practice belly breathing on your own as well. Barbara Wiegand, a breathing therapist in New York City, recommends lying on a bed or sofa with your upper body propped at a 30° angle, or semi-reclined. Breathe through your nose as you place one hand on your upper chest and the other on your abdomen. While you breathe, try to let the hand on your abdomen rise with each inhalation, and try to prevent your chest hand from moving.

Another approach, used by Dr. Rosemary Cluff, a physical therapist and former colleague of Lum's at Papworth Hospital, is to pause and relax intentionally for just an instant at the end of each exhalation. "This helps slow down the overall breathing rate," says Cluff.

People suffering from anxiety or phobias often improve just from learning to recognize the effects of their overbreathing. "When bad feelings come up, if a person can say, 'Okay, it's my breath-ing that's causing this,' it provides a sense of control, rather than fear," says Julie Weiner, a biofeedback therapist with the New York Pain Treatment Program at Manhattan's Lenox Hill Hospital. "The patient learns that by shifting to belly breathing, he or she can reduce those anxious feelings."

Many therapists employ biofeedback in teaching belly breathing. In one version, electrodes are used to monitor chest, neck and shoulder muscle tension. The patient breathes through a tube at a constant rate while trying to keep upper body tension low.

People who undergo breathing therapy often become less irritable and more social.

Even with professional therapy, muscle tension accumulated over a lifetime doesn't disappear overnight. Patients typically take one to six months to learn healthier patterns of breathing, plus another six months of practice to make them second nature. The benefits, however, are frequently permanent. "Only about one patient in 20 is an intractable case," says Lum.

Some of the people who have benefited most from breathing therapy are panic attack patients, who hyperventilate uncontrollably and may feel as though they are dying during attacks. These patients often go on to develop an unreasonable fear of the activity or situation that triggered the attack. "If the sequence isn't broken, the person can become a complete invalid in six months," explains Dr. William Gardner, a respiratory physiologist at King's College Hospital in London.

The question teasing researchers is: Which comes first, the panicky feelings or the hyperventilation? A number of lab experiments have shown that intentional hyperventilation will trigger panic attacks in a sizable portion of patients with the disorder. And in a survey of panic attack victims, Dr. Ronald Ley discovered that 80% said sensations of fear struck *after* a hyperventilation episode had begun.

Whatever the lab work finally reveals, panic disorder therapists have found that breathing therapy can virtually eliminate panic attacks; it's also effective in relieving a related disorder, agoraphobia (fear of public places). And preliminary studies suggest that overbreathing is implicated in sleep disturbances, migraine headaches, high blood pressure, epileptic seizures and heart attacks. A doctor in Israel recently reported that she had even cured a hyperventilating woman who had been misdiagnosed as a schizophrenic.

Gardner warns, however, against blaming too many ailments on the syndrome. "There are a lot of theories, but no firm conclusions yet," he says. "That's the state of the art. What we need to do now is take a more careful look at hyperventilation, cut through the theories and see what's really happening."

One thing clearly happening is that people who get their runaway breathing under control report improvements in their lives. Fried claims everyone can benefit from breathing training, even those who aren't clinically hyperventilating. "If you breathe more slowly, you'll feel more relaxed and have a greater sense of well-being," he says.

Weiner says patients who learn to breathe properly often become less irritable and get along better with others. "People often can't believe their behavior could be controlled by such a simple thing," she adds. "They'll say, 'I've been putting my family and friends through all this pain just because I'm breathing wrong?' But it's true."

Can we actually become nicer by breathing better? It's an enchanting idea—one to make anyone sigh with anticipation. Just make sure you do it slowly, please.

Mind Over Malady

Peter Jaret

Peter Jaret is a contributing editor.

Once a week they meet to talk, to cry, sometimes to laugh together. "Is the pain still worse in the mornings?" Margaret* asks Kate today.

A petite, graceful woman in her late forties, Kate shakes her head no. "It's getting bad all the time," she says in a voice raw with worry and fatigue. A few weeks ago she learned that the cancer that began in her breast had spread into her bones. Since then she's hardly slept. She knows, as do the other women in the group, that her prognosis isn't good. "Sometimes I'm afraid I'm not going to do that well because it all came on so fast," she tells them. "It's like being in the ocean and the waves are just coming too fast, and you can't get your breath."

They nod in tacit understanding, eight women sitting in a loose circle of chairs here in a small, sparely furnished room at Stanford University Medical Center. They know. All of them have been diagnosed with recurrent breast cancer.

"Sometimes I just cry and cry and cry," Linda tells the group. "I cry so hard I scare everyone in the family." Her admission brings small smiles of recognition.

"The worst part is the fear," Margaret says later. "That's what really makes it hard to enjoy the time we've got left."

So they gather here each Wednesday afternoon to talk with each other and to listen. It's a chance to discuss their fears and find some small comfort, a time to feel they're not alone. And in some way that no one has been able to explain, it may be keeping them alive.

Ten years ago, David Spiegel, the Stanford psychiatrist who runs these sessions, would have laughed at such a notion. The sixties and seventies had stitched a crazy quilt of alternative healing approaches—"wish-away-your-cancer" therapies, Spiegel calls them. Visualize your body filled with radiant light and be healed! Think happy thoughts and be well! Spiegel had heard it all. And he'd seen too many cancer patients,

desperate to live, go chasing after the latest New Age cure. One of his patients, a woman with breast cancer, had traveled a thousand miles for a course in visualization therapy, only to be asked by the therapist, when the technique failed to slow the disease, why she *wanted* her cancer to spread.

Spiegel had been furious. It was nonsense. Cruel nonsense. And in 1984, he had set out to prove it.

His method was simple. A few years earlier, he and his colleagues had conducted a study to evaluate the psychological

Stressed-out students catch
colds. Are they making themselves sick? Feisty cancer
patients live longer. Are
they making themselves well?

effect that emotional support groups have on cancer patients. They'd studied 86 women with breast cancer, all of whom were receiving conventional cancer therapies. Fifty women were randomly selected to take part in weekly discussion groups in which they shared their feelings and learned simple techniques to reduce stress. After a year, Spiegel had discovered, women in the support groups were less depressed, felt less pain, and had a more positive outlook than the women who received only conventional treatment.

---

* *The names of the women in the support group have been changed.*

By Peter Jaret. From *Health*, November/December 1992, pp. 87-88, 90, 92, 94. © 1992 by Hippocrates Partners. Reprinted by permission.

That in itself had been good news. It had suggested that support groups should be an important part of caring for patients with life-threatening illnesses. But the wish-away-your-cancer proponents went much further, claiming that a more positive outlook could actually help the body fight disease. If that were so, then women who took part in the support sessions should have fared better against the disease, and Spiegel didn't believe that for a moment. So he went back to see, confident that he would find no difference at all between the two groups.

What he found shocked him. The women who had received only conventional treatment had survived an average of 19 months after the study began. But women in the support groups had lived an average of 37 months—*nearly twice as long*. Forty months after the study began, Spiegel found, all the women in the control group were dead. One-third of the support group women were still alive.

"Believe me, if we'd seen these results with a new drug," he says, "it would be in use in every cancer hospital in the country today."

But it wasn't a new drug. It wasn't some high-tech experimental treatment. It was a group of women sitting around talking, sharing their fears, learning how to face a terminal illness.

And suddenly Spiegel found himself wondering if the wish-away-your-cancer types were on to something after all. Do negative thoughts make us more prone to illness? Can happy thoughts heal?

MOST OF THE WORLD'S traditional healing systems —from the practice of Ayurveda in ancient India to the Taoist teachings of China—have taught that states of mind can affect states of health. The father of modern medicine himself, Sir William Osler, declared at the turn of the century that the treatment of tuberculosis depended more on what was going on in a patient's head than in his chest. In the 1960s, psychiatrist George Solomon, then at Stanford University, argued that the crippling symptoms of rheumatoid arthritis occurred more often and with greater severity in women who were passive, self-effacing, and unable to express their anger. Could emotions, he wondered, affect the body's ability to fight disease?

But by then, few scientists were listening. Researchers studying the body's defenses were learning that they could take immune cells out of the bloodstream and culture them in the laboratory, and the cells would go right on killing viruses and tumor cells, even outside the body. The idea that happy or sad thoughts could somehow affect them seemed preposterous—the stuff of shysters and shamans, not serious scientists.

Then, in the mid-1970s, University of Rochester School of Medicine and Dentistry psychologist Robert Ader made a discovery that couldn't be so easily dismissed. Ader was conducting a simple variation of Pavlov's famous experiment in which dogs learn to salivate at the ringing of a bell. Instead of dogs and bells, Ader was giving rats a drink of sweetened water and then a shot of a drug that induces nausea. His plan was to study patterns in the way the animals, learning to associate an unpleasant stimulus with a pleasant taste, began to avoid the sweetened water.

But something went wrong. For no apparent reason, the rats began to sicken and die. Ader knew that the nausea-inducing drug he was using, called cyclophosphamide, could dampen immune responses. But the single shot most of the rats received was hardly enough to explain their deaths. And there was another mystery. The rats didn't seem to be getting sick in relation to how much cyclophosphamide they received—that would have implicated the drug itself—but instead to how much sweetened water they drank.

"I was lucky," Ader recalls with a mischievous smile, 15 years later. "I didn't know the first thing about immunology. So I was free to make up any story I wanted." The story he concocted made perfect sense to a psychologist: Not only had his rats come to associate the sweetened water with feeling nauseated, but they'd also come to associate the sweet water with the other action of the drug—its ability to dampen immune responses. In effect, the rats had learned how to shut down their own immune systems.

When Ader published his findings, immunologists howled. A learned immune response was impossible, they said, because the defense system was thought to operate under its own direction, shaping its strategies moment by moment, independent of any control from the brain or nervous system. How else to explain immune cells that went on destroying viruses and cancer cells even when outside the body?

But in a series of experiments conducted with immunologist Nicholas Cohen, Ader proved his guess was correct. The rats *were* learning to shut down their own immune systems, cued by the taste of sweetened water. And the discovery signaled a revolution. If such responses could be learned, there *had* to be specific connections between the brain and the body's defenses.

"Ader's discovery clinched it," says Solomon, whose own research in the area had gone largely ignored ten years earlier. In 1964, Solomon had proposed a new field, dubbed psycho-immunology, to study the interaction of mind and immunity. A decade later, Ader coined an even longer tongue-twister: psychoneuroimmunology. Since then, some researchers have jokingly suggested psychoneuroendocrinimmunology might be more accurate.

Call it PNI. As the term itself made clear, something was happening that couldn't be contained within the conventional categories of medicine. "Until recently, the mind belonged to psychiatrists, the brain to neurologists, the immune system to immunologists," says Solomon, now at the University of California at Los Angeles. "We understood the body by arbitrarily dissecting it into parts. But those divisions don't exist in the living, breathing body. The goal of psychoneuroimmunology is to put all those systems back into the body, to understand how they work together as a whole."

As word of Ader's findings spread, researchers around the country, many of whom had once scoffed at the notion that the mind could affect immunity, set about to understand the implications. If rats could learn to shut down their own immune systems, what powers might the human mind possess over health and sickness?

PSYCHOLOGIST Janice Kiecolt-Glaser and her husband, immunologist Ronald Glaser, had often talked about working together. But in the late 1970s it was hard to think of two fields with less in common than psychology and immunology. Then, at a conference in 1980, the Ohio State University researchers met Robert Ader and learned about his remarkable findings. "On the way home," says Kiecolt-Glaser, "we began to plan our experiment."

Their question was simple. "On an intuitive level, at least," Kiecolt-Glaser says, "many people seemed to think that stress could make them more vulnerable to illness. Find yourself in the middle of a rocky relationship and you'll be more likely to get sick. Get stressed out at work and you'll come down with a cold or flu." Several studies had shown that rates of illness were higher among people in the weeks and months after they suffered the severe emotional trauma of divorce or bereavement. The trick would be to show that more commonplace anxieties caused significant, measurable changes in immunity, something no one had ever done before.

So a month before final exams in 1981, the Glasers rounded up 75 medical students at the university. While Kiecolt-Glaser ran the students through psychological tests designed to measure stress, her husband checked their blood for indications of immune strength. Then, in the middle of the fingernail-biting anxiety of exam week, they repeated the tests.

Glaser was convinced the whole experiment was a waste of time. For years he'd been studying immune cells in glass dishes, watching them vigorously attack and destroy viruses and cancer cells. The idea that a little worry over exams could affect them seemed absurd.

But by every measure they used, the Glasers discovered the students' defenses slumped during the stress of exam week. The fighting power of natural killer cells—cells that appear to defend against viruses and cancer—had dropped significantly. In students who carried herpes, there were clear signs that the virus had become more active. Perhaps most surprising of all, the lonelier the students were, according to their psychological profiles, the bigger the drop in immune function.

"I was flabbergasted," says Glaser. Since then the researchers have studied people who are in the midst of divorce, bereavement, the trauma of caring for a loved one with Alzheimer's, and the inevitable tensions of married life among newlyweds. Ohio State University medical students still emerge bleary-eyed from a morning of exams to fill out psychological questionnaires and roll up their sleeves to give blood in an annual ritual that has come to be called, with the mordant humor of medical students, the Day of the Big Bleed.

In almost every case, the Glasers have shown, emotional stress seems to dampen the body's defenses in reliable, measurable ways.

Why? Part of the answer, researchers suspect, lies in the chemistry of emotions. Almost 30 years ago, George Solomon suggested that corticosteroids—hormones that flood into the bloodstream whenever we're alarmed or anxious—might affect the immune cells. Since then, scientists have found that some hormones, like cortisol, impair the cells' ability to multiply and function. Others, like prolactin, seem to give them a boost.

But since most of these substances have been studied only in laboratory dishes, no one really knows what effects they have as they pulse through the human body. Over the past few years, the researchers at Ohio State University have dogged a group of medical students during a 24-hour period of exam week, drawing blood every hour on the hour. In experiments with endocrinologist Bill Malarkey, they've invited newlyweds into the laboratory, coaxed them into bickering—all it usually takes is a question or two about in-laws or money—and then tapped blood specimens every 15 minutes. By matching stress levels and hormonal changes to the ups and downs of immune function, the Glasers hope to gain a better grasp of the shifting chemistry of mind and immunity.

The links between brain and immunity may be even more complicated. In 1981, Karen Bulloch at the University of California at San Diego traced nerves from the brainstem to the thymus, a gland tucked behind the breastbone where certain immune cells learn their functions or "go to school," as she puts it. Since then, researchers have identified an elaborate network of neurons that reaches from the brain into other organs of the defense system, including lymph nodes. Block those nerves, and immune cells lose much of their ability to produce antibodies or to attack and destroy invading cells.

Indeed, some scientists have come to think that the brain and the disease-fighting system, far from being separate and distinct, may actually speak the same biochemical language. In 1981, immunologist J. Edwin Blalock and his colleagues at the University of Texas Medical Branch at Galveston found something they weren't supposed to find: a substance called adrenocorticotropic hormone in a culture of immune cells. As far as anyone knew, this hormone was produced only by the pituitary gland in the brain, part of the body's reaction to stress. Since then, Blalock and other researchers have turned up dozens of neuropeptides—chemical messengers once thought to be synthesized only in the brain—that are produced and received by cells of the disease-fighting system. Nerve cells, meanwhile, have been found to manufacture chemical signals once thought to belong only to the defense system.

Scientists who have been deciphering this chemical language have been listening in on some surprising conversations. When immune cells encounter an invading virus or bacteria, they release a chemical called interleukin-1, which stimulates other defense cells to multiply. When molecules of this substance reach the brain, they tell the hypothalamus, the body's thermostat, to turn up the heat, creating a fever. The elevated temperature in turn appears to give immune cells an advantage in fighting infection.

Far more complex conversations are also taking place. In a variation of his original experiment, Robert Ader found that mice with an inherited form of the autoimmune disease lupus, in which an overactive system mistakenly attacks healthy tissues, are more likely than normal mice to go on drinking the sweetened water, despite the nausea associated with it. By doing so, they suppress their defenses and lessen the damage of the disease. In the end, they live longer. Somehow, Ader speculates, immune cells may signal the brain that something is wrong; the brain, in turn, alters the animals' behavior to compensate for the defect.

Such findings have made Blalock, for one, begin to wonder whether the illness-fighting system isn't really more like the body's sixth sense. "The immune system is designed to sense the things we can't hear or see or smell—infectious organisms like bacteria and viruses, tumor cells, foreign molecules," he says. "Whatever it finds is reported back to the brain. And the brain, in turn, exchanges information from other senses with the immune system. It's a totally integrated circuit."

Recently, Ader has suggested one unexpected way that circuit might be used to heal, by tapping the sort of learned responses he observed in rats and mice. Many useful drugs, Ader points out, have serious side effects. If people could be conditioned to associate only the beneficial effects of a drug with something harmless, say the sweet taste of a pill, then it might be possible to reduce doses of the drug and depend instead on learned immune responses. There's already evidence the approach might work. In 1984, researchers at the National Institutes of Health and the University of Alabama Medical School gave mice a whiff of camphor at the same moment they injected them with a drug that boosts natural killer cells. Later, when the mice again sniffed the camphor, the smell alone was enough to increase natural killer cell activity. More remarkable still, when these mice were injected with cancer cells and given occasional whiffs of camphor, on average they lived significantly longer than mice injected with cancer cells alone.

FOR PROPONENTS of the healing powers of the mind, the latest findings are heady stuff, indeed. At King's College School of Medicine and Dentistry in London, researchers have found that women who confront breast cancer with a fighting spirit survive longer than those who respond with stoic acceptance. Assertiveness and the ability to express emotions, according to psychologist Lydia Temoshok at the University of California at San Francisco, seem to improve melanoma patients' chances for survival. A lifetime of loneliness and isolation, on the other hand, increases the chances of illness and early death.

With each new finding, the popular press has been quick to trumpet the news. PESSIMISM LINKED TO POOR HEALTH! YOUR ATTITUDE CAN MAKE YOU WELL! Books proclaiming the healing powers of the mind have crowded the bookstores. In his enormously successful books, *Love, Medicine, & Miracles* and *Peace, Love, & Healing,* former Yale University surgeon and cancer specialist Bernie Siegel preaches the gospel to millions. "Your body is here to help you," he assures patients. "It's your gift. If you give it negative messages, it will die faster. If you give it positive messages it will fight for your life."

Lecturer and writer Louise Hay, the high priestess of the mind/body movement, has attracted converts and controversy with a far more radical message. Forget viruses and cancer cells; the real causes of disease, says Hay, are criticism, resentment, anger, and guilt. Polio is merely a symptom of paralyzing jealousy, farsightedness a sign of fear of the present. In her underground best-seller, *Heal Your Body,* Hay offers hundreds of medical mantras designed to overcome the ill effects of negative thoughts. Are you bothered by bunions? Intone three times a day: "I joyously run forward to greet life's wonderful experiences." Troubled by tumors? Then repeat after Hay.: "I lovingly release the past and turn my attention to this new day. All is well."

It's enough to give a scientist apoplexy. "This isn't PNI," Robert Ader grumbles, shaking a sheaf of the latest clippings announcing the miraculous healing powers of the mind. "It's deceit and utter nonsense."

Like many scientists charting the uncertain territory between mind and immunity, Ader worries that the rush to find larger meaning in the most isolated laboratory finding often leaves truth behind. "To claim that negative thoughts somehow cause disease or that happy thoughts can heal by helping the immune system is premature," Ader says. "There's simply not the slightest scientific evidence that it's true." During the past 15 years, Ader admits, PNI has gathered a scattering of provocative puzzle pieces; but the picture they trace is still far from clear.

Take those studies that find that patients with a fighting spirit survive longer. It may simply be that such patients push themselves harder to get up and become active after surgery. Or perhaps they're more motivated to follow doctors' orders. There's no proof yet that changes in immune power are responsible.

Or consider the evidence that stress weakens the body's defenses. True, the Glasers have shown again and again that many stressful situations lead to a decline in natural killer cell activity. Yet other studies have shown that the severe anxiety suffered during panic attacks can actually boost natural killer cells' fighting power. Sorting out the significance of such effects isn't easy.

Even if it were, says Ader, the jury is still out on whether all those ups and downs of immune response carefully noted by researchers really make a difference to anyone's health. The immune system is constantly changing. The number and activity of immune cells vary widely, even among people who are quite healthy.

Still, there's growing reason to wonder. During last year's Big Bleed, the Glasers gave their medical students vaccinations to protect against the serious liver ailment hepatitis B. The more stressed-out and anxious the students, the Glasers found, the more slowly they responded to the vaccine and the lower their levels of protective antibodies even when the series of three shots was completed. Had the students encountered the hepatitis B virus itself instead of the vaccine that mimics it, would the more anxious students have been slower to respond? Would they have become ill while calmer students stayed well? There's no easy way, short of locking subjects up in a sealed laboratory, to get at this point.

Which is precisely what scientists at the Common Cold Unit in Salisbury, England, did in a recent experiment. The researchers first evaluated stress levels of 394 subjects. Then they infected the volunteers, who were isolated in the live-in research facility, using a nasal spray laced with cold viruses. Seventy-four percent of those who ranked least stressed-out caught the bug, the scientists found, compared with 90 percent of the most stressed-out group. And who actually came down with the symptoms of a cold? Only 27 percent of the laid-back group, compared to 47 percent of their stressed-out counterparts. What's more, the scientists found a "dose response"— the higher a person's stress level the more likely that person was to become infected and sick. Remarkable. But like so much PNI research, the British experiment raised as many questions as it answered. The levels of both virus-fighting immune cells and cold-killing antibodies showed no differences between the stressed and the unstressed, leaving researchers to puzzle over why one group came down with more colds than the other.

If the power of negative thoughts is uncertain, proof that positive thoughts can heal is just as elusive. What, after all, *are* positive thoughts? Mental images of clear mountain streams? The support of friends and family? An optimistic outlook? A fighting spirit? Researchers have tried to measure the effects of stress reduction techniques on the immune system. But again, the results haven't always been clear-cut. When the Glasers taught residents of a retirement home such techniques, they found evidence of increased natural killer cell activity. But when medical students practiced similar exercises before exams, there seemed to be no effect at all on natural killers. Instead, helper T cells increased in number.

The most dramatic evidence to date of the effects of a more positive outlook comes from David Spiegel's startling study of women with breast cancer. And certainly it's tempting to think that emotional support therapy, by reducing stress, gave his patients' defense systems a fighting edge against the disease. But as Spiegel is quick to point out, that's mere conjecture. For one thing, his original study didn't include measures of immune function, so no one really knows whether the emotional support groups had any such effects at all. And, says Spiegel, there are other perfectly good explanations for what he found. "It may be just as likely, because women in the support group experienced less pain, anxiety, and depression, that they encouraged their doctors to be more aggressive in treating their cancers," he explains. "Or perhaps a more positive outlook helped them sleep and eat better, and that alone accounted for their longer survival. We just don't know." Still, Spiegel admits he finds it hard to believe that such explanations can account for results as dramatic as those he stumbled upon. In an ongoing series of experiments he is repeating his earlier study, this time around monitoring changes in his patients' immune systems.

There's already reason to think he'll find some difference. Researchers at the University of California at Los Angeles recently conducted an experiment that closely mirrors Spiegel's but included measurements of immune function. Eighty patients with melanoma were divided into two groups. Patients in both groups received standard treatment, but one group also took part in six weekly emotional support sessions. At the end of the six weeks, patients in the support groups felt better and had a more positive attitude. But their defenses, disappointingly, showed little change.

Six months out, however—long after the support groups had been discontinued—researchers found that there *were* differences. Almost two-thirds of the support group patients registered a rise of 25 percent or more in the number of one type of natural killer cells, the same cells that proved so vulnerable to stress in the Glasers' medical students. Only one patient in the control group registered so dramatic a jump.

Is a 25 percent rise in natural killer cells enough to matter? Again, no one really knows. The UCLA researchers are following the fate of their patients. If, like Spiegel's breast cancer patients, those who took part in support groups survive longer, it will offer, if not proof, at least one more tantalizing clue.

MEANWHILE, in the small meeting room at Stanford University Medical Center, the afternoon is waning. "I want you to imagine your body floating somewhere safe and comfortable," David Spiegel's voice intones—a lulling, reassuring murmur. "I want you to concentrate on a warm, tingling numbness that's penetrating your body."

Around the room, Kate, Margaret, and the others have closed their eyes.

"And now take a moment to filter out the pain," Spiegel gently urges. "Concentrate more and more on the pleasant numbness. Allow your body to feel as safe and comfortable as you can. Let the tension flow out of it . . ."

Someday, perhaps, researchers will know whether exercises like these really help us fight illness. Like many in the field, Spiegel worries that the exaggerated claims made by the so-called alternative healers will lead patients desperate for a cure to abandon conventional treatments. He's concerned, too, that wish-away-your-cancer therapies can end up making patients feel guilty when they don't get well. "It's easy for people to think that getting sick is their own fault," Spiegel says. "'If only I'd had a more positive attitude. If only I'd been able to meditate more.' That's nonsense. We don't die because we have a bad attitude. We die because we're mortal."

And no one's promising to conquer death. Among the 86 women in his original study, only three died of causes other than cancer. Still, Spiegel believes there's every reason to think that the chance to talk, to cry, even to laugh together may be just as important as the most aggressive chemotherapy or radiation. "We do know that patients in these groups experience about fifty percent less pain. They feel better about themselves in their condition. They can still find joy and pleasure, even in the face of death. If we're also helping them stay alive a little longer, great. But that alone isn't everything."

Indeed, for a moment or two in the hushed silence of the room, the fear and fatigue that have shadowed Kate's features all afternoon visibly lift. Her shoulders relax. And as she takes in a long, slow breath, it's easy to imagine that she's breathing in life itself.

How anger affects your health

Anger is a universal emotion, and when in the thrall of its physical symptoms—the pounding heart, the sweating palms, the rising blood pressure—most people can well believe that anger causes illness, particularly for those who live with chronic suppressed anger that boils over from time to time. Yet anger is not only universal, but can also be useful. For example, it can lead a person to struggle against injustice. It can get a voter to the polls. It can lead a parent to defend (or to instruct) a child. On the down side, it can lead to violent and antisocial behavior. For many years, scientists have looked for links between anger and heart attack, stroke, and high blood pressure, or between chronic hostility and cancer. Scores of studies have been carried out—some leading to dead ends. It's hard to isolate and study anger, which can result from real situations, such as hardship and poverty, or can sometimes seem groundless to the casual observer. Whether a person vents or suppresses anger may alter its effects.

Nevertheless, some plausible theories have begun to emerge. For example, recent research suggests that chronic anger may be more damaging to women than to men, at least in women who habitually suppress their anger. Yet when men are forced to suppress chronic anger day after day, their health suffers too. According to Dr. Leonard Syme of the University of California at Berkeley, the answer may well be that *a lack of control over the situations that cause anger,* rather than hostility itself, determines the long-term health effects of anger.

Hostility and the coronary arteries

The idea that personality and heart disease might be linked was formalized in 1969 with the concept of "Type A." Two California cardiologists, Dr. Meyer Friedman and Dr. Ray Rosenman, presented evidence that men with a certain kind of hard-driving, aggressive, competitive, tense, and hostile personality were at risk for chronic chest pain or angina (a word with the same root as anger) and for heart attack. The Framingham Heart Study, an important and large-scale investigation of the risk factors for heart disease—and one of the few that included women—also provided evidence that Type A personality puts a person at risk, not only men in white collar jobs, but women as well. But to the surprise of many researchers, subsequent studies were contradictory and failed to confirm the link between Type A behavior and heart disease. Careful study stripped away aggressiveness, tenseness, and competitiveness as risk factors for heart attacks. A recent 22-year follow-up by Dr. David Ragland and Dr. Richard Brand of the University of California at Berkeley indicated that Type A behavior was not related to heart attack deaths. Smoking and high blood pressure were far more important risks than personality or behavior.

Thus more than 20 years after Type A was introduced, most investigators have given up on it. What does continue to interest many of them, however, is just one component of Type A—anger, or more specifically the tendency to look at the world with cynicism and hostility. A recent study conducted by Dr. Redford Williams at Duke University Medical Center returned to the subject of heart attack and anger. It found that those identified as hostile personalities when they were 19 years old had significantly higher levels of total cholesterol and lower levels of beneficial HDL cholesterol at age 42 and were thus at higher risk for heart attack.

Dr. Williams and his colleagues hypothesized that hostility can actually affect blood cholesterol levels, or—a very different thing—that it simply leads to bad health habits. Other researchers, too, have conjectured that hostile people may adopt a "why bother" attitude: "Why be careful about my diet, why exercise, why take care of myself when things are so rotten anyhow?" And yet this line of thought hasn't panned out either. Williams's new evidence for a link between hostility and heart disease is called into question by equally good evidence that no such link exists. For example, a new study led by Dr. Dianne Helmer at the University of California at Berkeley found no significant link between hostility (as measured by standardized psychological tests among 158 people hospitalized for coronary angiograms) and heart disease. Hostility, the study concludes, does not predict heart disease. Other studies have had mixed results.

Women and anger: a taboo?

But other researchers are still on the trail. If not Type A or hostility, what about suppressed anger? If not heart disease, what about other diseases? And another question that remains alive is whether anger—if it poses health risks—might have different effects on women than on men. In 1985, in *The Dance of Anger,* Harriet Lerner of the Menninger Clinic in Topeka, Kansas, suggested that women's anger was a taboo topic for scientific investigators.

Some studies have appeared since then, however. For example, Dr. Mara Julius of the University of Michigan has reanalyzed the data from a long-term study of a Michigan community (the Tecumseh Community Health Study). How men and women in this study coped with anger had been measured by such questions as this: "If your spouse or an authority figure such as a policeman yelled at you for something you hadn't done, how would you react?" Possible answers ranged from "I wouldn't feel annoyed" to "I'd get angry and protest." Women—but not men—who suppressed their anger in such confrontations had a higher mortality rate over time. In fact, women who suppressed their anger in confrontations with their spouses had twice the mortality risk as other women, even when other factors such as high blood pressure and smoking were considered. Among couples, if both husband and wife suppressed anger, mortality rates went up among women but not men. Among men, only those who suppressed their anger *and* had high blood pressure had a higher risk of dying.

Thus Dr. Julius concluded that suppressing anger was a risk factor for heart disease and cancer in women. Her work also suggests that women may handle anger differently from men and thus be affected in special ways by suppressing it.

Blowing up may not help, either

But venting anger may not be any better than suppressing it. At the University of Tennessee, a small study of 87 middle-aged women investigated anger levels, and found that angry women tended to be pessimistic about themselves, to lack social support, to be overweight, to sleep poorly, and to lead sedentary lives. These women also believed that they could not control their problems and could do nothing about them. The angriest women were also more likely to have health problems already. It's not clear, of course, whether the anger results from this unhappy life-style, which is definitely not conducive to good health, or is simply another symptom of unhappiness. Researchers noted that many of the issues that made these women angry were not easy to modify. They also found that "contrary to popular wisdom, which recommends ventilation of anger," the women whose health seemed most adversely affected by anger were not suppressors of anger, but those who "directed it outward." In other words, blowing your stack may merely make you feel worse. And as a rule, no matter how justified the outburst, it doesn't promote social ties or provoke sympathetic reactions.

Thus for these women at least, the choice between suppressing or venting anger may be irrelevant. It may not be anger that makes people sick, or even the way they express it, but the inability to deal effectively with the situations that anger them. Recent studies of occupational stress have sug-

---

Managing anger: easier said than done

In 1989 Dr. Redford Williams of Duke University Medical Center wrote *The Trusting Heart*, subtitled *Great News About Type A Behavior*. In it he agreed that Type A behavior is not "toxic," but claimed that hostility is. He suggested several stress-management techniques to cope with anger, among them:

■ Monitor your cynical thoughts by keeping a log of situations that stir you up.

■ Try stopping cynical thoughts.

■ Put yourself in the other person's shoes.

■ Instead of yelling angrily, try to be assertive, calm, and clear about what's bothering you.

Good advice. But though the observation may be cynical, a person who can do all that is not too bad off to begin with. It's hard to develop a "trusting heart" if you have reasons not to be trustful. Whether to suppress or express anger, and how best to express it, depends inevitably on the circumstances and the other people involved. Managing uncontrollable angry outbursts in oneself or in a family member may require counseling, meditation, life-style changes, or other kinds of long-term psychological help.

Learning from the soaps

Some suggestions for managing anger from the Institute for Mental Health Initiatives (IMHI) may be helpful. A few years ago, recognizing that "people who have some skill at managing their anger are less likely to... suffer from emotional disorders such as depression, or grow up to be early victims of heart disease or stroke," IMHI undertook a study of how anger is handled on daytime TV soap operas. These shows have an audience of 20 million people, most of them women. In 1986 researchers analyzed how anger was presented on 12 daytime dramas on the three major networks. Finding that anger too often resulted in violence on the soaps, they drafted guidelines for producers and writers about healthier ways of portraying anger. No one knows just how effective these efforts have been, but according to surveys completed in 1990, IMHI found that anger has increasingly been portrayed on soaps not as an emotion felt by "bad" people but as a normal emotion that even likeable people exhibit and can deal with constructively. In addition, women have been increasingly portrayed as effective at handling anger. These ideas could conceivably be helpful for some viewers. Out of this research IMHI developed anger-management techniques that emphasize such tips as these:

■ Recognize your own anger and that of others.

■ Empathize with a person expressing anger.

■ Always listen carefully to what an angry person is telling you.

■ Try to express respect along with the anger.

■ Notice your own reactions, especially your physical reactions.

■ Focus your attention on the present problem, and avoid thinking of old grudges or wounds.

IMHI has developed pamphlets and workshop materials on anger for children, teenagers, and adults. For more about their programs, write to them at 4545 42nd Street NW, Suite 311, Washington, D.C. 20016, or call 202-364-7111.

gested that anger can loom large and can adversely affect health among men as well as women, especially when there's nothing they can do about their situation.

Men and anger: they are not immune

The health effects of anger on men may perhaps be gauged from some recent occupational research. Driving a big-city bus fits every criterion for a high-strain job (that is, one with high workload demands but little sense of control): pressure to meet a schedule, physical discomfort, high noise levels, unruly or hostile passengers to be dealt with, heavy traffic, the risk of a crash or breakdown. In addition, a virtual requirement of the job is some ability to suppress anger—to be courteous to the public under stressful conditions. According to a recent unpublished paper by Gary Evans of the University of California at Irvine, over 20 studies of bus drivers in various cities reveal that they have an elevated death rate from heart disease and are more prone to suffer from gastrointestinal disorders and musculoskeletal disorders, such as bad backs. They retire earlier than other civil servants, too, usually because of medical disabilities. A study of 1,428 San Francisco bus drivers (male, mostly nonwhite) supplied one puzzling piece of information: those who scored low on the stress scale—that is, who perceived their jobs as unstressful—tended to have high blood pressure more often than those who recognized the strain they worked under.

Human emotions are hard to study scientifically. Still, it does appear that suppression of anger—when a person has no other choice—is linked to ill health.

The Mindset of Health

THE WAY YOU THINK SENDS MESSAGES THAT INFLUENCE HOW YOUR BODY RESPONDS, SAYS A NOTED PSYCHOLOGIST IN THIS EXCERPT FROM HER BOOK *MINDFULNESS* (ADDISON-WESLEY).

ELLEN J. LANGER

Ellen J. Langer, Ph.D., is chair of the social psychology program at Harvard University and won the Distinguished Contributors to Psychology in the Public Interest Award from the American Psychological Association.

Consider this scenario: During a routine physical, your doctor notices a small lump in your breast and orders a biopsy as a cancer-screening measure. Your immediate reaction is fear, probably intense fear. Yet in some cases, a tiny breast lump or mole requires only a tiny incision, comparable to removing a large splinter. Fear in such a situation is based not on the procedure but on your interpretation of what the doctor is doing. You're not thinking splinters or minor cuts; you're thinking biopsy, cancer, death.

Our thoughts create the context that determines our feelings. In thinking about health, and especially in trying to change the consequences of an illness or the behavior that leads to it, an awareness of context—or what I have come to call a "mindfulness"—is crucial.

Understanding the Power of Context

"Is there a split between mind and body?" the comedian Woody Allen once asked. "And if so, which is better to have?" With these questions he penetrates to one of our most potent mindsets. From earliest childhood we learn to see mind and body as separate—and to regard the body as without question the more essential of the two. We are taught that "sticks and stones can break my bones, but names can never hurt me." And later, we

take our physical problems to one sort of doctor, our mental problems to another. But the mind/body split is not only one of our strongest beliefs, it is a dangerous and premature psychological commitment.

When we think of various influences on our health, we tend to think of many of them as coming from the outside environment. But each outside influence is mediated by context. Our perceptions and interpretations influence the ways in which our bodies respond to information in the world. If we automatically—"mindlessly"—accept preconceived notions of the context of a particular situation, we can jeopardize the body's ability to handle that situation. Sometimes, for the sake of our health, we need to place our perceptions intentionally, that is, mindfully in a different context.

Context can be so powerful that it influences our basic needs. In an experiment on hunger, subjects who chose to fast for a prolonged time for personal reasons tended to be less hungry than those who fasted for external reasons—for money, for example. Freely choosing to perform a task means that one has adopted a certain attitude toward it. In this experiment, those who had made a personal psychological commitment not only were less hungry on a subjective measure, but they also showed a smaller increase in free fatty acid levels, a physiological indicator of hunger. The obvious conclusion: State of mind shapes state of body.

Building Immunity Through Emotion

A wide body of recent research has been devoted to investigating the influence of attitudes on the immune system, which is thought to be the intermediary between psychological states and physical illness. The emotional context, our interpretation of the events around us, could thus be the first link in a chain leading to serious illness. And since context is something we can control, the clarification of these links between psychology and illness is good news. Diseases that were once thought to be purely physiological and probably incurable may be more amenable to personal control than we once believed.

Even when a disease may appear to progress inexorably, our reactions to it can be mindful or mindless and thus influence its effects. A very common mindset, as mentioned before, is the conviction that cancer means death. Even if a tumor has not yet had any effect on any body function, or how you feel physically, rarely will you think of yourself as healthy after having a malignancy diagnosed. At the same time, there are almost certainly people walking around with undiagnosed cancer who consider themselves healthy, and may remain so. Yet many doctors have noticed that, following a diagnosis of cancer, some patients seem to go into a decline that has little to do with the actual course of the disease. They appear, in a sense, to "turn their faces to the wall" and begin to die. But they needn't. By reinterpreting the context, they might avoid the unnecessary failure attributable to fear alone.

Harnessing the Power of the Mind

In recent years there has been much new research that now supports the value of a mindful approach in handling a variety of health situations such as:

Pain: Patients have been successfully taught to tolerate rather severe pain by seeing how pain varies depending on context (thinking of bruises incurred during a football game that are easily tolerated, versus the attention we require to nurse a mere paper cut).

This mindful exercise helped the patients get by with fewer pain relievers and sedatives and to leave the hospital earlier than a comparison group of patients. And the results seem to indicate more than a simple, temporary distraction of the mind, because once the stimulus — the source of pain — has been reinterpreted so that the person has a choice of context, one painful, one not, the mind is unlikely to return to the original interpretation. It has, in effect, changed contexts.

Hospitals: Part of the hospital context is its strangeness, a strangeness that has been found to be life-threatening in some cases. In a dramatic investigation, Klaus Jarvinen, lecturer in internal medicine at the University of Helsinki, studied patients who had suffered severe heart attacks and found that they were five times as likely to die suddenly when unfamiliar staff members made the rounds.

Had these patients been able to meet these staff members and helped to see the way they were much like the people the patients already knew and cared for, making the new staff seem less strange, the consequences might have been different.

Outsmarting Temptation

We all know people who have quit smoking "cold turkey." Do they succeed because their commitment to stop puts withdrawal symptoms into a new context? For many years I quit smoking from time to time, found it too difficult, and began again, as many people do. But when I stopped the last time, almost ten years ago, I surprisingly felt no withdrawal symptoms. There was no willpower involved. I simply did not have an urge to continue smoking. Where did it go?

Jonathan Margolis, a graduate student at Harvard, and I explored this question in two stages. First we tried to find out if smokers in a nonsmoking context experienced strong cravings for cigarettes. We questioned smokers in three situations that prohibited smoking: in a movie theater, at work, and on a religious holiday (Orthodox Jews are not permitted to smoke on the Sabbath). The results in each setting were very similar. People did not suffer withdrawal symptoms when they were in any of the nonsmoking contexts. But when they returned to a context where smoking was allowed—a smoke break at work, for instance—their cravings resurfaced.

All of these people escaped the urge to smoke in a mindless manner. Could they have achieved the same thing deliberately? Can people control the experience of temptation?

In designing a second experiment to answer this question, we assumed that a mindful person would look at addiction from more than one perspective. For instance, it is clear that there are actually advantages as well as disadvantages to addictions. But this is not the usual point of view of someone trying to break a habit.

People who want to stop smoking usually remind themselves of the health risks, the bad smell, the cost, others' reactions to their smoking — the drawbacks of smoking. But these effects are not the reasons they smoke, so trying to quit for those reasons alone often leads to failure. The problem is that all of the *positive* aspects of smoking are still there and still have strong appeal — the relaxation, the concentration, the taste, the sociable quality of smoking.

A more mindful approach would be to look carefully at these pleasures and find other, less harmful, ways of obtaining them. If the needs served by an addiction or habit can be satisfied in different ways, it should be easier to shake.

To test whether this dual perspective was at work when people quit smoking, we picked a group of people who had already quit and complimented each one for their success. We then paid careful attention to their responses to our compliments on their will power.

To understand our strategy, imagine being complimented for being able to spell three-letter words. A compliment doesn't mean much when the task is very easy. If you solve a horrendously difficult problem and then receive a compliment, it is probably most welcome.

We then asked these former smokers what factors they considered when they decided to stop smoking. Those who gave single-minded answers, citing only the negative consequences, were more likely to be the ones who accepted the compliment. Those who saw both sides usually shrugged it off, suggesting that quitting was easier for them. And months later, these people who did not experience a hardship when quitting were more likely to remain successful in staying off cigarettes.

Putting Addiction Out of Mind

Similar evidence of the importance of context in dealing with temptation comes from work on alcoholism and drug addiction, both often seen as intractable problems. For instance, even the degree of intoxication experienced can be changed by altering the drinker's expectations.

In one experiment, psychologists G. Alan Marlatt of the University of Washington and Damaris J. Rohsenow of the V.A. Medical Center in Providence, Rhode Island, divided a group of subjects according to whether they expected to receive an alcoholic drink (vodka and tonic) or a nonalcoholic drink (tonic alone). Despite the presumed physiological effects of alcohol on behavior, expectations were the major influence. What the people expected, tonic or vodka and tonic, determined how aggressively they behaved and how socially anxious and sexually aroused they became. In a similar study, researchers found that groups of men who believed they had been given alcohol, whether or not they had, showed a tendency for reduced heart rate, a condition associated with drinking.

These are just two of the many investigations showing that thoughts may be a more important determinant of the physiological reactions believed to be alcohol-related than the actual chemical properties of alcohol. The antics of high school kids at parties, generation after generation, are probably also influenced by context just as much as they are by the quantity of beer guzzled.

Here is another example. Informal reports from people who work with heroin addicts show that those addicts who are sent to prisons with the reputation of being "clean" (that is, the addicts believe there is absolutely no chance they will be able to get drugs there) did not seem to suffer withdrawal symptoms, while addicts sent to prisons whose reputations included easy access to drugs and who believed they would be able to get their hands on drugs — but didn't — experienced the pain of withdrawal.

Fooling the Mind

The deliberate nature of mindfulness is what makes its potential so enormous. And that potential has important precursors in methods we've developed to "fool" ourselves into better health. In the 1960s, experiments with biofeedback made it clear that it was possible to gain intentional control of such "involuntary" functions as heart rate, blood flow and brain activity. Through trial and error, people learned to control the workings of their own bodies and, for example, lower their blood pressure or counteract painful headaches.

Another method for harnessing the healing powers of the mind in a passive way is through the use of placebos, inert substances that in appearance resemble active drugs. Although inert, placebos are known to have powerful effects on health. But who is doing the healing? Why can't we just say to our minds, "Repair this ailing body." Why must we fool our minds in order to enlist our own powers of self-healing?

Placebos, hypnosis, autosuggestion, faith healing, visualization, positive thinking, biofeedback — these are among the ways we have learned to invoke our own powers. Each can be seen as a device for changing mindsets, enabling us to move from an unhealthy to a healthy context. The more we can learn about how to do this mindfully and deliberately, rather than having to rely on elaborate, indirect strategies, the more control we will gain over our own health.

The Mind's Active Placebo

Ever since we relied on our mothers to make a bruised knee better with a Band-Aid and a kiss, we have held on to the assumption that someone out there, somewhere, can make us

better. If we go to a specialist and are given a Latin name for our problem, and a prescription, this old mindset of that magical someone helping is reconfirmed.

But what if we get the Latin name without the prescription? Imagine going to the doctor for some aches and pains and being told you have Zapalitis and that little can be done for this condition. Before you were told it was Zapalitis, you paid attention to each symptom in a mindful way and did what you could to feel better. But now you have been told that nothing can be done. So you do nothing. Your motivation to do something about the aches, to listen to your body, has been thwarted by a label. With the loss of motivation eventually comes the loss of the skill of caring for ourselves, to whatever degree we otherwise would have been able.

In the past decade or so, a new brand of empowered patient/consumer movement has tried to restore our control over our own health. Many of the alternative therapies sought out by these people have as their most active ingredient the concept of mindfulness.

Whenever we try to heal ourselves and do not abdicate this responsibility completely to doctors, each step is mindful. We welcome new information, whether from our bodies or from books. We look at our illness from more than the single perspective of medicine. **We work on changing contexts, whether it is a stressful workplace or a depressing view of the hospital. And finally, when we attempt to stay healthy rather than to be made well, we become involved in the process rather than the outcome.**

In applying mindfulness theory to health, I have worked a good deal with elderly people. Success in increasing longevity by making more mental demands on nursing-home residents or by teaching meditation or techniques of flexible, novel thinking gives us strong reasons to believe that the same techniques could be used to improve health and shorten illness earlier in life. In a recent experiment we gave arthritis sufferers various interesting word problems to increase their mental activity. Compared to a group given a less stimulating task, the mindful patients not only reported increased comfort and enjoyment, but some of the chemistry of the disease changed as well.

There are two ways in which we have learned to influence our health: exchanging unhealthy mindsets for healthy ones and increasing a generally mindful state. The latter method is more lasting and results in more personal control. Understanding the importance of abandoning the mind/body dualism that has shaped both our thinking and the practice of medicine for so long can make a profound difference in both what we do and how we feel. The real value of fostering the idea of "active placebos" will come when people put them to work for themselves.

Consider how you learned to ride a bike. Someone older held on to the seat as you peddled to keep you from falling until you found your balance. Then, without your knowledge, that strong hand let go and you were riding on your own. You controlled the bicycle without even knowing you had learned how.

The same is true for all of us most of our lives. We control our health, and the course of disease, without really knowing that we do. But just as on the bike, at some point we all discover that we are in control. Now may be the time for many of us to learn how to recognize and use the control we possess over illness through mindfulness.

Drugs and Health

As a culture, Americans have come to rely on drugs not only as a treatment for disease, but as an aid for living normal, productive lives. This view of drugs has fostered both a casual attitude regarding their use and a tremendous drug abuse problem. The term drug abuse conjures up visions of derelicts, dark alleys, and wasted lives. In reality, this description is accurate for only a small minority of drug users. It is true that drugs are responsible for destroying many lives, but drug abuse has become so widespread that there is no way to describe the typical drug abuser, except to say that he or she could be anyone. What constitutes abuse varies, depending on the drug used and the circumstances in which it is used. Based on current trends, it seems likely that the problems of drug abuse will remain as long as attitudes toward drugs remain so casual.

What accounts for this casual attitude toward drug usage? There is no simple explanation for why America has become a drug-taking culture, but there is certainly evidence to suggest some of the factors that have contributed to this development. From the time we are children, we are constantly bombarded by advertisements about how certain drugs can make us feel and look better. While most of these advertisements deal with proprietary drugs, the belief is created that drugs are a legitimate and effective way to help us cope with everyday problems. Growing up, most of us probably had a medicine cabinet full of over the counter (OTC) drugs, freely dispensed to family members to treat a variety of ailments. The extensive use of OTC drugs by the American public, coupled with the protection limits of patent laws, has prompted several pharmaceutical companies to seek FDA approval for an OTC version of a prescription medication. The FDA has approved the reclassification from Rx to OTC for at least 45 prescription medications. The economic gains and widespread public support accompanying such moves are likely to trigger a wave of such products. One of the chief concerns regarding this change in status is that some of the reclassified candidates are powerful and potentially hazardous drugs. Larry Katzenstein's article "Rx to OTC" discusses the pros and cons of the switch. In the face of rising health care costs, many people are attempting to treat minor discomforts with OTC medications without sufficient knowledge of their possible side effects. While most of these preparations have little potential for abuse, they are not innocuous. "Ordinary Medicines Can Have Extraordinary Side Effects" addresses this problem. Most people know that taking prescription drugs in combination can produce some dangerous drug interactions, but they probably are not aware that some foods can also interact with and modify the action of drugs, producing dangerous side effects. "Foods and Drugs That Don't Mix" by Mark Fuerst

lists several drug-food interactions that consumers should be aware of.

Over the last few years, the FDA has come under increasing pressure to expedite its drug approval process so that experimental drugs used to treat conditions such as AIDS, Alzheimer's disease, and cancer can be made available to U.S. citizens much sooner than the typical 12-year waiting period. The FDA has responded by initiating an investigational new drug program (IND), which makes available to desperately ill patients experimental drugs that are still under review. This change in FDA policy may help save some lives, but it will most certainly raise many new questions regarding how new drugs are to be evaluated. The evaluation process is confounded even further when one considers recent findings concerning the placebo effect. These investigations have turned up new evidence that suggests that the placebo effect is twice as powerful as was previously thought, and they have prompted some researchers to call for stricter standards for testing new medications. How these findings will influence the FDA's approval process is unclear. Daniel Goleman's article "Placebo Effect Is Shown to Be Twice as Powerful as Expected" raises some interesting questions regarding the nature of drug testing and suggests that in certain instances, the placebo effect may be an important tool for bolstering the body's own healing powers.

Many people find it hard to understand why coffee, cigarettes, and alcohol are mentioned when the topic of discussion is drug usage, since as children they frequently observed parents and their friends drinking coffee, smoking cigarettes, and having an occasional alcoholic beverage. Despite the casual nature of our exposure to these substances, each contains a potent drug. Alcohol, nicotine, and caffeine are the most widely used and abused drugs in America, but they do not get nearly as much media coverage as do the more exotic and illicit drugs, such as cocaine, crack, PCP, and marijuana. Does this mean that these drugs are not as dangerous? When it comes to tobacco and alcohol, the answer is a resounding "no." Alcohol and tobacco are far and away the leading causes of death and disability related to drug usage. How can we as a society expect to significantly curtail drug usage in general, if we sanction the use of two drugs with such a deadly track record?

Of the drug problems facing this nation, alcohol use is clearly one of the most complex. This complexity stems from the ambivalence we feel regarding its use. While we deplore alcohol for the countless deaths and disabilities it accounts for each year, we openly sanction moderate use of alcohol in a variety of social situations. This ambivalence permeates even the scientific community. While it is clear that heavy alcohol use results in significant damage to a variety of organ systems, the same cannot be said of moderate use. In fact, the scientific community is currently wrestling with this issue regarding cancer and coronary artery disease. Several recent studies have reported that moderate alcohol use increases a woman's risk of breast cancer, but at the same time several studies have suggested that moderate alcohol use may help prevent coronary artery disease. What is the public to think in response to reports such as these?

Few people today continue to harbor any misconceptions about the health hazards caused by the prolonged use of tobacco. Most realize that this drug is associated with emphysema, lung cancer, strokes, and heart disease, but they may not be aware that smoking can cause retinal damage, impotence, cold fingers, and low back pains. Kristine Napier's article "Alcohol and Tobacco: A Deadly Duo" is particularly interesting because, in addition to presenting the health hazards of this dual addiction, it discusses why drinkers are heavier smokers. Given the amount of bad press that tobacco has had over the last few years, why is it that so many Americans continue to smoke? Perhaps the answer is nicotine. Recent studies indicate that nicotine is as addictive as heroin, and thus smoking is an addiction rather than merely a habit. "Saying Goodbye to an Old Flame" by Benedict Carey discusses the process of quitting smoking and examines several of the most popular smoking cessation programs.

America has finally conceded that the time has come to formally declare war on the drug problems of this country. How will we fight this war? Most experts agree that our strategy must include measures that reduce not only the supply, but also the demand, for drugs. This may be the most challenging aspect of all, and one that will require substantial funding for both educational and rehabilitative programs. This is a war that we must win, and one that will require a commitment on the part of all Americans if we are to succeed.

Looking Ahead: Challenge Questions

Do you think America has a drug problem? If so, why?

How do you feel about drug companies reclassifying medications from Rx to OTC? Who benefits and who loses when this occurs?

How might a person decide when drug use has become drug abuse?

What responsibility does the U.S. government have in the area of drug abuse?

What responsibility do communities have in the area of drug abuse?

Given society's ambivalence toward alcohol, how can we best curb the problem of alcohol abuse?

What restrictions, if any, should be placed on the use of tobacco products?

Recently the mass media has been charged with contributing to the growing drug problem by portraying drugs in an appealing manner. Do you feel this charge is justified? Why or why not?

Some states are considering passing laws that would make it a crime to abuse drugs during pregnancy. How do you feel about this?

One cancer you can give yourself.

Horrible isn't it?

AMERICAN CANCER SOCIETY

Ordinary medicines can have extraordinary side effects

CHRISTOPHER HALLOWELL

Elizabeth's cold was making her miserable—her throat was scratchy, her nose was so stuffed she could hardly breathe, and her head felt as if it were going to explode. After three days of suffering, she bought a popular over-the-counter decongestant and took the recommended dosage. "That night," she says, "though my congestion had let up, I felt as though my brain had been rewired. I was very jumpy and once I got to bed, I lay wide awake. I tossed and turned so much that my husband couldn't sleep either." The next morning she took another dose. "That day I felt even worse. I was so irritable I yelled at my kids over the littlest things."

It wasn't until her second sleepless night that Elizabeth began to suspect her medication as the cause. In the morning, she called her doctor, who explained that the preparation she'd been taking contained pseudoephedrine, a compound that can affect some people's nervous systems. The jumpiness, irritability and insomnia that Elizabeth experienced were direct reactions to the drug.

Elizabeth's story is not an unusual one, unfortunately. While we tend to hear about the physical side effects of certain drugs, we often are not informed that ordinary cold tablets, painkillers, allergy remedies and other common over-the-counter (OTC) and prescription medications can change our mood or affect our ability to think and function normally. Perhaps you, too, are being affected without even realizing it.

THE MENACE IN YOUR MEDICINE BOTTLE

It is still not known for sure exactly how medications cause mind- and mood-altering reactions—nor why some people experience them while others do not. But researchers do know that drugs are not always totally precise in performing their intended functions and that psychological side effects can result from a drug's unexpected interaction with the body's nerve circuitry. "Many drugs work by changing signals in the brain or the nerves, and problems can occur when they affect signals they weren't supposed to affect," says Bambi Batts Young, Ph.D., a scientist associated with the Center for Sci-

ence in the Public Interest, a Washington, D.C., consumer and research group. Dr. Young, who recently directed a Center-sponsored investigation into chemicals that affect the brain and nervous system, explains that adverse reactions also can result if, for some reason, the body is eliminating certain chemicals at a slower-than-normal rate.

Given the individuality of each person's chemical and neural makeup, it is all but impossible to predict who will be vulnerable to side effects from any given preparation. For the same reasons, it's hard to tell exactly what reactions may occur. Still, some medications do contain ingredients that have been known to cause problems. Fortunately, most of the side effects are temporary.

THE DANGERS OF DIET PILLS

Most over-the-counter diet pills contain a substance called phenylpropanolamine hydrochloride, or PPA for short, as the active ingredient. This compound is chemically related to amphetamine, a substance that is notorious for exciting the nervous system. Though the psychological reactions to OTC diet pills containing PPA are rarely severe enough to warrant medical intervention, they are sufficient to alter mood and behavior in some people. Typical is the case of former Congresswoman and Vice Presidential candidate Geraldine A. Ferraro. During a 1983 hearing on the safety and efficacy of OTC drugs before the House Subcommittee on Health and Long-Term Care, Congresswoman Ferraro reported that she began taking diet pills when she decided to lose weight. "I can recall . . . [that] my heart started beating very fast and I cleaned my house as if I was . . . the white tornado . . . ," she is quoted as saying in a transcript of the hearing. "I'd be up very early in the morning and I couldn't sleep at night. . . . I decided I didn't want to become a nervous wreck, so I stopped taking them . . . and immediately . . . the symptoms stopped."

PPA has been implicated in hundreds of similar reports, many of them emphasizing the feelings of nervousness, anxiety and irritability that overcome some people who take pills containing the ingredient. But PPA can also cause more serious psychological prob-

lems. The *Journal of the American Medical Association* cited the cases of seven women who were brought to a hospital emergency room suffering from hallucinations, dizziness and anxiety after taking PPA-containing tablets. Within several hours, all the women had recovered except one, who suffered a psychotic episode.

While such extreme reactions from PPA use are rare, feelings of euphoria are more common. These are thought to be the result of PPA's causing the release of chemicals in the brain in much the same way that amphetamines do. "Medications containing PPA used to be sold on the street as substitutes for amphetamines or 'speed,'" says Sorell L. Schwartz, Ph.D., a professor of pharmacology at Georgetown University School of Medicine in Washington, D.C. "I don't feel that there is any sound reason for supporting their use as diet aids."

CULPRITS IN COLD REMEDIES

The use of PPA is not restricted to diet pills. More than 100 OTC medications—including cough syrups, cold remedies and decongestants—contain the substance. The same mood shifts can occur with these preparations as with diet pills, but the threat is often doubled. In addition to PPA, these medications may contain ephedrine or pseudoephedrine, substances that relax air passages and constrict blood vessels not only in swollen nasal passages but also in the brain, thus affecting the nervous system. Among the common reactions are the ones Elizabeth experienced: nervousness, irritability and insomnia. Other possible side effects include dizziness and general malaise.

Children, because of their size and age, can be more severely affected than adults—even when the recommended dosages are followed. A report in the *British Medical Journal* warns that a frequently used over-the-counter cough medicine that contains pseudoephedrine and triprolodine (an antihistamine) can occasionally cause nightmares in children. Mood changes are also caused by the surprisingly high percentages of alcohol that many cold and cough medications contain. As one parent of a three-year-old girl recently said, "I gave my daughter

From *Redbook*, May 1987, pp. 132–134, 156, 159. © 1987 by Christopher Hallowell. Reprinted by permission of the author.

the recommended child's dose of a cough medicine I usually take. She lay in bed wide-eyed until midnight, when she suddenly started giggling about something. It helped fight her cough, but the next day she was tired and cranky."

THE PROBLEMS WITH PAINKILLERS

Aspirin and acetaminophen are two common remedies for minor pain; both are relatively safe. In large doses, such as might be taken to quell arthritic pain, however, aspirin can cause a ringing in the ears that may lead to feelings of disorientation.

For greater pain, prescription drugs are the best bet, but with their increased effectiveness also comes increased risk. The most frequently used of these are the synthetic opiates such as codeine, propoxyphene and meperidine. Their mood- and mind-altering side effects include irritability, disorientation, dizziness and drowsiness. And added to these problems is the possibility of addiction. "A person can easily become addicted to one of these drugs after three or four months of continued use," explains Charles Dackis, M.D., an expert on drug addiction and medical director of Hampton Hospital in Mount Holly, New Jersey. "Once addiction begins, psychological side effects become much worse. Personality changes, such as impulsive, irresponsible and antisocial behavior, are common. The person becomes less and less concerned with the relationships in his life."

ALLERGY TREATMENTS CAN SPELL TROUBLE

The symptoms of hay fever and other allergic reactions—itchy eyes, runny nose, etc.—are caused by histamine, a compound that is released from cells when allergy-inducing substances are present. Allergic reactions are often treated with antihistamines, which interfere with the effects of histamine by blocking its receptor sites.

But many antihistamines, such as chlorpheniramine, brompheniramine and diphenhydramine—to name but a few found in typical OTC and prescription antiallergy medications—are infamous for the drowsiness they can cause. Cheryl, a 35-year-old self-employed publicist, learned this the hard way. Although drowsiness is so common a reaction that physicians and pharmacists often caution patients about this side effect, Cheryl was given no warning when she purchased an OTC antihistamine to relieve a case of the sniffles. She took the drug in the morning, before going to the office. An hour later, during an important meeting with a potential new client, Cheryl felt so sleepy she could hardly concentrate on what she was saying. She cut the meeting short and lost the account as a result.

But drowsiness is not the only problem

a sexual TURNOFF

Among the most disconcerting side effects of some over-the-counter and prescription medications are a decrease in sexual desire and a lack of physical or emotional responsiveness to sex. "When an individual or a couple comes to me for help with a sexual problem, the first thing I want to know is what medications are being used," says Shirley Zussman, Ed.D., a New York City sex therapist. "Many common drugs diminish libido far more than anyone might expect."

For example, antihistamines can cause drowsiness and lack of concentration, so many allergy sufferers using these drugs find themselves too sleepy or unfocused for sex. Barry J. Klyde, M.D., an endocrinologist associated with Cornell University Medical College in New York City and a member of the staff at the New York Hospital, adds, "Because antihistamines interfere with the chemicals that carry nerve impulses—including those necessary for normal sexual function—they may hinder erection or lubrication, as well as orgasm in both men and women."

Tranquilizers also affect nerve impulses and so can induce similar reactions. Another way they can inhibit normal sexual responses is through their muscle-relaxing effects. And, adds Dr. Klyde, "Some sedatives have a depressive effect, which makes it even more difficult to become aroused or to reach orgasm."

Painkillers also can be a culprit. Dr. Klyde points out that people taking frequent doses of painkillers often experience a decrease in *all* their basic biological drives. According to Dr. Charles Dackis, these drugs suppress sexual desire and sometimes cause impotence.

Likewise, birth-control pills can reduce a woman's sex drive, says Dr. Zussman. This is due to the low estrogen levels in most pills prescribed today. Dr. Klyde explains: "The Pill can have effects similar to but not as severe as those experienced at menopause—thinning of the vaginal lining, decreased lubrication, painful intercourse and lessened desire." Women who notice such symptoms should speak to their gynecologists about changing to a Pill with slightly higher levels of estrogen.

Women may not always be aware of subtle changes in their sexual responsiveness, while with men the effects can be much more obvious. This is especially true with medications that often cause impotence, such as some prescription drugs used to treat high blood pressure, ulcers, heart disease and depression. "I know of more than two hundred drugs that cause sexual dysfunction in men," says E. Douglas Whitehead, M.D., a New York City urologist and a director of the Association for Male Sexual Dysfunction in New York City.

Changing a patient's prescription can often alleviate impotence, however, so it is important that a man alert his doctor to any problems he may be having. In fact, Dr. Zussman advises that anyone taking medication on a continual basis discuss its possible effects on sexuality with his or her doctor.

with antihistamines, says R. Michael Sly, M.D., chairman of allergy and immunology at the Children's Hospital National Medical Center and professor of child health and development at the George Washington University School of Medicine in Washington, D.C. "In some individuals, especially young children, antihistamines can have the opposite effect, causing restlessness, irritability and insomnia—side effects your doctor is less likely to mention." Nightmares are another, though rarer, reaction, he says.

A new prescription antihistamine called terfenadine does not appear to cause the side effects typically associated with antihistamines, although drowsiness may occur in some, adds Dr. Sly. And another fairly new drug, cromolyn sodium, is sometimes prescribed as an alternative to antihistamines because it has virtually no side effects. Used as a nasal spray in the treatment of allergies involving the nasal passages, the drug prevents the release of histamine from cells. "However, cromolyn sodium is not effective for everyone," cautions Dr. Sly.

The drugs used to treat asthma also cause a multitude of changes in mood and frame of mind. Among the most frequently prescribed are bronchodilators, which open constricted airways. Theophylline, the most common in this class of drugs, produces nervousness, insomnia, irritability, behavioral problems and difficulty in concentrating in many patients, according to Dr. Sly. Another group of bronchodilating drugs called beta-agonists—including albuterol, terbutaline and bitolterol mesylate—can cause some of the same side effects, although to a lesser degree than does theophylline, especially when they're inhaled through the mouth (via a nebulizer or metered-dose inhaler) rather than taken as tablets. (Albuterol is prescribed in tablet, liquid and inhaler form; terbutaline in tablet and inhaler form; bitolterol mesylate, only in inhaler form.) The reason inhaled drugs have fewer side effects than those taken in tablet, liquid or injected form: They're deposited directly at the site they're intended to treat (in this case, the airways) rather than absorbed through the bloodstream, which circulates the drug throughout the body. Also, less of the drug is needed when it doesn't have to take a roundabout route to reach its target. But unfortunately, inhaled drugs are not always effective in severe cases of asthma, because the airways may be too constricted for enough of the drug to penetrate.

Epinephrine (also know as adrenaline) is yet another beta-agonist drug. This one is associated with more side effects than the other drugs in this category—even when it is inhaled—according to François Haas, Ph.D., director of the Pulmonary Function Laboratory at New York University Medical Center in New York City and coauthor of *The Essential Asthma Book: A Manual for Asthmatics of All Ages* (Scribner, 1987). These include jitteriness, disorientation due to dizziness, and even anxiety, often resulting from the very rapid heartbeat the drug can bring on. "For this reason, epinephrine is usually limited to use in asthma emergencies, during which time it would most likely be injected," Dr. Haas says. Epinephrine *is* present in some OTC asthma medications, however, and he and other specialists warn against using these.

Finally, a class of drugs called steroids, prescribed both for asthma and persistent allergies involving severe inflammation, can cause feelings of euphoria and, in rare cases, psychotic behavior, according to Dr. Sly. Restlessness is another, although infrequent, reaction. But again, these side effects are usually associated with the tablet, not the inhaler form of the drug. Steroid sprays can be inhaled through the nose or, in the case of asthma, through the mouth.

UNEXPECTED EFFECTS OF TRANQUILIZERS

The usual preparations prescribed for anxiety include diazepam, lorazepam, oxazepam, prazepam, triazolam and chlordiazepoxide, all made from a class of compounds called benzodiazepines. These can cause drowsiness, depression or euphoria, dulled thinking and impaired motor coordination, according to Dr. Dackis. In addition, they can be addicting, he says. "Addiction can come on so quickly that many people are not even aware that they are addicted. And even after a few months of use, anxiety—the very problem these drugs are supposed to cure—can become much worse. Withdrawal causes additional problems: Irritability, increased nervousness and depression can result.''

The use of diazepam also can have another effect, one that worries Dr. Young. She is concerned about how it may affect a new-born infant. When the drug is given to a woman in labor, it quickly crosses the placental barrier via the umbilical cord. But because an infant's kidneys and liver are not completely developed at birth, the drug may not clear out of the baby's body for days. Dr. Young cites studies finding that babies born of mothers who took diazepam during labor showed a lack of responsiveness for up to several weeks. "We're not sure yet whether this is anything but a short-term effect, but it needs to be looked into," she says.

A new antianxiety medication on the market only a few months—buspirone—avoids many of the side effects of the benzodiazepines, according to John Feighner, M.D., associate clinical professor of psychiatry at the University of California Medical School in San Diego, who has tested the drug for seven years in his research institute. "Buspirone is a totally new type of compound that alleviates anxiety but is nonsedating," he says. He emphasizes, however, that it is most effective for long-term rather than occasional anxiety. "What is exciting," Dr. Feighner adds, "is that here is a drug that will not interfere with daily living. It is not addictive, produces no withdrawal symptoms, shows no complications with alcohol use and does not impair motor coordination or mental functioning." He does warn of possible side effects including restlessness and dizziness, but these reactions have occurred in less than ten percent of his patients.

HOW TO PROTECT YOURSELF

Because there is no government policy stipulating that drugs must be tested for their effect on mood, the mind and behavior, it is the consumer who must protect herself, advises Dr. Young. "Mental side effects are often so transitory or their origin so difficult to pinpoint that regulation against the chemical compounds in some drugs is slow in coming or is nonexistent. The Food and Drug Administration (FDA), the Federal Government agency that approves the sale of drugs, is likely to take action only if someone has a dramatic reaction or dies after having taken a recommended dosage," she says.

The FDA's stance concerning PPA is a case in point. In 1972 the agency began investigating PPA along with all other OTC drugs; in 1979 an advisory panel concluded that PPA was an effective dietary aid. Since then, scores of researchers as well as the American Medical Association and the influential *Medical Letter*—an authoritative and well-respected newsletter that keeps doctors abreast of the latest developments in drugs—have criticized it, but without effect in the marketplace. "Consumers assume that because a drug's sold over the counter, it must be safe," says Dr. Young. "But this is just not true." Though the FDA is continuing to investigate claims against PPA, it has made no move to restrict its sale.

What, then, can you do to avoid unnecessary psychological side effects from your medications? "While no magic potions exist, there are a large number of therapeutic alternatives to turn to if the adverse effects of one medication are too severe," says William Barr, Pharm.D., Ph.D., chairman of the department of pharmacy at the Virginia Commonwealth University in Richmond. "Given professional advice, most people can generally find something suitable for them." So be sure to report to your doctor any side effects you may be experiencing from a drug—whether it's a prescription or OTC remedy. Ask him if there's another suitable medication you might take instead. More advice from pharmacology experts:
• **Read package labels.** Package labels and inserts include warnings of any known possible adverse reactions that can occur with use.
• **Never exceed the recommended dosages.** Information about how much medication you should take can be found on the package labels of OTC drugs; if you're taking a prescription drug, make sure you understand your doctor's directions on the correct dose.
• **Question your doctor and pharmacist.** Survey after survey has shown that doctors write prescriptions far more freely than they offer information about what a drug may do besides bring relief. If you have any doubts as to whether a medication is appropriate for you, ask. Your pharmacist, as well as your doctor, is qualified to answer questions.
• **Consider switching pharmacists if you're not getting the information you need.** "Pharmacists are trained professionals," says Dr. Barr. "If yours won't take the time to answer questions about a medication, you should find a new one."

Being a well-informed consumer is probably the best defense against the potential side effects of any drug. Used carefully and sensibly, over-the-counter and prescription drugs can help us feel better—rather than worse.

Health

Foods & Drugs That Don't Mix

BY MARK FUERST

The possible side effects of most drugs are well known. What you may not know is that what you eat while on medication can cause even more problems.

Ordinary foods such as cheeses, oranges and cereals mixed with some medications can lead to nausea, headaches, even heart attacks, and may stop the medication from working. The wrong combinations can create new health problems too. Even vitamin supplements pose health risks.

In some cases, it's wise to eat certain foods in moderation or at least two hours after taking medications. But other foods must be avoided altogether. Ask your doctor or pharmacist what's right for your circumstances.

Other ways to protect yourself:
- **Read the package inserts** that come with nonprescription drugs and the labels on prescription medications.
- **Tell your doctor of any unusual symptoms** when you eat particular foods while on medication.
- **Eat a nutritionally balanced diet** from a wide variety of foods.

The elderly, those with chronic diseases and pregnant women are the most susceptible to side effects, but everyone on medication should be aware of the potential dangers.

Acne medicine Isotretinoin (Accutane)	**Vitamin A**	Can increase chance of side effects.
Antibiotics Tetracycline	**Calcium-rich foods:** Dairy products, soybeans, canned fish, green leafy vegetables, calcium pills and antacid tablets.	Reduce effectiveness.
	Zinc, iron and magnesium supplements	Prevent absorption.
	Vitamin A supplements	May induce severe headaches.
Anticoagulants Warfarin (Coumadin)	**Foods with Vitamin K:** Green, leafy vegetables, beef liver, dairy products	Counteract the drug.
	Vitamin A	High doses may slow effectiveness.
	Vitamin C	High doses can increase risk of bleeding.
Anticonvulsants Phenytoin (Dilantin)	**Folacin**	High doses can increase risk of seizures.
	Calcium-rich foods: See antibiotics	Prevent absorption.
Antidepressants MAO inhibitors	**Tyramine-rich foods:** Wine (Chianti), beer, aged cheeses, smoked or pickled fish, beef or chicken liver, dried sausages, Fava beans	Produce severe headaches, nosebleeds, high blood pressure and possibly strokes or heart attacks.
	Tryptophan supplements	Can cause hyperexcitability, headaches and hallucinations.
Lithium	**Salty foods:** Potato chips, salted nuts, seafood	Large amounts may reduce drug response.
Antihypertensives Various drugs	**Natural licorice***	Elevates blood pressure.
Asthma drugs Theophylline	**Charcoal-broiled foods**	Speed drug through the body, reducing effectiveness.
	Caffeine: Coffee, tea, cola drinks, chocolate	May accelerate side effects of nervousness and insomnia.
Potassium-sparing diuretics Various drugs	**Potassium-rich foods:** Beef, oranges, bananas, dates, avocados, lima beans, flounder, halibut, potatoes, salt substitutes, potassium supplements	Can lead to muscle weakness and abnormal heart rhythms. (Some diuretics are potassium-wasting and should be taken *with* potassium-rich foods.)
	Natural licorice*	See antihypertensives.
Heart drugs Digitalis	**Bran fiber**	Reduces drug absorption.
Levodopa (L-Dopa)	**Protein-rich foods:** See asthma drugs, plus amino acid supplements (tryptophan, tyrosine, phenylalanine)	Inhibit the body's response to the drug.
	Vitamin B$_6$-rich foods: Avocado, bacon, beans, beef liver, tuna, peas, pork, vitamin B$_6$ supplements	Reverse drug activity.

*Most licorice in the United States is artificial and harmless. Imported licorice from Europe is often natural.

From *Woman's Day,* September 22, 1992, p. 48. © 1992 by Mark Fuerst. Reprinted by permission of Mark Fuerst, a freelance health writer in New York.

R̟ to OTC

Who Pays and Who Profits When Prescription Drugs Go Over the Counter

Larry Katzenstein

Larry Katzenstein is a Senior Editor of AMERICAN HEALTH

You may well have contributed to some of the biggest drug success stories of the past few years: You have if you've taken Advil, introduced in 1984 and now, with annual sales of $275 million, second only to Extra-Strength Tylenol as America's best-selling pain-killer. Or Benadryl, the leading nonprescription anti-histamine. Or Tinactin, the leading athlete's foot remedy.

They all owe their existence to Food and Drug Administration (FDA) decisions allowing the active ingredients they contain—previously available only by prescription—to be sold over the counter (OTC). And more such switches can be expected.

Marketers of some of the best-selling prescription drugs, such as Tagamet, Zantac, Seldane and Naprosyn, are now working to get FDA approval for nonprescription versions. Over the next five years, drug companies reportedly plan to submit more than 50 prescription ingredients to the FDA for switch approval.

Drug companies still make their reputations on breakthrough drugs for serious and sometimes life-threatening conditions. But increasingly, they're making their *profits* in the nonprescription market. One pharmaceutical analyst predicts that the early to mid 1990s will see "the biggest wave ever of drug switches from Rx to OTC."

Though the wave has yet even to appear on the horizon, the prospect of it is already churning up controversy. Some switch candidates are quite potent and potentially hazardous if misused. Will their unsupervised use jeopardize public safety? Is the FDA too eager to approve switches—or too cautious? And just who really benefits from these switches—drug companies or consumers?

O VER THE LAST 15 years the FDA has allowed about 45 prescription ingredients to be marketed over the counter. The most successful of all switches occurred in 1960, when a pain reliever available only in liquid form for children gained approval for nonprescription sale in adult strength. The product that resulted, Tylenol tablets and capsules, became the most successful over-the-counter drug of all time.

For the drug industry, most switches have proved to be low-cost, high-profit investments. By the time FDA approval is granted, much of a company's expense to establish safety and effectiveness has been amortized. And once the switch is made, savvy marketing can almost ensure profitability.

You've been hearing the televised slogans for years: *The same medicine in the prescription brand Motrin . . . You don't need a prescription, just a cold . . . Doctors have prescribed it for children more than any allergy medication ever.* A brand's prescription heritage suggests strong medicine—more effective than any of the other pain relievers, antihistamines or cough/cold remedies it will compete against.

A second reason for the marketers' desire to switch is the fact that patents on many best-selling prescription drugs—Tagamet, Seldane and Naprosyn, to name a few—will expire in the next few years. Prescription drugs reap most of their profits during the 10 or more years their patents protect them from imitators; but earnings erode as soon as lower-priced generics—drugs with the same active ingredient—appear. Switches to over-the-counter versions before patents expire are one way to head off the competition from generics.

The patent on the anti-ulcer prescription drug Tagamet, the world's third largest-selling drug, will expire in 1994. For the past several years SmithKline, the maker of Tagamet, has been carrying out clinical studies needed to win FDA approval for a lower-dose version that would be marketed OTC as an indigestion aid rather than an ulcer cure.

If the new version is approved, a 1984 law will compensate SmithKline for its efforts to bring it OTC by protecting the product for up to three years from nonprescription competitors. During that time, OTC Tagamet would surely capitalize on its prescription heritage to carve out a share of the antacid market. And when generic competitors do appear, they'll have quite a lot of catching up to do in the public consciousness.

"Generics have a major impact on prescription sales, but a minimal effect on OTC drugs," says pharmaceutical

From *American Health*, April 1991, pp. 49-53.

analyst Hemant Shah of HKS & Co. in Warren, N.J. "Most consumers don't know there are inexpensive, generic versions of Tylenol, or even that Bayer is aspirin that can be bought generically for a tenth of the price."

Tagamet's patent expiration will allow other popular OTC drugs to be formulated so that they contain the drug's active ingredient—but they'll have trouble overcoming its head start. And since trademarks don't have expiration dates, a skillfully marketed switched brand that builds strong name recognition can look forward to virtually limitless success.

The trend toward drug switching can benefit consumers, too. "It's really symbiotic, because everyone makes out well," says Kenneth Palmer, manager of international regulatory affairs at Schering-Plough, an industry leader in drug switching. "The companies make more money and consumers save more money."

Consumers do save—but not necessarily because the switched product costs less than its prescription version. Contrary to what many people think, the new nonprescription drug may cost more. At least it did in a limited price survey conducted by AMERICAN HEALTH in February.

We compared prescription and nonprescription prices for Gyne-Lotrimin, a cream for treating vaginal yeast infections. It received switch approval last December, but some outlets still sell the prescription version. In our survey of 10 New York City pharmacies, the average prescription price was $18.63, while the same-size, same-strength OTC version averaged $20.21.

Surveys involving other drugs might well find a price edge for the OTC drug. But whatever the differences, the biggest cost savings from switches come not from effects on drug price but through a less direct route.

Because drug switches account for most of the new products that can be sold without a prescription, they offer consumers more options for self-medication—and fewer trips to the doctor's office. Rather than spend time and money ($38 on average) for a visit to the doctor to get a prescription, consumers can simply buy the drug at a pharmacy or supermarket. In this era of increasing self-care, those savings can be considerable.

One recent study looked at nationwide savings stemming from a single switch: $1/2$% hydrocortisone, a topical anti-itch product most commonly sold under the name Cortaid. In the three years after hydrocortisone became available in 1979, the study found that consumers saved more than $1 billion on doctor visits.

Not surprisingly, doctors don't always look kindly on drug switches. Recent surveys found that only 57% of doctors favored switches, compared with 73% of the general adult population. Loss of business isn't the only reason. A drug switch means that doctors lose control over a weapon in their medical arsenal. It's a loss some apparently resent. Others doubt that the public has the requisite knowledge to self-medicate. Still others fear patients will feel cheated if they leave a physician's office with a recommendation for an OTC drug rather than a prescription.

Surveys find that medical resistance to drug switches

Recent switches...and some in the pipeline

Recent Switches

▶BENADRYL brand of diphenhydramine hydrochloride, an antihistamine tablet or capsule, approved in January of 1985.

▶IMODIUM-AD brand of loperamide hydrochloride, an antidiarrheal caplet or liquid, approved in May of 1988. It reportedly rivals the prescription antidiarrheal Lomotil in effectiveness.

▶LOTRIMIN AF brand of clotrimazole, an antifungal cream for athlete's foot, jock itch and ringworm, approved in October of 1989.

▶NIX brand of permethrin, a cream rinse for treating head lice, approved in May of 1990.

▶GYNE-LOTRIMIN brand of clotrimazole, the first nonprescription treatment for vaginal yeast infections,

approved in December of 1990. To make sure they're treating the right condition, women should use the drug only if they've had a previous yeast infection that has been diagnosed by a physician.

Down the Line

▶MONISTAT, a topical yeast infection treatment similar to Gyne-Lotrimin. FDA approval is expected within a few months.

▶1% TOPICAL HYDROCORTISONE for rashes, insect bites and other skin inflammation problems. The ½% hydrocortisone products, available since 1979, reportedly don't work well for some users, for whom the 1% strength would be more effective.

▶TOPICAL ERYTHROMYCIN antibiotic for acne.

▶SELDANE nonsedating antihistamine. This popular prescription drug has been available OTC in Canada and Great Britain for several years. FDA approval has been delayed because of reports that Seldane can interact with the antiyeast drug ketoconazole to cause an abnormal heart rate. Approval is not expected until 1993.

▶NICORETTE, the nicotine chewing gum that helps smokers quit.

▶NAPROSYN, a nonsteroidal anti-inflammatory drug that is similar to ibuprofen.

▶The manufacturers of four of the six prescription ulcer drugs are working to convert their brands to over-the-counter status, probably for use as indigestion aids. The four are PEPCID, ZANTAC (the world's best-selling drug), TAGAMET and CARAFATE.

comes mainly from primary-care physicians. Specialists tend to take a more favorable view, since OTC drugs can satisfy patients who might otherwise take up their time with minor complaints.

Among the clearest beneficiaries of switches are insurance companies, which generally don't reimburse patients for nonprescription drugs. But for some people enrolled in such plans, switches can be downright detrimental.

Consider a woman who, under her company's health plan, pays only $1 per prescription for Gyne-Lotrimin cream, which was approved for OTC sale last December. Her insurer—and most others, including Medicaid—won't pay for nonprescription drugs. Unless her doctor is willing to prescribe a different antiyeast drug—Mycostatin, for example,—the woman now must pay about $20 for a tube of OTC Gyne-Lotrimin. (She'll still be covered, however, if she takes Motrin, the prescription brand of ibuprofen, in 300 mg, 400 mg, 600 mg or 800 mg tablets for, say, severe menstrual cramps. Ibuprofen has been switched—but only in the 200-mg dosage form used in Advil, Nuprin, Motrin IB and other brands.)

For people on Medicaid, or those who need expensive prescription drugs for chronic illnesses, loss of reimbursement through a drug switch can be particularly distressing. For just this reason the National Cystic Fibrosis Foundation recently urged the FDA not to switch pancreatin, a digestive aid widely prescribed for people with the disease.

Prescription drugs treat serious health problems such as infections, epilepsy and heart disease. They offer major therapeutic benefits, so some severe side effects are allowable. But OTC drugs usually have the more modest aim of relieving symptoms: the aches, pains, coughs, stomach upsets and fevers that regularly afflict us. For that reason, only minor adverse effects are tolerated. That's also true for switched drugs, whose recommended doses are usually smaller than their prescription-only predecessors.

Take Advil, for example, whose 200-mg capsules of ibuprofen are intended for treating symptoms such as headache, muscle pain and fever. By contrast, Motrin and other prescription ibuprofen brands provide at least 300 mg of ibuprofen and are typically prescribed for treating arthritis or severe pain.

A savvy consumer can convert Advil to prescription strength by exceeding the recommended dose—as the FDA is perfectly aware. Before approving Advil or any other switch, the FDA must be convinced that the benefits of making it available to the public without a prescription far outweigh the risks.

As long as a drug is prescription-only, doctors and pharmacists help ensure that it's used safely by the people who need it. But these safeguards vanish when a drug goes over the counter. There's no doctor to prescribe it, no pharmacist to dispense it, and the drug becomes available at thousands of outlets, from supermarkets to gas stations. "You're allowing a drug to be used without any supervision," says drug analyst Shah. "If something should go wrong, it could affect millions of people."

No wonder the FDA often deliberates years before approving a switch, which must meet a number of conditions, including the following:

► The prescription drug must have a history (three years at a minimum) of heavy-yet-safe use. Once the drug goes

OTC, the agency says, adverse reactions are rarely detected and hardly ever reported.

► Misuse or abuse of the switched drug should not cause serious side effects.

► The consumer must be able to self-diagnose the health problem that the drug claims to treat. (A cough/cold remedy stands a much better chance of switch approval than a drug for treating hypertension.)

► The health problem being treated should readily respond to self-care.

Such caution reflects the agency's mandate to protect public health as well as its desire to avoid embarrassment. "No one at the FDA gets awards for approving something," says Arthur Kibbe, scientific director at the American Pharmaceutical Association (APhA). "The last person at the FDA to win an award was Frances Kelsey, in 1962—and that was for *not* approving thalidomide. The attitude at the agency is, 'If we're wrong, we get in a lot of trouble. But if we don't let something on the market, we avoid trouble because no one will know.' "

THE ONCE-ANTICIPATED WAVE of drug switches probably won't crest any time soon. If recent history is a guide, a steady trickle seems more likely. Switch approvals have fallen from nearly four per year from 1985 through 1987 to an average of just over one per year from 1988 through 1990. William Gilbertson, head of the FDA's over-the-counter drug division, describes the agency's current attitude toward switches as "very conservative."

That caution has created what the Nonprescription Drug Manufacturers Association (NDMA) calls a "nonprescription drug lag." The NDMA contends that at least 34 drug ingredients—available only by prescription in the U.S., if available at all—can be bought without a prescription in other countries.

While the industry clamors for more approvals, the FDA must also contend with critics such as Representative Ted Weiss (D.-N.Y.) and Dr. Sidney Wolfe, head and co-founder with Ralph Nader of the Health Research Group. In 1989, Wolfe and Weiss pressured the FDA to reverse its decision on Phenergan, a leading prescription cough/cold remedy for children that the FDA had tentatively approved for switching. They claimed the misuse of Phenergan to treat infants could result in Sudden Infant Death Syndrome—a charge that Wyeth-Ayerst, the drug's manufacturer, strenuously denies.

Such opposition to switches may well intensify. Many of today's switch candidates are more potent than their predecessors—and more likely to pose hazards if misused. Opposition to the four ulcer drugs that are now in the switch pipeline—Tagamet, Zantac, Carafate and Pepcid—is already building.

"I'm totally opposed to making Tagamet or the other ulcer drugs over the counter," says Dr. Gary Holt, an assistant professor of pharmacy at the university of Wyoming. A specialist in self-medication, Holt says the drugs would be approved only for symptomatic relief—of acid indigestion, for example—and not for treating stomach ulcers. But he's skeptical that they'd be used accordingly.

"People know these drugs have historically been used to

treat ulcers," says Holt. Making the drugs available without a prescription, he explains, would invite consumers to treat the more serious problem. "There are certain conditions that should never be treated without at least some professional supervision, and a gastric ulcer is one of them." In addition, says Holt, unsupervised use of potent ulcer drugs could mask symptoms of stomach cancer.

To minimize such risks, the American Pharmaceutical Association favors the creation of a new drug category for recently switched drugs. Available without a prescription, they would be dispensed only by licensed pharmacists, who would ensure that consumers use them for the right reasons and who would discuss possible side effects. Switches that prove safe could eventually become available without restriction; those found to cause adverse reactions could return to prescription status. According to an APhA official, legislation calling for a transitional drug class will probably be introduced during this session of Congress.

The U.S. system of only two drug classes is unique; many other countries have multiclass systems. But the FDA shows no interest in changing the status quo. And the nonprescription drug industry actively opposes the idea—for economic reasons. Drugs in a third category could be sold only in the nation's 50,000 pharmacies, not in the 700,000 outlets where such drugs are now sold.

Drug switches will continue to affect the drug market—and the millions of consumers who take advantage of them for self-care. The FDA's track record in approving them is sound: More effective medicines are available for consumers, and so far there have been no disasters. But keep in mind that any drug—whether newly switched or an old standby such as aspirin—can cause side effects ranging from mild to fatal. The best way to make it work for you is to take it with a healthy dose of common sense.

Placebo Effect Is Shown to Be Twice as Powerful as Expected

Daniel Goleman

"Hurry, Hurry—use the new drugs while they still work!" a 19th-century French physician urged his colleagues. He may not have known why faddish drugs work on credulous patients, but the fact that they do has been borne out by scientists studying the power of the placebo to cure.

New findings show that the placebo effect—in which patients given an inactive treatment believe it can cure them—is most powerful when a trusted physician enthusiastically offers a patient a new therapy. In a study of more than 6,000 patients being given experimental treatments for asthma, duodenal ulcer and herpes, two-thirds improved, at least temporarily, even though rigorous tests later found the treatments medically useless. They were then abandoned.

Some argue that the placebo effect should be exploited to help the patient.

The old rule of thumb among medical researchers was that only about one-third of patients will show some improvement when given a placebo. The results of the new studies reveal the effect to be twice as powerful as was thought.

These and other findings that the placebo effect can be far stronger than had been widely assumed are leading some researchers to call for stricter standards for testing new medications. Others are proposing that physicians try to capitalize on the placebo effect in treating their patients in order to marshall the body's own healing powers.

"I argue that instead of just trying to control for placebo, we should try to maximize it," said Dr. Frederick Evans, a psychologist at the Robert Wood Johnson School of Medicine in New Brunswick, N.J. "If a doctor believes in what he's doing and lets the patient know that, that's good medicine."

While many people think a "placebo" is simply a sugar pill or other medicine with no active ingredients, the term has a broader meaning. The "placebo effect" includes any improvements in a patient not specifically due to a particular ingredient in a treatment, like a drug or surgical procedure. These "nonspecific," or placebo, effects, may be due to causes ranging from a patient reporting relief from symptoms in an unconscious effort to please a well-liked physician, to actual biological improvement.

TESTING THE PLACEBO EFFECT

To assess the potency of the placebo effect during the burst of enthusiasm for a new medical treatment, researchers reexamined data from initial clinical trials of five procedures which had at first seemed highly promising, and then later were shown to be useless. The procedures included surgical removal of the glomus, a structure near the carotid arteries in the neck, to treat asthma; and gastric freezing for duodenal ulcers. They also included three treatments for herpes simplex virus—the drug levamisole, organic solvents like ether and exposure of dyed herpes lesions to fluorescent light.

"In these studies, the doctors treating were also those evaluating the symptoms, which is what happens in a typical physician's office," said Dr. Alan H. Roberts, a psychologist at the Scripps Clinic and Research Foundation in La Jolla, Calif., who led the research. The results were published in the current issue of Clinical Psychology Review.

The physicians, who offered the treatments as part of an early clinical trial and believed in their efficacy, told their patients the various approaches were new and promising. With both physicians and patients having high hopes for a cure, the resulting placebo effect was potent. Because these were very early trials of new drugs, no control groups were used.

Of a total of 6,931 patients receiving one or another of the five treatments, 40 percent were reported to have excellent results, another 30 percent had good outcomes and only 30 percent were reported to have "poor" results, Dr. Roberts and his colleagues found.

Yet in later trials, when patients who received the treatments were methodically compared with control groups of patients who received placebos or nothing at all, "the effectiveness disappeared," said Dr. Roberts.

Dr. Roberts believes that for relatively mild medical problems, under the best conditions the placebo effect will produce positive results in roughly two-thirds of patients. The effects would not be nearly as strong for serious diseases such as AIDS or cancer, he said: "In the more severe disorders, the placebo effects would be mainly in terms of patient's subjective complaints, not their physical symptoms."

PSYCHOLOGICAL FACTORS

In Dr. Robert's view, the improvements associated with placebos are caused by factors like patients unconsciously exaggerating improvements of

From *New York Times*, August 17, 1993, p. C3. © 1993 by The New York Times Company. Reprinted by permission.

their symptoms in order to please their doctors, and doctors who hope for positive results skewing their evaluations of symptoms favorably.

The notion that the placebo effect is due to biological changes from patients' hopes being raised is met with skepticism by Dr. Roberts. But other researchers disagree.

"Could an enthusiastic physician and a believing patient create a clinical improvement in a patient?" said Dr. Ronald Glaser, a virologist at Ohio State University Medical School. "That question has haunted drug studies. But there may well be a psychological effect with a significant biological outcome, if you extrapolate from data showing that psychological factors like stress can affect viruses like herpes. It's definitely one possible explanation."

The herpes virus is one of Dr. Glaser's specialties; with his wife, Janice Kiecolt-Glaser, a psychologist, he has studied the effects of people's emotional swings on the replication of herpes virus.

"We've found herpes viruses are responsive to stress, improving or worsening depending on a patient's emotional state," said Dr. Kiecolt-Glaser. "Since herpes virus is quite responsive to psychological influences, the first wave of physicians' enthusiasm could well have a beneficial medical effect."

Dr. Roberts is not the first researcher to find that the placebo effect can account for improvements in more than one-third of patients, a ratio proposed in the 1950's by Dr. Henry Beecher, one of the first to do research on the placebo.

PATIENTS MOST LIKELY TO BENEFIT

"The range for placebo recovery I've seen varies from zero to 100 percent," said Dr. Arthur K. Shapiro, a psychiatrist at Mt. Sinai Medical Center in Manhattan. "Different factors combine to produce the magnitude of a placebo. For example, in my own research with 1,000 patients, those who like their physician most and who were most anxious showed the greatest improvement from placebo."

Such findings on the power of the placebo are bringing calls for revising the way in which new treatments are tested. In order to be sure the benefits attributed to experimental treatments are not simply due to placebo, tests of new medications now use a "double-blind" design, in which neither the physician nor the patient knows what medicine is being given, and some patients are given a nonactive treatment.

"There is a false sense of security about the scientific tests of drugs, particularly psychiatric drugs," said Dr. Roger Greenberg, a psychologist at the State University of New York Health Science Center at Syracuse.

One of the main problems with the standard double-blind test, said Dr. Greenberg, is that patients and physicians alike can very often tell who is getting the active medication and who is getting the placebo, because only the true medication has side effects. This can lead to placebo enhancement of the seeming effectiveness of the medication being tested.

"In instances when researchers have asked patients and physicians to guess whether they were using the active medication or the placebo, the results are sobering—in one such study, 78 percent of patients and 87 percent of their physicians could tell," said Dr. Greenberg. "That means the so-called 'double-blind' is not really blind."

For that reason, Dr. Greenberg proposes that in addition to the medication being tested and the usual inert placebo, tests of new drugs should include an "active" placebo which produces side effects but has no medical consequence. And, in the most rigorous test, a physician other than the one giving the medicines would make the evaluations of improvement.

In a meta-analysis of 22 studies of antidepressants, Dr. Greenberg and colleagues found that if, in addition to the new drug being tested, some patients were given an older antidepressant as a control, the new drug was only one-quarter to one-half as powerful as was reported in studies without the comparison drug, in which the new drug was pitted only against an inert placebo.

The research finding, published last year in the Journal of Consulting and Clinical Psychology by Dr. Greenberg and colleagues, concludes that current standard practices for drug testing often exaggerate the potency of new medicine.

"In general," said Dr. Greenberg, "the better a study is controlled, the blinder it becomes and the smaller the difference becomes between the real drug and the placebo."

SAYING GOODBYE TO AN OLD FLAME

How smokers quit—and how you can help.

Benedict Carey

Benedict Carey is a staff writer.

It's a Tuesday afternoon, and the 14 men and women in Gerry Reilly's quit-smoking class are shifting in their chairs, trying to sit through an educational video starring former United States Surgeon General C. Everett Koop. Severe and righteous, Koop is reciting a list of frightening statistics: "Smoking kills 300,000 Americans a year . . . Smokers are ten times more likely to develop lung cancer than nonsmokers; two times more likely to develop heart disease . . . Smoking a pack a day takes six years off a person's life . . . Seventy-five percent of unaided smokers who try to quit fail within the first three months, and . . ."

That does it. As the film winds down, the people in the small audience are starting to walk out, one at a time, probably for a smoke.

Nothing against the former Surgeon General, but these people *know* the bad news. In this class, a five-week program at San Francisco's Kaiser Permanente Hospital, one man, Duane, 50, has heart trouble. Mike, a smoker in his sixties, has

the beginnings of emphysema. And a number of the others are short of breath. This is why Reilly, herself a former smoker, doesn't dwell on the Koop video as more than a quick source of information in an otherwise upbeat, humorous series of classes. "We know scare tactics just don't work," says Reilly.

So why do smokers decide to quit?

A real-life example, say the sight of a friend dying of lung cancer, or a smoker's own brush with serious illness, can do it. More often, says Rhode Island psychologist James Prochaska, people one day simply get so disappointed and angry with themselves for smoking that they decide to do something about it. "They say 'I'm fed up with this. I'm sick of being controlled by it. I want out,' " he says.

Here's how a few members of Reilly's class put it:

"I'm just bored with it anymore," says Mike, a smoker since he was 15. 'It's mostly habit. I don't even enjoy it very much."

"I can't stand the control it has on me," says Don, a four-pack-a-day smoker who lives by himself. "I always smoke in the kitchen, with the fan on, drinking coffee. I spend most of my life in there."

"I'm sick and tired of it," says Kay, who's smoked 48 of her 69 years. "I'm tired of being a slave."

How can I get someone to stop smoking?

"GET OFF THEIR BACKS," says Susan Curry, an investigator at Seattle's Center for Health Studies. "I don't think nagging does any good at all. Instead," she says, "try telling someone, 'I care about you, I enjoy spending time with you, and I'd like to do that without smoking getting in the way.' " If this sort of talk doesn't work, try telling the person you're simply worried— about her persistent cough, or his frequent colds, her trouble breathing on hikes, or his difficulty keeping up on the basketball court.

In the end, says Curry, smokers will quit only when *they* decide they're ready,

Nicotine is one of the most addictive drugs there is.

and are convinced it's something they need to do for themselves. But it doesn't hurt to remind somebody that quitting is possible, no matter how bad the habit.

Why is quitting so hard?

BECAUSE NICOTINE is one of the most addictive drugs there is. It mimics a body chemical called acetylcholine, which stimulates the nervous system, forming a physical addiction. But in larger doses nicotine *numbs* the nervous system, producing a feeling of calm.

"It has this remarkable ability to both relax people when they're anxious and jack them up when they're tired," says Reilly. This is why people light up when they're stressed or satisfied, angry or bored. It's why cigarettes go so well with food, coffee, reading, driving, working, just hanging around—anything.

Smoking becomes not just a diversion, but a way of interacting with the world, a psychological addiction as well as a physical one. "Take away tobacco," Reilly says, "and smokers have to learn to do everything all over again—how to drive to work, how to talk on the phone, how to read the paper, without the aid of a cigarette." That's one reason why the discomfort of early withdrawal seems to fill every waking moment.

How do people quit?

NINE IN TEN former smokers say they quit without professional help, and some of them simply dropped the habit and never looked back. But most succeed, says Prochaska, only after trying again and again, slipping in and out of smoking for seven to ten years before finally making a clean break.

"If it didn't work the first time, or the

second time or third," says Clifford Carr, a smoking cessation researcher at the University of California at Los Angeles, "it does work on the fourth or fifth try. They get better at it."

Do group quit-smoking programs help?

THEY CAN, YES. These courses range from weekly group sessions conducted by nonprofit organizations such as the American Lung Association and the American Cancer Society, to moderately priced commercial programs such as SmokEnders and Smokeless, to pricey, fancy live-in clinics complete with doctors, hot tubs, and special menus.

Harry Lando, a University of Minnesota psychologist who's studied group programs, says most unhook between 20 and 30 percent of their clients, with some of the more expensive programs tending to have slightly higher rates—possibly because paying more creates a greater investment in quitting.

Most formal programs, like Reilly's at Kaiser Permanente, draw from the same catalogue of quitting strategies, all of which can be useful for people trying to go it alone. For example:

Set a quit date: In most groups people quit together, usually a week or two from the first session. Committing to a date allows them to give proper warning at work and at home about their decision, and to solicit some help.

"Quitting is not something you want to do when you're under stress," says Linda Ebright, who gives quit-smoking classes at Northwestern University in Chicago. "If you're going through a divorce, forget it. It's too much to handle."

Get to know the habit: It's very common for smokers in formal programs to keep a diary for several days, recording every cigarette they light, the time of day, how they feel, and what they expect to get from each smoke.

Mike, the smoker in Reilly's class who decided to quit because he was bored with his 40-year-old habit, boldly listed one 10:15 P.M. cigarette as "the last one of the day." The one he smoked 15 minutes later was identified as "a treat," followed 20 minutes later by "another treat." Others in the class had similarly weak reasons for lighting up: "habit," "for something to do," "pissed at a bad driver," "bored."

"The first thing people see when they keep a diary," says Michael Eriksen, a

former smoker who runs stop-smoking classes at the M.D. Anderson Cancer Center in Houston, "is exactly where smoking fits into their lives."

Tinker with routine: The next step, often, is to change the usual smoking pattern a little—exchanging regulars for menthols, say, or vice versa. Then, smokers may move to brands lower and lower in tar and nicotine and, finally, cut down on the number of cigarettes they smoke a day. According to the American Cancer Society, most smokers really crave only five or six of the daily cigarettes they light up. "If they can get down to around ten a day or less," says Eriksen, "they're ready."

Quit: In many programs, the approach of the quit date is a little like a religious holiday. The day before everyone does a sort of ritual cleaning: of house, car, office, teeth—anywhere that the smoking habit has left its mark.

Nicotine withdrawal can set in within 25 minutes of the last cigarette. The symptoms range from mild headaches and sleeplessness to migraines, confusion, and what Lisa, in Reilly's class, refers to as an "everyone's-stupid, life's-boring" attitude—extreme irritability and impatience.

But a few report that they find the experience bizarrely blissful. "I felt giddy for a week," says a woman named Carol in Reilly's class, "like I was high on air. I was kind of disappointed that it ended."

Don, the four-pack-a-day smoker, was weak, almost anemic, and unable to concentrate at work for at least a month after his last smoke. "For a while I thought it was permanent brain damage from all those years of smoking," he says.

Withdrawal can linger from three days to three weeks or longer. No single technique or gimmick will relieve the sharp cravings in the beginning, but every quit-smoking program offers people a whole bag of tricks that can help: Stay away from friends who smoke, and avoid parties and bars. Drink lots of water. Take a shower. Run, walk, play tennis—get any kind of exercise. Suck on a cinnamon stick, or grab a yo-yo—anything to keep hands and mouth busy. Review your reasons for quitting. Say a prayer, call a friend. "Take deep breaths," says Herb, one of the people in Reilly's class. "It sounds hokey, but it works."

Because smokers often reach for a cigarette rather than handling a difficult emotion or situation, some programs offer exercises to help people learn constructive ways to express anger, for instance, or to assert themselves.

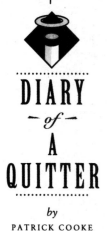

DIARY
—of—
A
QUITTER

by
PATRICK COOKE

WEDNESDAY, AUGUST 21:
Tomorrow I will do something I haven't done for nearly two decades—try to live 24 hours without a cigarette. I am terrified that the morning's hypnosis session won't work. I am also terrified that it will. Either way I'm a wreck, so tonight I'm chain-smoking.

It's been almost 20 years to the day since I lit up for the first time. Ever since, I've been merrily justifying the habit away, by the carton, by the year.

For instance, I remember standing on a broad beach in Northern California not too long ago, smoking and watching a flock of hang gliders float down out of the nearby mountains. What is the difference, I thought, between dying on one of those contraptions and dying smoking cigarettes? Bungee jumping, skydiving, deep-sea diving, mountain climbing. People die all the time doing these heroic things; they are deaths as clearly preventable as deaths from smoking.

Eventually, though, the logic didn't ring true any more. Sure, the climber's rope frays, the diver's tank punctures, the parachutist fails to notice the tatter. But those horrible images weren't as real as this one: I am sitting on a doctor's examination table, ridiculous in that silly gown, listening to the verdict vibrate in the little room.

Lung cancer. It's doubtful that comparing smoking with hot air ballooning is going to be much comfort then. All that would matter is how foolish I'd feel for having reduced this perfectly good body to a blackened husk.

THURSDAY, AUGUST 22: I am nearing the on-ramp to the Golden Gate Bridge. When I reach the middle of the bridge I light a cigarette. It may, or may not, be the last one I ever smoke. I want to go home and forget this hypnosis mumbo jumbo.

The cigarette, a nasty menthol number, rock-bottom in both tar and nicotine, is hard to enjoy. I have been smoking these for more than a week, following the telephone advice of my hypnotist, D.H.

This past week I also designated the bathroom as the only room in which I could smoke, and I cut down from nearly three packs of cigarettes a day to about a pack (isn't that progress enough?!).

By the time I reach the hypnotist's office my last cigarette has been snuffed. When D.H. meets me at the door, I hand her the remainder of the pack.

For the next hour we chat about my smoking habits: the cigarettes I most enjoy (only three or four a day, as it turns out), when I find myself smoking the most (when don't I?), what I really want (a magic pill).

Suddenly it's Showtime. I lie down on a white sofa in a darkened room. Eyes closed. D.H. talks me through several minutes of muscle-relaxing exercises.

What gradually begins to occur can best be described as a kind of descent: As she counts backwards from 100, I become more and more relaxed, breathing deeply. "Picture yourself in a tranquil place," says D.H. I light on a long-ago memory, a snowy New Hampshire woods in moonlight.

D.H. is recording her voice during the session; I will take the tape with me when I go in order to rehypnotize myself as needed over the coming weeks.

Once I have arrived in a presumably suggestible state, D.H. walks me through a typical day in my future. No cigarettes with coffee, no cigarettes after lunch or dinner, no cigarettes while working. She makes the future actually sound inviting. "You no longer need them," she keeps saying. "You no longer need them." The message is surprisingly simple.

"Ninety-one, ninety-two . . . " The long ascent back up.

Then it was over. The session had taken about two and a half hours. There were no swinging watches, no twirling eyeballs; being hypno-tized was a little like a dream. I was never so far gone that I clucked like a chicken—at least I don't think I did. Even in the deepest moments, in fact, my skepticism never entirely vanished.

Afterward I felt slightly drugged and a little dislocated, as though the world were moving faster than I was. As I left the office, the sun broke through the clouds.

There was a strange emptiness in the house when I arrived home, as if someone I had lived with for a long time had gone away without leaving an explanation or any way to get in touch. There was a quiet and a kind of sadness.

FRIDAY, AUGUST 23: Hell day. Listened to the tape at least four times. There is no doubt that it helps, but the tape alone is not enough to offset the terrible craving for a smoke. I now realize that withdrawal is a full-time job.

Finally went jogging and was astonished at how much it helped. Maybe it reinforces the trancelike state, and the resolve to stick with it. Thank God it kills time.

SATURDAY, AUGUST 24: Friends have been kindly calling to ask how I feel. *How do I feel?! I'll tell you how I feel . . .* They mean well, but jeez, this hurts like hell. I now live for marking off the days on the calendar, but time is only crawling along.

Listened to the hypnosis tape for what seemed like the entire day. It helped. Also stretched out for a while in the local park—it's impossible to work—and found myself doubting the whole process. Do hypnotists and other stop-smoking practitioners take money knowing that the only "service" they actually provide is watching you accomplish something you desperately wanted to do anyway?

Attended a dinner party. Big challenge. First social setting without cigarettes. Easier than I thought it would be.

SUNDAY, AUGUST 25:
Unexpected side effect of quitting

is vivid dreaming. However, almost everyone in my dreams is smoking. Last night's cast included General H. Norman Schwartzkopf, my nephew Davin, a rattletrap Volkswagen bug I owned in college, and my mother. It was horrible.

Surprisingly, I'm feeling better today. For the first time since Thursday I'm not barking at the wallpaper. It's a little as if a fever has broken. I go jogging in the morning with nice results. Check off another day.

D.H. called to see how I was getting on. Feeling a little bad now about doubting her. She says it's still going to be hard for a few days. I thank her from the bottom of my heart for this information.

D.H. recommends ordinary gum as a cigarette substitute. Others use Lifesavers or toothpicks. I am supplanting my urges by chewing on swizzle sticks. They're cheap, plentiful, and risk-free—at least until the Surgeon General issues the Swizzle Stick Report.

POSTSCRIPT, FEBRUARY 22: This past New Year's Eve I fired up a fat cigar. It was the first tobacco I'd lit in nearly six months and it tasted pretty good. But after a few moments I began to feel warmly mesmerized by the old sight of smoke. I panicked and chucked the thing out.

That uneasy peace with smoking is the way I suspect things will be for the rest of my life. I can't promise that I won't relapse, but then again, I don't know that I will.

All I know is that if you had told me six months ago that I could survive a single day without a cigarette, I'd have laughed my head off. Now, with the help of the people who care what happens to me, I'm stringing the days together into weeks and months, maybe years.

Who knows, in time I may feel free to nag other people about their smoking. That's when I'll know the cure has taken.

Patrick Cooke is a contributing editor.

Is there a drug that relieves cravings?

FOR THE TIME BEING, only one—nicotine. Taken in non-cigarette form nicotine not only cools the lust for a smoke, it also softens withdrawal symptoms, which is enough to get many smokers over the hump. At the outset, quitters need a continuous flow of the drug in their systems, at a level low enough so that they can go off nicotine altogether after the withdrawal has passed.

Some programs recommend that people ask their doctors about a prescription for either nicotine chewing gum or the newer nicotine patch, which releases the substance through the skin. Neither of these products works unless used exactly as prescribed, and neither should be relied on for more than three months.

Can hypnotism or acupuncture help?

HYPNOTISTS USE all sorts of techniques, but their aim is almost always the same: To plant suggestions that make smokers repulsed by the habit and increasingly confident they can do without cigarettes (see "Diary of a Quitter").

Acupuncturists operate on the principle that placing needles at certain points on the ear helps soothe cravings for some drugs, including heroin, cocaine, and nicotine. Although there's no complete Western explanation for exactly how this works, studies have shown that acupuncture stimulates the release of endorphins, brain chemicals that block the perception of pain, and may therefore ease withdrawal.

Some hypnotists and acupuncturists claim astronomical success rates—70 percent, 80 percent, and higher—but if these rates were accurate, smokers would be on the Sierra Club's list of endangered species. Both treatments work best when combined with the sort of strategies and ongoing support offered in most quit-smoking programs. "Smoking is a way of life," says UCLA's Clifford Carr. People who've given up cigarettes have to learn new ways of coping with the world.

What about weight gain?

SINCE SMOKING speeds up metabolism, smokers do burn off an extra 100 to 200 calories a day, and those who quit often develop a sweet tooth. But according to the American Cancer Society's statistics, people who kick the habit average a gain of only six pounds.

The *fear* of weight gain is a big problem, however, particularly among women. Though as a group they smoke fewer cigarettes a day than men, women seem to have a harder time quitting. No one's sure exactly what social and psychological pressures account for this difference, but a fear of getting fat is certainly part of it. This sort of thinking has helped produce a deadly statistic: By 1995, if current trends continue, the United States will become the first country in which female smokers outnumber male.

Make no mistake: Compared to smoking a pack a day, the health risk of gaining pounds—even ten or 15—is minuscule.

When's the hardest part over?

THREE MONTHS, more or less. A quarter of the quitters who make it this far quit for good. The cravings become milder with time, but they still linger. "After eighteen years, I still dream about cigarettes," says Eriksen. And even the strongest resolve can break in a crisis. The loss of a job, a death in the family—any serious shakeup—can make people long for a smoke as they would for an old friend.

"You have to anticipate the crisis, imagine the worst thing that could happen," says Reilly. "And then tell yourself that smoking is not an option. Period."

FIVE WEEKS AFTER the quit date, four of the 14 people in Gerry Reilly's class had slipped off the program and gone back to smoking. But nine of the faithful turned up at the first reunion, a potluck dinner held in their old classroom, and it was a changed group.

Lisa was coping with the help of "parrot food" (sunflower seeds), and Kay was now hooked on brisk morning walks. Everyone seemed pleased, increasingly confident of a new status: They didn't smoke anymore.

At the three-month mark, eight of the 14 still weren't smoking. Some found their resolve growing stronger as the time passed.

"Forget about it," said Duane. "It's not something I do. I'm a nonsmoker. I didn't go through that first week of climbing the walls for nothing, and I'm not going through that again."

ALCOHOL and TOBACCO:

A Deadly Duo

Kristine Napier

Kristine Napier, M.P.H., R.D., is a Cleveland-based freelance writer. She studied alcohol/tobacco interactions during her graduate work.

Cancer of the upper respiratory and alimentary tracts claimed over 23,000 lives in 1989 and 57,000 additional cases were diagnosed. The majority of individuals who fall prey to this type of cancer are males who abuse both alcohol and tobacco.

THE RISK

The fact that the risk of developing cancer of the esophagus, lip, tongue, mouth, pharynx or larynx, increases dramatically in people who are heavy users of alcohol and tobacco is substantiated by 30 years of collective research. Studies demonstrate that the risk to individuals dually addicted far outweighs the risk to individuals who abuse only one substance. This confirmed link between alcohol and tobacco abuse and an increased risk in upper alimentary and respiratory tract cancer makes this type of disease among the most preventable.

THE CORRELATION BETWEEN SMOKING AND DRINKING

It has been observed that individuals who drink alcohol have a greater tendency to smoke than non-drinkers. One of the first studies to establish and quantify the degree of association between drinking and smoking was reported in 1972. The investigation compared 130 alcoholic men hospitalized for alcohol withdrawal to 100 non-alcoholic psychiatric outpatients. Ninety-four percent of the alcoholic men smoked one or more packs of cigarettes per day, as compared to only 46 percent of the non-alcoholics, who smoked one or more packs per day.

Another study, which compared male and female alcoholics enrolled in an army drug and alcohol rehabilitation program to non-alcoholic army personnel and their relatives, affirmed the smoking-drinking association. The report found that individuals who were alcoholics smoked an average of 49 cigarettes per day, but that the non-alcoholic subjects smoked only 13 cigarettes per day. In addition, the study established a high correlation between the number of cigarettes smoked and the grams of alcohol consumed by alcoholics, as opposed to a very weak association for the non-alcoholic control group.

In a similar report, 58 percent of the non-drinkers were non-smokers, but the individuals who were alcoholics did not abstain from smoking. The finding that smokers who did not drink smoked significantly less than smokers who did drink was further substantiated in additional studies.

WHY DO MANY DRINKERS SMOKE MORE?

Studies released in the late 1950s, correlating heavy coffee consumption with smoking and drinking, suggested that a strong oral drive caused drinkers to smoke more frequently. However, new evidence suggests that a strong oral drive is not the culprit.

In one study, alcoholics who had successfully stopped drinking demonstrated no appreciable increase in smoking. In fact, some even smoked less with alcohol abstinence. If a strong oral drive was responsible for the drinking-smoking association, one would expect an increase in smoking during periods of alcohol abstinence.

An alternative theory claimed that drinkers smoked more due to social pressure. However, a study showing that alcoholics who drank alone smoked just as much as alcoholics who drink in the company of other people

Reprinted with permission from *Priorities* magazine, Spring 1990, pp. 6-7. Published by the American Council on Science and Health.

dispelled this theory. The most plausible explanation is that drinkers smoke more than non-drinkers due to a greater physiological need for nicotine.

Nicotine, the main psychoactive component of tobacco, is a potent chemical. It has a stimulating effect on the nervous system, causing, among other things, increased heart rate and mental stimulation. Once addicted to **nicotine, a person may experience tremors or shakiness as** blood levels of nicotine decrease to critically low levels. The smoker will crave another cigarette as blood levels reach this threshold to avoid these uncomfortable symptoms. Alcohol apparently causes blood levels of nicotine to fall more rapidly in smokers by activating enzymes in tissues which metabolize drugs. For example, rats pretreated with ethanol cleared nicotine from their blood more rapidly than rats not receiving ethanol. This research, coupled with numerous independent observations, strongly suggests that drinkers must smoke more in order to maintain the blood nicotine levels upon which they have become dependent.

WHY IS THERE MORE CANCER AMONG ALCOHOL AND TOBACCO USERS?

Investigations are under way to find an answer to this question. Laboratory studies have shown that alcohol enhances the metabolism of several tobacco associated carcinogens, including nitrosamines. It is known that tobacco and its smoke contain many classes of chemical carcinogens which must be activated to react with DNA and initiate steps towards carcinogenesis. Important in this activation process are cytochrome P-450 enzymes, which are induced by alcohol in heavy drinkers. Thus, alcohol and smoking are synergistic in increasing cancer risk.

Since alcohol increases the metabolism and hence the need for nicotine, it follows that the success of smoking cessation programs will be improved if drinking habits of patients are controlled. Treatment of incipient alcoholism thus becomes a prerequisite for the ultimate success of behavior modification aimed at the elimination of smoking.

Alcohol in perspective

True or false?

1. An ounce-and-a-half of 80-proof vodka or whiskey contains more alcohol than a 12-ounce can of beer.
2. A woman gets more intoxicated than a man from the same amount of alcohol.
3. Most Americans drink little or no alcohol.
4. Fatalities caused by alcohol-impaired driving are declining.
5. Measured in real dollars, the cost of alcoholic beverages has risen steadily during the last 40 years.

Answers

1. False. They contain the same amount. So does a five-ounce glass of wine.
2. True. The box on page 5 explains why.
3. True. Abstainers account for about 35% of the adult population, and light drinkers another 35%. Light drinkers, in the official definition, are those consuming two drinks a week or less. Moderate drinkers, who average one-half to two drinks a day, account for another 22%. Heavier drinkers—8% of us—consume more than two drinks a day.
4. True. The percentage of road crashes involving alcohol declined from 57% to 49% over the past decade. And the greatest decline was among teens and young adults. This is attributed to new laws setting the minimum drinking age at 21 in all states and to widespread educational efforts.
5. False. It cost less (in inflation-adjusted dollars) to drink in 1992 than it did in 1951. That's not a good thing—see below.

Double messages

Alcohol, a natural product of fermentation, is probably the most widely used of all drugs. It has been a part of human culture since history began and part of American life since Europeans settled on this continent. "The good creature of God," colonial Americans called it—as well as "demon rum." At one time, beer or whiskey may have been safer to drink than well water, but there have always been many other reasons for drinking: the sociability of drinking, the brief but vivid sense of relaxation alcohol can bring, and the wish to celebrate or participate in religious and family rituals where alcohol is served. In some cultures, abstention is the rule. In others, the occasional use of alcohol is regarded as pleasurable and necessary—but such use is carefully controlled and intoxication frowned upon. Tradition and attitude play a powerful role in the use of this drug.

Some people, unfortunately, drink because of depression and/or addiction to alcohol. Apart from such needs, powerful social and economic forces encourage people to drink. For starters, alcoholic beverages are everywhere—from planes and trains to restaurants and county fairs. Also, drink is cheap. The relative cost of alcohol has declined in the last decades. Since 1967 the cost of soft drinks and milk has quadrupled, and the cost of all consumer goods has tripled, but the cost of alcohol has not even doubled. This is because the excise tax on alcohol is not indexed to inflation. Congress has raised the federal tax on beer and wine only once in 40 years (in 1990). The tax on hard liquor has been increased only twice—small raises in 1985 and 1990. Opinion polls have shown that the public is in favor of raising federal excise taxes on alcohol, but the alcohol industry successfully fights increases. Furthermore, about 20% of all alcohol is sold for business entertainment and is thus tax deductible, making it that much less costly to whoever pays the bar bill.

Finally, the alcohol, advertising, and entertainment industries tirelessly promote the idea that it's normal, desirable, smart, sophisticated, and sexy to drink. In print, on television, and at the movies, we see beautiful, healthy people drinking. Beer ads associate the product with sports events, fast cars, camaraderie, and sex. Hollywood's stars have always imbibed plentifully, on and off camera: "Here's looking at you, kid," echoes down the ages. Among modern American male writers, alcoholism has been a badge of the trade: Hemingway, Fitzgerald, and Faulkner were all alcoholics. In *The Thirsty Muse*, literary historian Tom Dardis cites the deadly effect of alcohol on male American writers, many of whom made a credo of heavy drinking.

Considering all these pro-drinking forces, it is amazing that 35% of us over 18 never drink, and another 35% drink lightly and only occasionally. It's equally amazing that our drinking levels have been declining for the past 10 years. But it's estimated that only 8% of us consume more than half of all the alcohol. Still, out-and-out alcoholism is only one factor in the grief caused by drinking, and alcohol problems are not a simple matter of the drunk versus the rest of us.

Alcohol's toll

It's a rare person in our society whose life goes untouched by alcohol. Alcohol causes, or is associated with, over 100,000 deaths every year, often among the young. In 1990, alcohol-related traffic crashes killed more than 22,000 people—almost the same number as homicides. Half the pedestrians killed by cars have elevated blood alcohol levels. At some time in their lives, 40% of all Americans will be involved in an alcohol-related traffic crash. Alcoholism creates unhealthy family dynamics, contributing to domestic violence and child abuse. Fetal alcohol syndrome, caused by drinking during pregnancy, is the leading known cause of mental retardation. After tobacco, alcohol is the leading cause of premature death in America. The total cost of alcohol use in America has been estimated at $86 billion annually, a figure so huge as to lose its meaning. But money is a feeble method for measuring the human suffering.

In a free society, banning alcohol is neither desirable nor acceptable. But government, schools, and other institutions could do more than they do to protect the public health, teach the young about the dangers of alcohol, and treat alcoholics. As individuals and as citizens, we could all contribute to reducing the toll alcohol exacts on American life.

Alcohol and the body: short-term effects

Five ounces of wine, 12 ounces of beer, and 1.5 ounces of 80-proof spirits—all average servings—put the same amount of pure alcohol (about 1/2 to 2/3 ounce) into the bloodstream. But how fast it gets into the blood depends on many things. Some alcohol is absorbed through the stomach lining, enabling it to reach the bloodstream very quickly. If the stomach is empty, absorption is even faster: food slows it down. Aspirin in the stomach can hasten alcohol absorption. Since the alcohol in beer and wine is less concentrated, it tends to be absorbed more slowly than straight whiskey (and presumably you drink beer and wine more slowly than a shot of whiskey). But downing two beers in an hour raises blood alcohol concentration (BAC) more than one drink of whisky sipped for an hour. It's the alcohol that counts. A BAC of 0.10 is defined as legal intoxication in most states (0.08 in California, Maine, Oregon, Utah, and Vermont). It's hard to predict BAC accurately, since so many factors affect it. But a 150-pound man typically reaches a BAC of 0.10 if he has two or three beers in an hour. Any BAC impairs driving ability.

It takes the body about two hours to burn half an ounce of pure alcohol (the amount in about one drink) in the bloodstream. Once the alcohol is there, you can't hurry up the process of metabolizing it. You can't run it off, swim it off, or erase the effects with coffee. Leaner, larger people will be less affected by a given amount of alcohol than smaller ones with more fatty tissue—women, for instance. The effects of a given BAC are also greater in older people than in younger.

Every cell in the body can absorb alcohol from the blood. Of the short-term effects, none is more dramatic than those on the central nervous system. At first the drinker gets a feeling of ease and exhilaration, usually short-lived. But as BAC rises, judgment, memory, and sensory perception are all progressively impaired. Thoughts become jumbled; concentration and insight are dulled. Depression usually sets in. Some people get angry or violent. Alcohol induces drowsiness but at the same time disrupts normal patterns of sleeping and dreaming. It also adversely affects sexual performance.

The most unpleasant physical after-effect of too much alco-

Different for a woman

The alcohol industry has tried for some time to hitch a ride on women's quest for equality. Liquor ads promote the idea that if a woman can work like a man, she can, and indeed should, drink like a man. Nothing could be further from the truth.

Today 55% of women drink alcoholic beverages, and 3% of all women consume more than two drinks a day. But the ads don't tell a woman that she'll get more intoxicated than a man from the same amount of alcohol. Alcohol is distributed through body water, and is more soluble in water than in fat. Since women tend to be smaller than men and have proportionately more fatty tissue and less body water than men, the blood alcohol concentration resulting from a given intake will be higher for a woman than for a man of the same size. Recent research also shows that the stomach enzyme that breaks down alcohol before it reaches the bloodstream is less active in women than in men.

This may explain why excessive drinking seems to have more serious long-term consequences for women. They develop cirrhosis (liver disease) at lower levels of alcohol intake than men, for instance, and alcohol also puts them at increased risk for osteoporosis.

Finally, pregnant women who drink heavily risk having babies with fetal alcohol syndrome—characterized by mental retardation, structural defects of the face and limbs, hyperactivity, and heart defects. Because no level of alcohol consumption during pregnancy is known to be safe, pregnant women (as well as women planning pregnancy or having unprotected intercourse) are advised not to drink and to continue to abstain while breastfeeding. The amount of alcohol that passes into breast milk is smaller than the amount that crosses the placenta during pregnancy, but recent studies suggest that even a small amount can inhibit motor development in an infant. The idea that drinking beer promotes milk supply and benefits the baby is a myth.

hol is a hangover: dry mouth, sour stomach, headache, depression, and fatigue. Its cause is over-indulgence—not, as some believe, "mixing" drinks or drinking "cheap booze." No remedy has ever been found for hangovers.

The heart effect: worth drinking for?

Much recent research shows that moderate drinkers have a lower risk of developing heart disease. Supposedly, this beneficial effect comes from alcohol's ability to raise HDL cholesterol, the "good" type that protects against atherosclerosis. Some researchers have suggested that only one kind of beverage—for example, red wine—is protective. But it's more likely to be alcohol itself. Still, it's only moderate drinking that's helpful, and some people can't stick to moderation, while others (pregnant women) shouldn't drink at all. Few doctors suggest that nondrinkers begin drinking to protect their hearts.

Heavy drinking: long-term effects

Chronic, excessive use of alcohol can seriously damage nearly every organ and function of the body. When alcohol is burned in the body it produces another, even more toxic substance, acetaldehyde, which contributes to the damage. Alcohol is a stomach irritant. It adversely affects the way the small intestine transports and absorbs nutrients, especially vitamins and minerals. Added to the usually poor diet of heavy drinkers, this often results in severe malnutrition. Furthermore, alcohol can produce pancreatic disorders. It causes fatty deposits to accumulate in the liver. Cirrhosis of the liver, an often fatal illness, may be the ultimate result. Though alcohol is not a food, it does have calories and can contribute to obesity.

The effects of heavy drinking on the cardiovascular system are no less horrific. For many years doctors have observed that hypertension and excessive alcohol use go together, and according to a number of recent studies, heavy drinkers are more likely to have high blood pressure than teetotalers. Heavy alcohol consumption damages healthy heart muscle and puts extra strain on already damaged heart muscle. And it can damage other muscles besides the heart.

Some of the worst effects of alcohol are directly on the brain. The most life-threatening is an acute condition leading to psychosis, confusion, or unconsciousness. Heavy drinkers also tend to be heavy smokers and are also more likely to take and abuse other drugs, such as tranquilizers. Excessive drinking, particularly in combination with tobacco, increases the chance of cancers of the mouth, larynx, and throat. Alcohol appears to play a role in stomach, colorectal, and esophageal cancers, as well as possibly liver cancer.

What causes alcoholism?

Alcoholism is a complex disorder: the official definition, recently devised by a 23-member committee of experts, is "a primary, chronic disease with genetic, psychosocial, and environmental factors influencing its development and manifestations. The disease is often progressive and fatal. It is characterized by impaired control over drinking, preoccupation with the drug alcohol, use of alcohol despite adverse consequences, and distortions in thinking, most notably denial."

Alcohol use, by itself, is not sufficient to cause alcoholism. Medical science cannot yet explain why one person abstains or drinks rarely, while another drinks to excess—or why some heavy drinkers are able to stop drinking, while others continue until they die of cirrhosis. One area currently under intensive investigation is heredity. Are children of heavy drinkers more likely to fall victim to alcohol than others?

The answer is yes, but not just because these children were raised in an adverse environment. Studies have shown that, even when raised in nonalcoholic households, a significant number of children of alcoholic parents become alcoholics. This suggests that the ability to handle alcohol may be in part genetically

Strong laws and community action

What legislative proposals concerning alcohol should you support—through voting, or even by writing to your representatives in Congress and the state legislature? What can communities do to decrease problems caused by alcohol? The following ideas make sense:

1. Alcoholic beverages should be labeled to provide accurate information about ingredients, calories, percentage of alcohol, and number of drinks per container (a drink being defined as 12 ounces of beer, 5 ounces wine, or 1.5 ounces of 80-proof liquor). Every container should carry a toll-free telephone number for information on alcoholism and related problems. A bill with these provisions has been introduced in Congress by Representative Patricia Schroeder of Colorado.

2. Broadcast and print ads should carry warnings that alcohol may be addictive, impairs driving ability, interacts with other drugs, and may harm a fetus—among other health and safety messages. Bills are currently before Congress to require such labeling (H.R. 1443, and S. 664). If you want to support them, let your representatives know.

3. Promotions aimed at minors, such as high school and college students, should be ended, as well as alcohol industry sponsorship of sporting and entertainment events. Malt liquors (beers with high alcohol content) such as Colt 45 and King Cobra have consistently been aimed at the young and others who suffer disproportionately from drug and alcohol problems. The Bureau of Alcohol, Tobacco, and Firearms has been petitioned to exercise its regulatory power to prevent this. For more information, write to the Center for Science in the Public Interest, 1875 Connecticut Avenue NW, Suite 300, Washington, DC 20009-5728.

4. Alcohol advertising in public places—especially billboards—often target Latino and African-American neighborhoods. For example, one recent survey in Milwaukee showed that billboards advertising alcohol and cigarettes were heavily concentrated where young people, African-Americans, and the poor were most likely to see them. In Chicago, researchers recently noted that of 233 billboards in one Latino neighborhood, 176 advertised alcohol and 40 tobacco. In many cities, neighborhood groups have formed to remove this advertising. The Outdoor Advertising Association of America has proposed "voluntary limits" on the number of billboards advertising products that cannot be sold to minors, and "exclusionary zones" near schools and hospitals. For information on how to organize a community program, write to Makani Themba, Marin Institute, 24 Belvedere Street, San Rafael, California 94901.

5. Tax laws should be revised so that alcohol is no longer a deductible business expense.

6. A hike in federal excise taxes could provide revenues for education and research. There's evidence that higher prices would reduce alcohol consumption (and alcohol-impaired driving) among the young, in particular.

determined. Not long ago, researchers claimed to have located an alcoholism gene, setting off a bitter controversy and raising the possibility of testing children, job applicants, and even fetuses for latent alcoholism. But if there are alcoholism genes, they remain to be identified, and a test for potential alcoholism is a long way off. Researchers point to differences in blood enzymes among alcoholics and non-users—but do not know whether the difference is responsible for the alcoholism or the result of it. Perhaps the chemistry of the body will prove to be the key to whether a person can drink moderately or not. Though most investigators believe that alcoholism has genetic, as well as environmental, causes, this does not mean that any individual is "doomed" to be an alcoholic. Alcoholic parents don't always produce alcoholic children. And many alcoholics come from families where no one ever drank.

Alcoholism is treatable

One problem in treating alcoholism is that it is hard to recognize. A person who is chronically drunk in public is obviously an alcoholic. But not all alcoholics display their problem by falling down in the street, losing their jobs, causing traffic crashes, or getting arrested. Many drink secretly or only on weekends, only in the evening, or even only once a month. Some may drink from depression, while others are sensation-seekers. They may successfully hold down a job or practice a profession. Yet at some point, whatever their drinking patterns, they have lost their ability to control their use of alcohol.

Many of the serious physical and personal consequences of alcoholism can be halted or reversed if drinking is discontinued soon enough. There are many different approaches to alcoholism: Alcoholics Anonymous and similar 12-step programs, individual or group psychotherapy, hospitalization and detoxification, and other methods. No single system will work for everyone. For some people, a combination of methods can help. Others may do as well with individual counseling. Family therapy may help others. The families of alcoholics also need therapy and other forms of social support. Scientific data about treatment are inconclusive. The crucial factor, most experts agree, is for the drinker to recognize that a problem exists and to seek the kind of treatment he or she needs.

Nutritional Health

The wellness movement has had a significant impact on the way Americans view their responsibility toward health maintenance. Today it is generally recognized that an individual's lifestyle is the primary determinant of health and longevity. This new attitude has fostered tremendous consumer interest in the area of nutrition. The food industry has responded by introducing new products and promoting old ones on the basis of exaggerated health benefits. The challenge for the consumer is to make wise nutritional choices when confronted and bombarded with seductive and often unsubstantiated health claims. Unfortunately, this is not an easy task because much of the nutritional advice we receive is conflicting and controversial.

From the mid-1970s through most of the 1980s, nutrition experts encouraged Americans to reduce their salt intake as a way to prevent hypertension. Today, however, most nutrition experts agree that only a minority of the population would actually benefit from a sharp reduction in sodium intake. "To Salt or Not to Salt" by Mary McMann examines the salt issue and concludes that broad dietary recommendations advocating salt restriction are not only contrary to current scientific data but may prove hazardous for certain individuals.

Examples of conflicting nutritional advice are rampant, largely because nutritional science is in its infancy, and thus is fraught with contradictions and controversies. Until nutritional science reaches maturity, advice coming from nutrition experts will be tentative at best. Given these limitations, this unit presents current thinking on a variety of nutritional issues. The article "Are You Eating Right?" addresses many of the current controversial nutritional issues and attempts to eradicate some of the confusion, based on the recommendations and advice of 68 nutritional experts.

Nothing better illustrates the controversial nature of nutritional advice than the debate among nutrition experts over revisions of the basic four food groups. The role of the "basic four" was to serve as a fundamental dietary guideline for planning nutritionally sound meals. In addition, these four food groups also represented the major lobbying organizations within the American agricultural system. A great deal has been learned about the role that each of the food groups should play a in healthy diet, and the findings have not pleased the meat and dairy groups. The U.S. Department of Agriculture has replaced the "basic four" with what it terms the "eating right pyramid." This new dietary guideline breaks all foods into six groups that graphically represent the relative amount that each group should contribute to a person's diet. According to this new dietary guideline, Americans should eat 11 to 20 servings of plant foods a day, compared to only 4 to 6 servings of animal foods. Not surprisingly, the meat and dairy councils have rejected the eating right pyramid on the basis that it slights their products. Surprisingly, the eating right pyramid was adopted in spite of the political lobbying against it by the meat and dairy councils. Given these changes, it is not surprising that a growing number of Americans are eliminating animal products from their diets and becoming vegetarians. While it is quite possible to meet all of a person's nutritional needs from a strict vegetarian diet, to do so may necessitate the taking of vitamin and mineral supplements, since some essential micronutrients occur mainly or exclusively in animal foods.

For years the majority of Americans paid little attention to nutrition, other than to eat three meals a day and, perhaps, take a vitamin supplement. While this dietary style was generally adequate for the prevention of major nutritional deficiencies, medical evidence began to accumulate linking the American diet to a variety of chronic illnesses. The most ominous finding was the link between dietary fat and coronary heart disease. This connection has been the focus of numerous studies, and the role that dietary fat plays in the process of atherosclerosis has been well documented. Recommendations based on these studies strongly suggest that Americans should reduce their intake of saturated fats and substitute monounsaturated or polyunsaturated fats whenever possible. This appears to be particularly true for individuals under stress. The article "New Thinking About Fats" discusses why the type of fat eaten may be as important as the amount when it comes to preventing heart disease.

The National Research Council (NRC) currently recommends that Americans trim back their dietary fat intake so that it constitutes no more than 30 percent of total caloric intake. The NRC also recommends that saturated fats be limited to less than 10 percent of the total daily intake. While these recommendations may be prudent, compliance with them can be challenging. Major obstacles blocking compliance are the misconceptions that consumers have about them. The most common misconception is that any food that derives more than 30 percent of its calories from fat should be eliminated from the diet. The NRC diet is not concerned with the percentage of fat calories found in specific foods, but instead with the importance of keeping the total daily diet at or below the 30 percent fat ratio. "Eating Right: It's Easier Than You Think" demonstrates how with minor modifications, typical meals can be modified to comply with the NCR recommendations concerning dietary fat.

As a result of all the bad press about dietary fats, millions of Americans are making a concerted effort to cut the fat content of their diets. Snack food is one food category in which they have been least successful. Americans currently spend over $13.4 billion a year on snack foods, and with an eager market for low-fat alternatives to the most popular snack foods, the food industry has responded by introducing reduced-fat versions of many of the most popular snack foods. Most challenging has been the production of low-fat potato chips and candy bars that retain the flavor and texture of the originals. It is too early to tell how well these low fat versions will be accepted by consumers, but the food industry is banking on the belief that consumers will settle for less crunch and flavor if the tradeoff means significantly less fat. Another way in which food companies have attempted to maintain their market share in the face of all the negative press regarding dietary fat has been to substitute monounsaturated and polyunsaturated fats for tropical oils and animal fats. "Snack Attack" by Patricia Long examines the fat content of various snack foods and suggests that the problem with snacking is not the eating between meals, but rather the food choices that are made at such times.

While fats have increasingly come under scrutiny as a source of health problems, carbohydrates have been given high ratings for health. Nutritionists generally agree that Americans should eat more carbohydrates, particularly the complex type, as they are a good source of vitamins, minerals, and fiber. While complex carbohydrates generally receive high marks for their nutritional value, highly refined forms such as sugar do not fare nearly as well. Over the last 20 years, dietary sugar (sucrose) has been linked to the etiology of obesity, heart disease, diabetes, dental caries, and periodontal disease. As a result, millions of Americans have made the switch to artificial sweeteners. Does this switch represent a positive change? Health authorities now generally agree that while sugar is a source of empty calories, the only demonstrable health hazards it poses appear to be dental.

Over the past few years, dietary fiber has become a hot issue. Several studies reported that individuals eating high fiber diets demonstrated a lower incidence of colon cancer and lower blood cholesterol levels. In response to these findings, several noted health authorities have encouraged Americans to increase their consumption of dietary fiber. The food industry also responded by marketing several new high-fiber products and emphasizing the fiber content of their other products. Researchers have recently reinterpreted the data of earlier studies and have come to some interesting conclusions. While it is true that the individuals who ate high-fiber diets did have lower rates of both colon cancer and cardiovascular disease, these health benefits could also be explained by the fact that individuals eating high-fiber diets simply consumed fewer dietary fats. These findings suggest that dietary fiber, while beneficial, is probably not as valuable as previously thought.

The use of dietary supplements is another highly controversial topic. Today approximately 33 percent of Americans take a vitamin supplement regularly. For some, this consists of a simple multiple vitamin; others, however, rely on megadosing. Should individuals take vitamin supplements? If so, which ones? How many and how much? Is there a difference between natural and synthetic vitamins? These questions remain largely unanswered by the scientific community. Numerous studies have been initiated in an attempt to resolve them, but definitive conclusions cannot be drawn from the data now available. This creates a confusing situation for the health consumer who is trying to make informed decisions regarding the use of dietary supplements. Most nutritional experts agree that eating a varied and balanced diet is the single best way to meet all a person's nutritional needs, but not everyone eats a balanced diet, and for those who do not, supplements may be necessary.

Another nutritional concern that has received considerable attention in the last few years is the problem of osteoporosis, particularly in women. Currently, most authorities agree that many Americans do not get sufficient amounts of dietary calcium. There is, however, considerable debate on how this deficit is best corrected.

Looking Ahead: Challenge Questions

Given the controversies that abound in the area of nutrition, what guidelines should an individual use to make dietary decisions?

If you were asked to advise someone on how they might reduce the fat content of their diet, what advice would you give them?

Given what we now know about the link between salt and hypertension, do you think it is a good idea for the National Research Council to continue its widespread advocacy of dietary salt restrictions? Explain.

What dietary changes could you make to improve your diet? What is keeping you from making those changes?

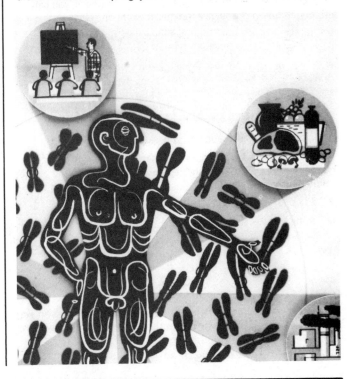

How's Your Diet?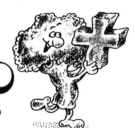

The 40 questions below will help you focus on the key features of your diet. The (+) or (–) numbers under each set of answers instantly pat you on the back for good habits or alert you to problems you may not even realize you have.

The Grand Total rates your overall diet, on a scale from "Great" to "Arrgh!"

The quiz focuses on fat, saturated fat, cholesterol, sodium, sugar, fiber, and vitamins A and C. It doesn't attempt to cover everything in your diet. Also, it doesn't try to measure precisely how much of these key nutrients you eat. (For that, we recommend the *DINE nutrition software.* [Contact CSPI at (202) 332-9110.])

What the quiz will do is give you a rough sketch of your current eating habits and, implicitly, suggest what you can do to improve them.

And don't despair over a less-than-perfect score. We didn't get a +117 either.

INSTRUCTIONS

■ Under each answer is a number with a + or – sign in front of it. Circle the number that is directly beneath the answer you choose. That's your score for the question. (If you use a pencil, you can erase your answers and give the quiz to someone else.)

■ Circle only one number for each question, unless the instructions tell you to "average two or more scores if necessary."

■ *How to average.* In answering question 18, for example, if you drink club soda (+3) and coffee (–1) on a typical day, add the two scores (which gives you +2) and then divide by 2. That gives you a score of +1 for the question. If averaging gives you a fraction, round it to the nearest whole number.

■ If a question doesn't apply to you, skip it.

■ Pay attention to serving sizes. For example, a serving of vegetables is ½ cup. If you usually eat one cup of vegetables at a time, count it as two servings.

■ Add up all your + scores and your – scores.

■ Subtract your – scores from your + scores. That's your GRAND TOTAL.

QUIZ

1. How many times per week do you eat unprocessed red meat (steak, roast beef, lamb or pork chops, burgers, etc.)?

(a) 0   (b) 1 or less   (c) 2-3   (d) 4-5   (e) 6 or more
  +3   +2   0   –1   –3

2. How many times per week do you eat processed meats (hot dogs, bacon, sausage, bologna, luncheon meats, etc.)? *(OMIT products that contain one gram of fat or less per serving.)*

(a) 0   (b) less than 1   (c) 1   (d) 2-3   (e) 4 or more
  +3   +2   0   –1   –3

3. What kind of ground meat or poultry do you usually eat?

(a) regular or lean ground beef   (b) extra lean ground beef
         –3   –2
(c) ground round   (d) ground turkey   (e) Healthy Choice
       –1   +1   +3
(f) don't eat ground meat
       +3

4. Do you trim the visible fat when you cook or eat red meat?

(a) yes   (b) no   (c) don't eat red meat
  +1   –3   0

5. After cooking, how large is the serving of red meat you usually eat? *(To convert from raw to cooked, reduce by 25 percent. For example, 4 oz. of raw meat shrinks to 3 oz. after cooking. There are 16 oz. in a pound.)*

(a) 8 oz. or more   (b) 6-7 oz.   (c) 4-5 oz.   (d) 3 oz. or less
       –3   –2   –1   0
(e) don't eat red meat
       +3

6. What type of bread, rolls, bagels, etc., do you usually eat?

(a) 100% whole wheat   (b) whole wheat as 1st or 2nd ingredient
       +3   +2
(c) rye, pumpernickel, or oatmeal   (d) white, French, or Italian
       +1   –1

7. How many times per week do you eat deep-fried foods (fish, chicken, vegetables, potatoes, etc.)?

(a) 0   (b) 1-2   (c) 3-4   (d) 5 or more
  +3   0   –1   –3

8. How many servings of non-fried vegetables do you usually eat per day? *(One serving = ½ cup. INCLUDE potatoes.)*

(a) 0   (b) 1   (c) 2   (d) 3   (e) 4 or more
  –3   0   +1   +2   +3

9. How many servings of cruciferous vegetables do you usually eat per week? *(ONLY count kale, broccoli, cauliflower, cabbage, Brussels sprouts, greens, bok choy, kohlrabi, turnip, and rutabaga. One serving = ½ cup.)*

(a) 0   (b) 1-3   (c) 4-6   (d) 7 or more
  –3   +1   +2   +3

10. How many servings of vitamin-A-rich fruits or vegetables do you usually eat per week? *(ONLY count cantaloupe, apricots, or cooked carrots, pumpkin, sweet potatoes, spinach, winter squash, or greens. One serving = ½ cup.)*

(a) 0   (b) 1-3   (c) 4-6   (d) 7 or more
  –3   +1   +2   +3

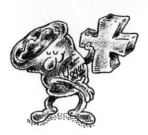

11. How many times per week do you eat at a fast-food restaurant? *(INCLUDE burgers, fried fish or chicken, croissant or biscuit sandwiches, topped potatoes, and other main dishes. OMIT plain baked potatoes, broiled skinned chicken, or low-fat salads.)*

(a) 0   (b) less than 1   (c) 1   (d) 2   (e) 3   (f) 4 or more
+3   +1   0   −1   −2   −3

12. How many servings of grains do you eat per day? *(One serving = 1 slice of bread, 1 large pancake, 1 cup cold cereal, or ½ cup cooked cereal, rice, pasta, bulgur, wheat berries, kasha, or millet. OMIT heavily-sweetened cold cereals.)*

(a) 0   (b) 1-3   (c) 4-5   (d) 6-8   (e) 9 or more
−3   0   +1   +2   +3

13. How many times per week do you eat fish or shellfish? *(OMIT deep-fried items, tuna packed in oil, and mayonnaise-laden tuna salad– a little mayo is okay.)*

(a) 0   (b) 1   (c) 2   (d) 3 or more   (e) 0 (vegetarians)
0   +1   +2   +3   +3

14. How many times per week do you eat cheese? *(INCLUDE pizza, cheeseburgers, veal or eggplant parmigiana, cream cheese, etc. OMIT low-fat or fat-free cheeses.)*

(a) 0   (b) 1   (c) 2-3   (d) 4 or more
+3   +1   −1   −3

15. How many servings of fresh fruit do you eat per day?

(a) 0   (b) 1   (c) 2   (d) 3   (e) 4 or more
−3   0   +1   +2   +3

16. Do you remove the skin before eating poultry?

(a) yes   (b) no   (c) don't eat poultry
+3   −3   0

17. What do you usually put on your bread or toast? *(AVERAGE two or more scores if necessary.)*

(a) butter or cream cheese   (b) margarine   (c) peanut butter
−3   −2   −1

(d) diet margarine   (e) jam or honey   (f) 100% fruit butter
−1   0   +1

(g) nothing
+3

18. Which of these beverages do you drink on a typical day? *(AVERAGE two or more scores if necessary.)*

(a) water or club soda   (b) fruit juice   (c) diet soda
+3   +1   −1

(d) coffee or tea   (e) soda, fruit "drink," or fruit "ade"
−1   −3

19. Which flavorings do you most frequently add to your foods? *(AVERAGE two or more scores if necessary.)*

(a) garlic or lemon juice   (b) herbs or spices   (c) olive oil
+3   +3   −1

(d) salt or soy sauce   (e) margarine   (f) butter   (g) nothing
−1   −2   −3   +3

20. What do you eat most frequently as a snack? *(AVERAGE two or more scores if necessary.)*

(a) fruits or vegetables   (b) yogurt   (c) crackers
+3   +2   +1

(d) nuts   (e) cookies or fried chips   (f) granola bar
−1   −2   −2

(g) candy bar or pastry   (h) nothing
−3   0

21. What is your most typical breakfast? *(SUBTRACT an extra 3 points if you also eat bacon or sausage.)*

(a) croissant, danish, or doughnut   (b) whole eggs
−3   −3

(c) pancakes or waffles   (d) cereal or toast
−2   +3

(e) low-fat yogurt or cottage cheese   (f) don't eat breakfast
+3   0

22. What do you usually eat for dessert?

(a) pie, pastry, or cake   (b) ice cream
−3   −3

(c) fat-free cookies or cakes   (d) frozen yogurt or ice milk
−1   0

(e) non-fat ice cream or sorbet   (f) fruit   (g) don't eat dessert
+1   +3   +3

23. How many times per week do you eat beans, split peas, or lentils?

(a) 0   (b) 1   (c) 2   (d) 3   (e) 4 or more
−3   0   +1   +2   +3

24. What kind of milk do you drink?

(a) whole   (b) 2% fat   (c) 1% low-fat
−3   −1   +2

(d) ½% or skim   (e) don't drink milk
+3   0

25. Which items do you choose at a salad bar? *(ADD two or more scores if necessary.)*

(a) nothing, lemon, or vinegar   (b) fat-free dressing
+3   +2

(c) low- or reduced-calorie dressing   (d) regular dressing
+1   −1

(e) croutons or bacon bits
−1

(f) cole slaw, pasta salad, or potato salad
−1

26. What sandwich fillings do you eat most frequently? *(AVERAGE two or more scores if necessary.)*

(a) regular luncheon meat   (b) cheese   (c) roast beef
−3   −2   −1

(d) peanut butter   (e) low-fat luncheon meat
0   +1

(f) tuna or chicken salad   (g) fresh turkey breast or bean spread
+1   +3

(h) don't eat sandwiches
0

27. What do you usually spread on your sandwiches? *(AVERAGE two or more scores if necessary.)*

(a) mayonnaise   (b) light mayonnaise
−2   −1

(c) catsup, mustard, or fat-free mayonnaise
+1

(d) nothing
+2

28. How many egg yolks do you eat per week? *(ADD 1 yolk for every slice of quiche you eat.)*

(a) 2 or less   (b) 3-4   (c) 5-6   (d) 7 or more
+3   0   −1   −3

29. How many times per week do you eat canned or dried soups? *(OMIT low-sodium, low-fat soups.)*
(a) 0   (b) 1-2   (c) 3-4   (d) 5 or more
+3   0   −2   −3

30. How many servings of a rich source of calcium do you eat per day? *(One serving = 2/3 cup milk or yogurt, 1 oz. cheese, 1 1/2 oz. sardines, 3 1/2 oz. canned salmon (with bones), 5 oz. tofu made with calcium sulfate, 1 cup greens or broccoli, or 200 mg of a calcium supplement.)*
(a) 0   (b) 1   (c) 2   (d) 3 or more
−3   +1   +2   +3

31. What do you usually order on your pizza? *(Vegetable toppings include green pepper, mushrooms, onions, and other vegetables. SUBTRACT 1 point from your score if you order extra cheese.)*
(a) no cheese with vegetables   (b) cheese with vegetables
+3   +1
(c) cheese   (d) cheese with meat toppings
0   −3
(e) don't eat pizza
+2

32. What kind of cookies do you usually eat?
(a) don't eat cookies   (b) fat-free cookies
+3   +2
(c) graham crackers or ginger snaps   (d) oatmeal
+1   −1
(e) sandwich cookies (like Oreos)
−2
(f) chocolate coated, chocolate chip, or peanut butter
−3

33. What kind of frozen dessert do you usually eat?
(SUBTRACT 1 point from your score for each topping you use—whipped cream, hot fudge, nuts, etc.)
(a) gourmet ice cream   (b) regular ice cream
−3   −2
(c) frozen yogurt, ice milk   (d) sorbet, sherbet, or ices
0   +1
(e) non-fat frozen yogurt or fat-free ice cream
+1
(f) don't eat frozen desserts
+3

34. What kind of cake or pastry do you usually eat?
(a) cheesecake, pie, or any microwave cake
−3
(b) cake with frosting   (c) cake without frosting
−2   −1
(d) unfrosted muffin, banana bread, or carrot cake
0
(e) angelfood or fat-free cake   (f) don't eat cakes or pastries
+1   +3

35. How many times per week does your dinner contain grains, vegetables, or beans, but little or no animal protein (meat, poultry, fish, eggs, milk, or cheese)?
(a) 0   (b) 1-2   (c) 3-4   (d) 5 or more
−1   +1   +2   +3

36. Which of the following "salty" snacks do you typically eat? *(AVERAGE two or more scores if necessary.)*
(a) potato chips, corn chips, or pre-popped popcorn
−3
(b) tortilla chips, reduced-fat potato chips, or microwave popcorn
−2
(c) salted pretzels   (d) light microwave popcorn
−1   0
(e) unsalted pretzels   (f) fat-free tortilla or potato chips
+1   +2
(g) homemade air-popped popcorn   (h) don't eat salty snacks
+3   +3

37. What do you usually use to sauté vegetables or other foods? *(Vegetable oil includes safflower, corn, canola, sunflower, and soybean.)*
(a) butter or lard   (b) margarine   (c) vegetable oil
−3   −2   −1
(d) olive oil   (e) broth   (f) water or cooking spray
+1   +2   +3

38. What kind of cereal do you usually eat?
(a) whole grain (like oatmeal or Shredded Wheat)
+3
(b) low-fiber (like Cream of Wheat or Corn Flakes)
0
(c) sugary low-fiber (like Frosted Flakes)   (d) regular granola
−1   −2

39. With what do you make tuna salad, pasta salad, chicken salad, etc?
(a) mayonnaise   (b) light mayonnaise   (c) non-fat mayonnaise
−2   −1   0
(d) low-fat yogurt   (e) non-fat yogurt
+2   +3

40. What do you typically put on your pasta? *(ADD one point if you also add sautéed vegetables. AVERAGE two or more scores if necessary.)*
(a) tomato sauce, with or without a little parmesan
+3
(b) white clam sauce   (c) meat sauce or meat balls
0   −2
(d) Alfredo, pesto, or other creamy or oily sauce
−3

YOUR GRAND TOTAL

+59 to +117	GREAT!	You're a nutrition superstar. Give yourself a big (non-butter) pat on the back.
0 to +58	GOOD	You're doing just fine. Pin your Quiz to the nearest wall.
−1 to −58	FAIR	Hang in there. Tape CSPI's Nutrition Scoreboard poster to your refrigerator for a little friendly help.
−59 to −116	ARRGH!	Stop lining the cat box with *Nutrition Action Healthletter*. Empty your refrigerator and cupboard. It's time to start over.

ARE YOU EATING RIGHT?

In a candid survey, 68 nutrition experts told us what they really think about diet and health

*H*ow much harm is done to health by our one-sided and excessive diet no one can say. Physicians tell us that it is very great.

Those words were written in 1894 by W. O. Atwater, of the U.S. Department of Agriculture. The first Government official to offer Americans dietary advice, Atwater sounded a warning on fatty, sugary foods and advocated a diet low in fat, moderate in protein, and high in complex carbohydrates. A century later, it's still advice Americans need to hear.

Since Atwater's time, the sense of concern over our national diet has deepened as the value of a low-fat, high-carbohydrate diet has become even more clear. Such a diet is the centerpiece of nutrition recommendations put forth by the Government and by health groups such as the American Heart Association. The nation's eating and drinking habits have been implicated in 6 of the 10 leading causes of death—heart disease, cancer, stroke, diabetes, atherosclerosis, and chronic liver disease and cirrhosis—as well as in several nonfatal but potentially disabling disorders, such as osteoporosis and diverticulosis. Yet many Americans are still confused, misinformed, or apathetic about the connection between diet and health.

If Americans are uncertain about how to choose a nutritious diet, it may be partly due to the crosswinds of scientific debate that blow through the popular news media. A third of adults are "confused by all the reports which give dietary advice," according to an American Dietetic Association survey. It's little wonder: In the past year alone, we've been advised to use oils sparingly but to load up on olive oil; to avoid overweight, yet somehow avoid "yo-yo" dieting; to drink red wine because the French have fewer heart attacks but to refrain from alcohol because the French have more liver disease. The food industry has profited from the confusion by marketing a wide range of products with dubious nutritional claims and by saturating the market with products that follow the nutritional fad of the moment.

To find out what dietary advice we can truly bank on, we conducted a survey among 94 nutrition professionals—scientists, clinicians, registered dietitians, and educators—who had served as members of Federal advisory boards relating to nutrition, or on nutrition committees of professional organizations. They are among the most widely respected experts on nutrition in the country. Sixty-eight of them completed a comprehensive 18-page questionnaire.

Expert advice
We first asked these experts to assess the strength of the scientific evidence for each of 44 presumed connections between nutrition and health (such as the link between saturated fat and coronary heart disease). In many cases, we found, expert opinion about the strength of the evidence is still split. But despite conflicting evidence on many specific points, these experts agree there's good reason to change the typical American diet—and to change some aspects of it dramatically.

We asked our experts to define a "reasonable" diet: "Given the realities of food choices, dietary habits, and so on," we asked, "what guidelines would you feel comfortable recommending to the American public?" The "reasonable" diet they agree on—one relatively low in fat and high in fruits, vegetables, and grains—closely matches the Government's latest dietary recommendations as well as the guidelines issued by panels on which the experts had previously served.

The experts' responses were more revealing when we asked their candid opinion of what makes an "ideal" diet. We asked, "What do you feel would be a theoretically ideal diet to promote good health and reduce the risk of chronic disease, if personal preference, cost, and the difficulty of dietary change were not at issue? Imagine, in other words, that you could magically persuade the American people to adopt the perfect diet—what would that be?"

Our experts came up with an "ideal" diet very different from the current American diet—and different in some significant ways from other standard public-health recommendations. The experts said the ideal diet should:

Provide only 25 percent of calories, or less, from fat. Three-fourths of the experts believe this restriction is necessary to an ideal diet. Americans now get about 36 percent of their calories from fat; the standard recommendation has been to cut back to 30 percent.

Include seven or more servings of fruits and vegetables a day. Fifty-five percent of the experts endorse this recommendation as ideal—and virtually all the rest recommend five servings or more. Standard nutritional advice has been to eat five or more servings of fruits and vegetables a day, a good deal more than most Americans now eat.

Include no more than three 3-ounce servings of red meat a week. Three-fifths of the experts endorse this limit on the number of servings and the portions of red meat. That's about half as much red meat as Americans now eat on the average, and about one-quarter as much as many men eat. (A three-ounce serving of meat is roughly the size of a deck of playing cards; that's a smaller portion than many Americans are used to.)

This is the first time, to our knowledge, that a group of this stature has endorsed a specific limit on red-meat intake. Other groups have merely proposed guidelines for an eclectic "meat group," which also includes poultry, fish, and beans. Lobbying by beef producers has dissuaded Government agencies from suggesting limits on red meat explicitly, even though it is a major source of fat, saturated fat, and cholesterol.

The experts' ideal diet, though very different from what most Americans eat, does define a goal that most people could readily move toward. In that regard, our experts agree with the kinds of changes outlined in the Dietary Guidelines for Americans—a joint venture of the U.S. Department of Agriculture and the Department of Health and Human Services—although our experts often recommend a greater degree of change than do the Guidelines. The Guidelines advise Americans to cut

HOW MUCH FAT?

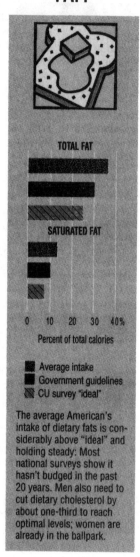

TOTAL FAT

SATURATED FAT

0   10   20   30   40%

Percent of total calories

■ Average intake
■ Government guidelines
▨ CU survey "ideal"

The average American's intake of dietary fats is considerably above "ideal" and holding steady: Most national surveys show it hasn't budged in the past 20 years. Men also need to cut dietary cholesterol by about one-third to reach optimal levels; women are already in the ballpark.

back on fats and cholesterol, to use sugars, salt, and alcohol in moderation, and to eat more fruits, vegetables, and grains. Such changes are attainable; most of our nutrition experts say they follow such guidelines in their own diets.

Eating right: Good medicine

Nutrition scientists can't always say precisely which foods affect the risk of which diseases, and to what degree. Establishing the connection between diet and disease is a complicated business. Some studies have

compared countries that differ in both diet and disease rates, but such research can't establish cause and effect. Other studies have compared the diets of individuals with a particular disease, such as cancer or heart disease, to those of healthy people; but those studies rely on their subjects' ability to recall eating patterns from years ago. Clinical trials that require people to change their diets over a long period of time are more conclusive, but are difficult and expensive to perform. Finally, diet is only one component in the development of disease; heredity, environment, and lifestyle all join in the equation, and interact with diet in ways that are not completely understood.

Despite the many contradictions in nutrition research, the lines of evidence have converged to suggest an approach to eating that's consistent with overall good health and protection from a range of chronic diseases. "This is a nice coincidence," says Dimitrios V. Trichopoulos, chairman of epidemiology at the Harvard School of Public Health. "Although there's plenty of disagreement about what causes specific diseases, we all come to the same conclusion with respect to a healthy diet."

The kind of diet outlined by our experts represents precisely that consensus. Cutting back on high-fat

STILL SAYING 'CHEESE'

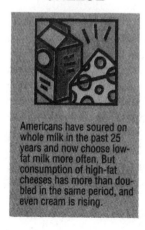

Americans have soured on whole milk in the past 25 years and now choose low-fat milk more often. But consumption of high-fat cheeses has more than doubled in the same period, and even cream is rising.

foods makes room for high-carbohydrate foods and also lowers calories. A low-fat, high-carbohydrate diet should also provide the vitamins and minerals you need in amounts that meet the U.S. Recommended Daily Allowances, or U.S. RDAs, set by the Government.

The sections that follow cover our recommendations for major parts of an "ideal" diet, based on what our experts said and our own review of the literature. The accompanying report ("Eating Right, It's Easier Than You Think") gives some practical advice on ways to meet these dietary goals.

FAT: NUTRIENT NON GRATA

Recommendations: *Keep total fat intake at or below 20 to 25 percent of calories and saturated fat at 7 percent of calories or less. As a second priority, try to keep dietary cholesterol at or below 200 to 300 milligrams per day.*
The Governments's Dietary Guidelines and other major health advisories aim to whittle the amount of calories from fat in the average American's diet to 30 percent. But that standard seems to have been established by pragmatic considerations as much as by science.

Our nutrition experts believe that the 30 percent limit on fat is far from ideal. Most of them believe that fat

FEWER HENS A-LAYING

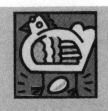

Eggs have been on a down-hill roll for 45 years due to their high cholesterol content. But chickens and other poultry are in greater demand than ever as a substitute for higher-fat red meat.

WHO WE SURVEYED

The experts we surveyed included members of the following committees and groups, which have been highly influential in setting nutrition policy over the last decade.
■ Committee on Diet and Health, National Research Council
■ Senior editorial advisors, The Surgeon General's Report on Nutrition and Health
■ Food and Nutrition Board committees for the Tenth Edition of the Recommended Dietary Allowances
■ Dietary Guidelines Advisory Committee, U.S. Department of Agriculture and Department of Health and Human Services
■ American Cancer Society, work study group on diet, nutrition, and cancer
■ American College of Nutrition, officers and directors
■ American Dietetic Association, nutrition research group
■ American Heart Association, nutrition committee of the scientific councils
■ Council of the American Society of Clinical Nutrition

should be cut to 25 percent of calories or less, and more than two-fifths of them would aim for 20 percent or less. The experts are especially stern on the subject of saturated fat, which is found primarily in meat and dairy products, and they recommend restrictions on dietary cholesterol, which comes almost entirely from those foods.

Several lines of scientific evidence support those recommendations. First, our nutrition experts believe there is strong evidence that high-fat foods are a significant cause of weight gain. The experts also believe that a high-fat diet boosts the risk of cancer, but there is disagreement on the evidence as to whether or not reducing fat intake would lower the cancer risk.

That uncertainty mirrors the state of research on fat and cancer. For the U.S. and other countries where fat contributes a large proportion of calories, overall cancer rates are high. That's particularly true for cancer of the breast, colon, and prostate. But studies comparing groups of individuals haven't shown a consistent link between fat and cancer. Two major

studies now being planned—one by the National Institutes of Health, one by a group of European researchers—will provide more precise data, but not before the end of the century.

The most extensive research on the hazards of a high-fat diet has focused on heart disease, and our experts' advice to cut back on fat clearly leans heavily on this work. Our experts agree the evidence is very strong that a diet high in total fat, saturated fat, and cholesterol increases the risk of coronary heart disease. In essence, the theory says that those dietary factors can increase the level of blood cholesterol, which can clog the arteries; and blockages in the coronary arteries, which supply the heart muscle with blood, can cause a heart attack. Here's how our nutrition experts evaluate the evidence on those three factors:

Saturated fat. Our experts, like most nutritionists, firmly believe that cutting back on saturated fat can lower heart-disease risk. Reducing saturated fat has been shown to lower blood-cholesterol levels, and studies using drug therapy show

PYRAMID POWER

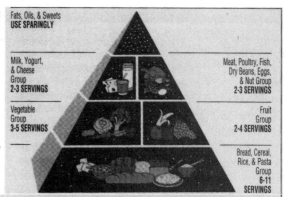

Fats, Oils, & Sweets
USE SPARINGLY

Milk, Yogurt,
& Cheese
Group
2-3 SERVINGS

Meat, Poultry, Fish,
Dry Beans, Eggs,
& Nut Group
2-3 SERVINGS

Vegetable
Group
3-5 SERVINGS

Fruit
Group
2-4 SERVINGS

Bread, Cereal,
Rice, & Pasta
Group
**6-11
SERVINGS**

Last spring, the U.S. Department of Agriculture officially launched the Food Guide Pyramid, right, to give visual punch to the Government's latest dietary guidelines. Below, with help from an American Dietetic Association representative, we've taken the Pyramid a step further: Within each food group we've listed items that are a good choice anytime, foods that nutritionists advise eating once in a while, and foods that should be considered an indulgence or eaten in very small amounts. Foods are categorized with the goal of keeping fat and cholesterol low, limiting excess sodium and sugar, and providing adequate levels of vitamins, minerals, and fiber. All foods in the "Choose often" column get fewer than 30 percent of calories from fat. We've listed no foods from the tip of the Pyramid, which represents salad dressings and oils, butter, margarine, soft drinks, candies, and desserts—high-calorie foods that should all be kept to a minimum. For more advice on choosing foods, see page 117.

Choose often	Choose sometimes	Choose rarely (or in very small amounts)
MILK, YOGURT, & CHEESE GROUP: 2 to 3 Servings		
Skim and 1% lowfat milk	2% lowfat milk	Whole milk
Buttermilk made with skim or 1% lowfat milk	Buttermilk made with 2% lowfat milk	
Yogurt made with skim or 1% lowfat milk	Yogurt made with 2% lowfat milk	Yogurt made with whole milk
	Hot cocoa or chocolate milk from skim or 1% milk	Hot cocoa or chocolate milk from 2% milk
	Puddings made with skim or 1% milk	Puddings made with 2% or whole milk
1% lowfat or dry-curd cottage cheese	2% cottage cheese	Creamed or regular (4% fat) cottage cheese
Cheeses with 2 or fewer grams of fat per ounce	Cheeses with 3 to 5 grams of fat per ounce	Cheeses with more than 5 grams of fat per ounce
Frozen dairy desserts with 2 grams of fat or less per item or per ½-cup serving	Frozen dairy desserts with 3 to 5 grams of fat per item or per ½-cup serving	Ice cream and frozen dairy desserts with more than 5 grams of fat per item or per ½-cup serving
MEAT, POULTRY, FISH, DRY BEANS, EGGS, & NUTS GROUP: 2 to 3 Servings		
Beef: Eye of round, top round	Beef: Tip or bottom round, sirloin, chuck arm pot roast, top loin, tenderloin, flank, T-bone steak	Beef: Porterhouse steak, brisket, chuck blade roast, rib-eye, ribs, short ribs, ground beef (even "lean" or "extra lean"), liver, corned beef, pastrami, bologna, salami, frankfurters
Veal: All cuts except loin, rib, and ground	Veal: Loin, rib chop, ground	
Pork: Tenderloin	Pork: Sirloin chop, top or center loin chop, rib chop, ham, Canadian bacon	Pork: Blade steak, bacon, pepperoni, sausage, frankfurters, bologna, salami
Lamb: Foreshank	Lamb: Shank half, leg, sirloin half, loin chop	Lamb: Rib chop, arm, blade, shoulder, ground lamb
Chicken breast without skin; turkey breast or leg; turkey wing without skin; ground turkey without skin	Chicken breast with skin; chicken leg, thigh, or wing without skin; turkey wing with skin	Chicken leg, thigh, or wing with skin; chicken liver; ground turkey with skin; duck and goose; poultry frankfurters
Poultry cold cuts with up to 1 gram of fat per ounce	Poultry cold cuts with 2 grams of fat per ounce	Poultry cold cuts, 3 or more grams of fat per ounce
All fresh fish and shellfish	Smoked fish	
Canned fish, water-packed, drained	Canned fish, oil-packed, drained	
All dried beans, peas, and lentils	Soybeans, tofu	Nuts, peanuts, and other nut butters
Egg whites	Egg substitutes	Whole eggs or yolks
VEGETABLE GROUP: 3 to 5 Servings		
Fresh vegetables or frozen vegetables without sauce	Canned vegetables, vegetable juices	Frozen vegetables in sauce
FRUIT GROUP: 2 to 4 Servings		
All fresh fruit (except avocado and olives)	Dried fruit, fruit juices	Avocado, olives
	Canned fruit in its own juice	Canned fruit in heavy syrup
Unsweetened applesauce		Sweetened applesauce
BREAD, CEREAL, RICE, & PASTA GROUP: 6 to 11 Servings		
Bread, bagels, pita	Egg breads, such as challah and egg bagels; French toast; pancakes; waffles	Bread stuffing, croissants
Muffins, biscuits, or rolls with 2 or fewer grams of fat (e.g., English muffins, hamburger buns)	Muffins, biscuits, and rolls with 3 to 4 grams of fat each	Muffins, biscuits, and rolls with more than 4 grams of fat each
Unbuttered air-popped popcorn, pretzels, rice cakes, bread sticks		Oil-popped and/or buttered popcorn
Corn tortillas	Flour tortillas	
Crackers with 1 gram or less of fat per ½ ounce: Melba toast, matzoh, flatbread, saltines	Crackers with 2 grams of fat per ½ ounce, such as graham crackers	Crackers with 3 or more grams of fat per ½ ounce, such as Ritz crackers
Cold cereals with 2 or fewer grams of fat and 6 or fewer grams of sugar per serving (e.g., Cheerios, corn flakes, shredded wheat, Grape Nuts)	Cold cereals high in sugar or fat (e.g., granola)	
Hot cereals		
Rice, barley, bulgur wheat, couscous, kasha, quinoa		
Pasta	Egg noodles	

WHAT'S IN A SERVING? Here's how the USDA calculates serving sizes. **Milk, yogurt, and cheese:** 1 cup of milk or yogurt, 1½ ounces of natural cheese, or 2 ounces of process cheese. **Meat:** 2 to 3 ounces of cooked lean meat, fish, or poultry; 1 to 1½ cups of cooked dry beans, 2 to 3 eggs, and 4 to 6 tablespoons of peanut butter. **Vegetables:** 1 cup of raw, leafy vegetables, ½ cup of other vegetables (cooked or chopped raw), or ¾ cup of vegetable juice. **Fruit:** 1 medium apple, banana, or orange; ½ cup of chopped, cooked, or canned fruit; ¾ cup of fruit juice. **Bread, cereal, rice, and pasta:** 1 slice of bread, 1 ounce of ready-to-eat cereal, or ½ cup of cooked cereal, rice, or pasta.

Consultant: Gail A. Levey, M.S. R.D., spokesperson, American Dietetic Association

that reducing blood cholesterol does reduce the risk of heart attack. Our experts' recommendation is, ideally, to restrict saturated fat to 7 percent of total calories—less than the 10 percent advised by other nutrition committees—and to sharply limit intake of red meat, a major source of saturated fat in the diet, to no more than three small servings per week.

Total fat. The heart-disease risk posed by a high total fat intake is somewhat ambiguous. Nevertheless, our nutrition experts do recommend strict limits on total fat, to prevent heart disease as well as obesity and cancer. Reducing overall fat will generally also lower the amount of saturated fat in the diet. And several studies have shown that even a moderately low-fat diet—one that supplies 30 percent of calories from fat—can reduce blood-cholesterol levels by about 10 percent, which translates into a 20 percent reduction in heart-disease risk.

In follow-up interviews, several experts said they were particularly impressed by recent studies that use X-rays to directly measure changes in the size of arterial blockages. These studies show significantly fewer new blockages in people eating a low-fat diet.

Cholesterol. Cholesterol from food is known to have less impact on heart disease than does saturated fat. Generally, the more cholesterol you eat, the less your body produces, a feedback mechanism that helps keep blood-cholesterol levels in check. For about one out of five people, however, that process doesn't work efficiently: When fed cholesterol-rich meals that are low in fat, these people still have a significant rise in the body's cholesterol count.

Since there's no easy way to determine who is a cholesterol "responder," public-health officials recommend limiting dietary cholesterol to 300 milligrams a day, a little more than the amount in one egg yolk. Our nutrition experts generally endorse that limit, or an even lower one: About half of them recommend less than 200 milligrams of cholesterol a

day and no more than three egg yolks a week. Overall, however, our experts' own assessment of the evidence suggests that reducing dietary cholesterol is less crucial than cutting back on total fat and saturated fat.

Recently, several independent studies have suggested that people with total cholesterol levels below 160—a very low level for Americans—have a higher-than-normal risk of death from a number of causes, including hemorrhagic stroke, liver cancer, lung disease, suicide, and alcoholism. These connections are still much less well established than the link between high cholesterol and heart disease, however, and the cause-and-effect relationship between low cholesterol and these causes of death remains unclear.

Two of the studies showing a risk from low blood cholesterol have been published since our survey. When our experts answered the questionnaire, however, they believed the evidence linking low cholesterol levels to cancer or violent death was very weak—weaker than almost all of the other proposed diet-health connections we asked them to evaluate.

'GOOD' FATS: NO FISH STORY

Recommendations: *Obtain most of the fat you eat in the form of unsaturated fats. Eat fish at least twice a week—but skip fish-oil capsules.*

For decades, researchers have known that a diet high in polyunsaturated fats—the kind that predominate in most vegetable oils—can lower blood-cholesterol levels when substituted for saturated fats. Even so, they have been reluctant to recommend a dramatic increase in polyunsaturates. Very high proportions of polyunsaturated fats in the diet have been linked to cancer in animal studies. Because no country's diet is naturally high in these fats, and because no large population has ever been on a high-polyunsaturate diet for long, there's no way to know if such a diet would pose any risk to people eating it over a lifetime.

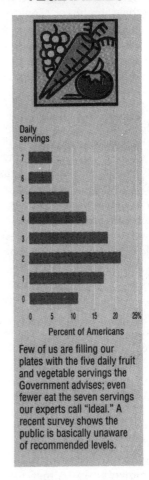

FRUITS & VEGETABLES

Daily servings

Percent of Americans

Few of us are filling our plates with the five daily fruit and vegetable servings the Government advises; even fewer eat the seven servings our experts call "ideal." A recent survey shows the public is basically unaware of recommended levels.

On average, Americans now get about 7 percent of their calories from polyunsaturated fats, and that seems to be a fairly good benchmark. Our nutrition experts generally believe the evidence linking polyunsaturates to cancer is weak, and they see little reason to worry. There's also widespread agreement in the nutrition community that monounsaturated fat—the kind of fat that predominates in olive and canola oil—helps lower blood cholesterol when it is used in place of saturated fats. Diets that are relatively high in monounsaturated fat, such as the traditional Mediterranean diet, appear to be safe.

In recent years, much attention has focused on a special kind of polyunsaturated fat: omega-3 fatty acids, found in some fish oils. The omega-3s first came under scrutiny with the discovery that heart disease is rare among the Greenland Eskimos, who dine liberally on fatty fish and whale blubber. Many studies later, we know that omega-3 fatty acids reduce blood levels of triglycerides—fats that contribute to heart disease—and reduce the body's tendency to form blood clots, which can trigger a heart attack.

Those findings have piqued interest in fish-oil capsules to prevent heart disease. But taking enough fish oil to keep up with the Eskimos would be costly, and it could leave you vulnerable to hemorrhagic stroke and bleeding disorders. Nearly all our nutrition experts said fish-oil supplements weren't necessary.

A solid majority of our experts do recommend eating fish two or more times a week. In addition to being a natural source of omega-3s—which are particularly high in salmon, mackerel, whitefish, shad, bluefish, and canned white tuna—fish is a good source of protein and low in saturated fat. (Women who are pregnant or planning to become pregnant should probably avoid salmon, swordfish, bluefish, and lake whitefish, which tend to accumulate toxic contaminants like mercury and PCBs; see CONSUMER REPORTS, February 1992.)

CARBOHYDRATES: PRAISE FOR POTATOES AND BROCCOLI

Recommendations: *Eat at least seven servings of fruits and vegetables a day. Eat at least six servings of grain products a day. Obtain more than half your daily calories from carbohydrates.*
Last July, with much fanfare, the National Cancer Institute launched a five-year, $18-million effort to encourage Americans to eat at least five servings of fruits and vegetables daily. A majority of our experts believe seven a day would be a better goal. A serving can be as small as a medium-sized banana or a half-cup of cooked vegetables. (See "What's in a serving?").

Fruits and vegetables have emerged as heroes of the healthy diet. Despite justified concerns over pesticide residues, which demand strict regulation, the health benefits of eating fresh produce vastly outweigh any pesticide risk.

Our experts believe there is moderate to very strong evidence that a diet rich in fruits and vegetables reduces the risk of certain cancers. They also believe that cruciferous vegetables such as broccoli and cauliflower can be especially helpful in preventing cancer. A recent review of 156 studies, published in the journal Nutrition and Cancer, supports their views. In 128 of the studies, fruits and vegetables offered significant protection against cancers of the lung, colon, breast, cervix, esophagus, oral cavity, stomach, bladder, pancreas, and ovaries.

Fruits and vegetables are thought to provide cancer protection on several fronts: They're good sources of antioxidant vitamins; several seem to contain other, specific anticancer compounds; and all are good sources of dietary fiber. The last benefit is one that they share with other high-carbohydrate foods, the grains and legumes.

Fiber, the indigestible portion of plants, can be divided into two basic types, soluble and insoluble. Every plant food contains a mixture of both kinds of fiber, though one type often predominates.

Soluble fiber made headlines a few years ago when oat bran—a good source of soluble fiber—was reported to reduce blood-cholesterol levels, a claim that food companies rapidly exploited. Hype aside, our nutrition experts say that there's moderately strong evidence that a diet rich in soluble fiber—also found in strawberries, brussels sprouts, beans, and lentils, among other foods—can reduce blood-cholesterol levels. But the degree of benefit may be modest. An analysis of 10 clinical trials, published recently in the Journal of the American Medical Association, showed that eating oat-bran cereal or oatmeal every day can lower blood cho-

lesterol by 2 to 3 percent on average.

Insoluble fiber, abundant in wheat-bran cereals, whole-grain breads, and the skins of fruits and root vegetables, can prevent or help relieve constipation by adding bulk to waste and speeding it through the intestines. That effect could also help explain the purported link between a high-fiber diet and a low rate of colon cancer. However, our experts generally believe the evidence on fiber and cancer prevention is less strong than the evidence that fiber can help prevent heart disease.

Half our experts endorse the National Cancer Institute's recommendation that Americans eat 20 to 35 grams of fiber a day. But ultimately, it's less practical to count grams of fiber than to follow the more general advice to eat large amounts of fruits, vegetables, and grains.

PROTEIN: PRO AND CON

Recommendation: *Don't worry about protein one way or the other.*
Most Americans eat at least as much protein as they need: The average American gets somewhat more than the U.S. RDA of 65 grams. Even vegetarians consume plenty of protein, as long as they take in enough calories and eat a varied diet, including whole grains, legumes, seeds, nuts, and vegetables.

Scientists have recently been more concerned about the risks of eating too much protein than about protein deficiency. The concern comes largely from studies showing that populations eating large amounts of animal protein have a high incidence of coronary heart disease and colon or breast cancer. The evidence is inconsistent, and confounded by the fact that high-protein foods, meat and dairy products, for example, are often high in fat and saturated fat as well. Nevertheless, a possible risk from excess animal protein can't yet be ruled out.

Our nutrition experts agree that Americans should not increase the amount of protein they eat—and any significant decrease in the average protein intake would bring it below the U.S. RDA. In short, protein is one nutrient that most people get in just about the right amount.

VITAMINS AND MINERALS: GETTING THE ESSENTIALS

Recommendations: *Eat grains, certain vegetables, fish, poultry, and occasionally meat for iron; low-fat dairy foods for adequate calcium; and a variety of fruits and vegetables, especially those high in antioxidants. Some women of childbearing age may need iron supplements. Women at risk for osteoporosis should consider calcium supplements.*

In general, our experts believe it's possible to get sufficient amounts of key vitamins and minerals—iron, calcium, and antioxidant vitamins—from a well-balanced diet alone. However, they acknowledge that iron and calcium supplements may help some people.

Iron. This mineral is a key component of hemoglobin, the compound in the blood that ferries oxygen to the organs and muscles. If the mineral is lacking in the diet, the body's iron reserves dwindle, and iron deficiency eventually sets in. As the iron deficiency deepens, hemoglobin production drops, resulting in anemia, with loss of energy and appetite, weakness, and shortness of breath. The capacity for physical work diminishes and concentration flags.

Iron deficiency is considered to be the nation's most common nutritional deficiency. According to a national survey, iron deficiency affects up to 9 percent of infants; 12 percent of adolescent boys, who need extra iron for growth spurts; and up to 14 percent of women aged 15 to 44, who lose iron in menstrual blood. Surveys of food consumption show an even wider problem: In a 1985–86 survey, more than 90 percent of infants and premenopausal women, and half of young children, were getting less than the Government's recommended levels of dietary iron. Although the body can compensate for a low iron intake to some degree,

SOURCES OF IRON

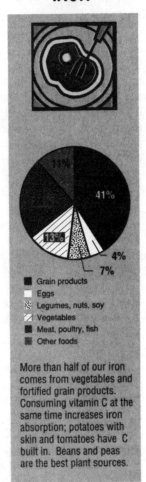

- ■ Grain products
- □ Eggs
- ▓ Legumes, nuts, soy
- ◿ Vegetables
- ▨ Meat, poultry, fish
- ▦ Other foods

More than half of our iron comes from vegetables and fortified grain products. Consuming vitamin C at the same time increases iron absorption; potatoes with skin and tomatoes have C built in. Beans and peas are the best plant sources.

a chronically low intake increases the risk that clinical deficiency can develop.

Our nutrition experts believe it's possible for most people to satisfy their iron requirements through diet alone—even a diet that plays down red meat. Poultry and fish also provide iron in a form readily absorbed by the body. And just a small amount of meat, fish, or poultry in a meal, or some vitamin C, will boost the absorption of iron from sources like beans, grains, and green leafy vegetables. Our experts do acknowledge that iron supplements at U.S. RDA levels may be necessary for some people with above-average iron needs—women with excessive menstrual bleeding, pregnant or lactating

women, and people with certain medical conditions.

Calcium. Recommendations for calcium intake have ping-ponged in the past decade, reflecting inconsistencies in the research on calcium and bone loss. Two facts are clear, however: Chronic low calcium intake is almost certainly connected to osteoporosis, severe bone loss that affects 15 to 20 million Americans and that accounts for 1.3 million fractures a year. And many of the people most vulnerable to osteoporosis, especially women, are getting far less calcium than they need.

In the past few years, scientists have recognized the importance of getting high levels of calcium during the years that bones grow larger and heavier, up to about age 35, to help bones reach their maximum mass. After age 35, bones gradually lose

LOW ON CALCIUM

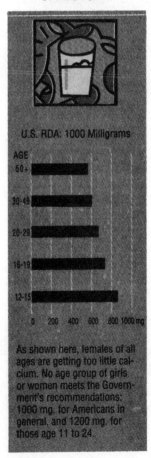

As shown here, females of all ages are getting too little calcium. No age group of girls or women meets the Government's recommendations: 1000 mg. for Americans in general, and 1200 mg. for those age 11 to 24.

heft, as the normal process of bone-tissue breakdown accelerates. In women, bone loss speeds up significantly after menopause. Soon after menopause, additional calcium does little for bone strength unless it is accompanied by estrogen replacement therapy. But one recent study of women at least five years past menopause found that a daily calcium supplement did slow bone loss.

As with iron, calcium supplements may be necessary for some groups of people. The National Institutes of Health now recommends 1500 milligrams of calcium a day—an amount 50 percent higher than the U.S. RDA, and a level virtually impossible to achieve without supplements—for post-menopausal women who have risk factors for osteoporosis: women who are thin, who smoke, who drink large amounts of alcohol, who get little weight-bearing exercise, or who have a family history of the disease. White and Asian women are at higher risk than are African-American women.

Our experts' recommendation is even a bit broader. By a slight majority, they recommend supplements to bring daily calcium intake above 1000 milligrams for all women at special risk for osteoporosis, whether or not

INVISIBLE SALT

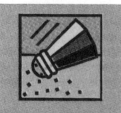

Ounce for ounce, some ready-to-eat cereals have almost three times as much sodium as salted potato chips. Luncheon meats, process cheeses, and canned soups and vegetables are also high. Restaurant menus signal high-sodium items with terms such as smoked, barbecued, and marinated.

they have yet gone through menopause. They do not recommend calcium supplements for the public at large, but they strongly advise everyone to get enough calcium in the diet, presumably by relying on low-fat dairy products.

Antioxidants. Nutrition researchers have recently focused attention on substances known as antioxidants, including beta-carotene and vitamins C and E. Laboratory studies have shown that these substances may play a role in protection from cancer, heart disease, and other disorders. Population studies show that groups eating foods high in these substances tend to have lower rates of those diseases, and some small clinical studies have also shown benefits from antioxidant supplements.

Some researchers have recently suggested that the greatest benefit may come from taking in more antioxidants than the U.S. RDA specifies. (The U.S. RDA is 60 milligrams for vitamin C and 30 IU for vitamin E; there is no U.S. RDA for beta-carotene, but 6 milligrams is equivalent to the U.S. RDA for vitamin A.) Our experts aren't convinced that the evidence warrants taking antioxidants in pill or capsule form as supplements. However, almost half of them do advise trying to get higher-than-RDA levels by eating fruits and vegetables that are rich in antioxidants, such as sweet potatoes, spinach, broccoli, kale, cantaloupe, strawberries, and citrus fruits.

SUGAR, SALT, COFFEE, AND ALCOHOL: NO TABOOS

Recommendations:
Sugar: Don't avoid it obsessively—but do go easy on high-sugar foods.
Salt: If you have or are at risk for developing high blood pressure, cut back on salt to minimize your risk.
Coffee: If your blood-cholesterol level is high, drink only drip-filtered coffee to be on the safe side.
Alcohol: One or two drinks a day is fine, but more is not better—and there's no reason to start if you're not a drinker.
These American favorites have been

THE NATION'S SWEET TOOTH

We've cut back on refined sugar in favor of artificial sweeteners, but corn syrups are liberally added to many processed foods. The use of caloric sweeteners has increased more than 16 percent on a per-person basis in the past two decades.

implicated in ills ranging from heart disease to juvenile delinquency. But they don't deserve such a shady reputation.

Sugar. It has long been accused of causing diabetes, depression, obesity, hyperactivity, and even criminal behavior. In fact, for most people, the only real problem sugar contributes to is tooth decay.

While sugar is not a nutritional demon, however, there are good reasons to eat it in moderation. Each year, the average American eats tens of thousands of calories' worth of sugars in candy, sweetened snacks, soft drinks, and such. These sugars provide "empty" calories that contribute energy but nothing else. And many sweet foods such as ice cream and cookies are also high in fat, which is a major player in weight gain. For those reasons, Government guidelines continue to urge people to rein in their taste for sweets, and our experts tend to agree. Half of them recommend reducing the average intake of added sugars to 5 percent of calories, from the current average of 11 percent.

Salt. An antisalt sentiment has been part of public-health guidelines for two decades. The sodium in salt is clearly a problem for about half of the 60 million people in the U.S. with high blood pressure, whose blood pressure changes in response to the amount of sodium in their diet. Since sodium can also interfere with the action of blood-pressure drugs, even patients who aren't naturally salt-sensitive may benefit from cutting back on salt if they are taking medication.

Most of our experts agree with the National Research Council, which advises all Americans to reduce salt intake to less than 6 grams a day (about 1½ teaspoons), which contains 2400 milligrams of sodium—roughly half the current national average intake. Half our experts believe an ideal level would be only 4.5 grams of salt.

Increasingly, however, medical authorities are soft-pedaling such recommendations, as evidence shows that salt may not be the widespread health threat once believed. Although salt does pose problems for certain high-risk groups, there's little evidence that salty diet can cause high blood pressure in people who are not already prone to it, or that restricting salt will prevent it. Four years ago, the 32-nation Intersalt Study—a rigorous investigation of more than 10,000 people—found that salt intake had only a minor influence on blood pressure in most populations, except those whose overall salt consumption is very low.

While there's no apparent harm in restricting salt intake as our experts suggest, CU's own medical consultants believe that cutting back on sodium is beneficial only for people who have hypertension or are at risk of developing it—those who have a family history of the disease, or are overweight or elderly. African-Americans also have a higher-than-average genetic risk of salt-sensitive high blood pressure. Chances are that everyone else can safely keep the salt shaker on the table.

Coffee. Over the past three decades, some studies have linked America's favorite morning beverage to high blood-cholesterol levels, while other reports have failed to find a link. Recent research may explain why: Studies showing the most con-

sistent link between coffee and cholesterol have come from Norway, where people prepare coffee by boiling it. When researchers compare the effects of boiled coffee to filtered coffee, as several studies now have, only boiled coffee raises blood cholesterol. Apparently, filtering removes some still-unidentified component that has potent cholesterol-raising effects. Most studies now show that moderate amounts of filtered coffee—up to five cups a day—are safe. (Unfortunately, no major studies have yet been done on cholesterol and percolated or instant coffee.)

Our experts agree there's little evidence that drinking coffee—caffeinated or not—increases the risk of coronary heart disease. A slight majority believes it would be ideal to limit caffeinated coffee to two cups a day, but that's not an urgent goal for most people. You probably don't need to skip coffee breaks—unless caffeine gives you the jitters or you have medical problems such as stomach ulcers or an irregular heartbeat.

Alcohol. One of the most consistent research findings in the diet-health arena has the medical community in a quandary: It seems that having one or two alcoholic drinks a day reduces the risk of heart disease. (One drink is equivalent to 12 ounces of beer, 5 ounces of wine, or 1½ ounces of spirits.) Alcohol appears to raise levels of HDL cholesterol, the protective component of blood cholesterol that is difficult to improve by other dietary means. However, research has not been conducted to show that raising HDL levels actually reduces heart-disease risk. And alcohol abuse is a major public-health problem.

For those reasons, no one is eager to advise the public to take up drinking for health. Although half of our experts believe there is strong evidence for the health benefits of moderate alcohol intake, virtually none recommend that people purposely start drinking, even in moderation, to reduce heart-disease risk.

"If we recommend a drink or two a day, people will think four or five are better," says Peter Kwiterovich,

chief of the lipid research and atherosclerosis unit at the Johns Hopkins School of Medicine. But like many clinicians, he tells patients who already take one or two drinks a day that it probably won't hurt and may indeed help. All our experts agree, however, that pregnant women and people with a personal or family history of alcohol abuse should abstain.

WEIGHT CONTROL: WHO SHOULD SCALE DOWN?

Recommendations: *Consider losing weight if you fall above the ranges recommended in the Dietary Guidelines for Americans, if your waistline is larger than you hip measurement, or if you have a medical problem that might be helped by losing weight.*

The extra pounds many Americans carry can increase the risk of hypertension, diabetes, and other disorders. Scientists disagree about how many pounds are really extra, and whether or not it's harmful to gain small amounts of weight as you age. Several tables of recommended weights for people of different heights have now been developed. By a small margin, our nutrition ex-

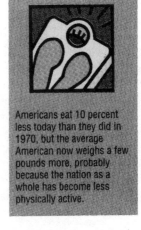

EATING LESS, WEIGHING MORE

Americans eat 10 percent less today than they did in 1970, but the average American now weighs a few pounds more, probably because the nation as a whole has become less physically active.

SUGGESTED WEIGHTS FOR ADULTS

Height [1]	Weight in pounds [2]	
	19 to 34 years	35 years and over
5' 0"	97-128	108-138
5' 1"	101-132	111-143
5' 2"	104-137	115-148
5' 3"	107-141	119-152
5' 4"	111-146	122-157
5' 5"	114-150	126-162
5' 6"	118-155	130-167
5' 7"	121-160	134-172
5' 8"	125-164	138-178
5' 9"	129-169	142-183
5' 10"	132-174	146-188
5' 11"	136-179	151-194
6' 0"	140-184	155-199
6' 1"	144-189	159-205
6' 2"	148-195	164-210
6' 3"	152-200	168-216
6' 4"	156-205	173-222
6' 5"	160-211	177-228
6' 6"	164-216	182-234

The higher weights in the ranges generally apply to men, who tend to have more muscle and bone; the lower weights more often apply to women, who have less muscle and bone.

[1] Without shoes.
[2] Without clothes.
Source: Dietary Guidelines for Americans.

perts prefer the tables that are presented in the Dietary Guidelines for Americans, which allow higher weights for people age 35 and above (see chart).

It's hard to lose a substantial amount of weight, however, and dieting poses risks of its own. So before you try to lose weight, try to determine how great a risk your weight really poses to your health, and how much weight you need to lose to lower that risk. Research shows that people who add bulk around the waist face a greater risk of chronic disease than do those who bulge at the hips and thighs. And people with diabetes and high blood pressure are particularly likely to improve their health when they shed extra pounds. Diabetes and hypertension often improve dramatically with a weight loss of 10 percent or

less. If you have one of these conditions, you may be able to improve your health even if you don't quite reach the weight the tables recommend.

Heredity and metabolism contrive to keep some people overweight despite their best efforts to reduce. For such people, striving to attain a "recommended" weight may be futile and even damaging to health. Nonetheless, like everyone else, such people would do well to follow a high-carbohydrate, low-fat diet and to exercise regularly. (Inactivity may play an even greater role in weight gain than a high-calorie diet does.) Those measures will both improve the odds of losing weight effectively and help maintain health at whatever weight one finally attains.

"It's important to realize that we can't all be skinny, but we can all try

to be healthy," says psychologist John Foreyt, director of the nutrition research clinic at Baylor College of Medicine in Houston. For people with a chronic weight problem, he says, "It's better to focus on healthy habits and get on with your life."

SUMMING UP: WHY IT'S WORTH THE EFFORT

Public-health officials underscore the dangers of eating high-fat, high-calorie foods by reminding us that diet is implicated in one-third of cancer deaths and a large proportion of heart attacks. For any individual, however, the risk in eating a typical American diet is less certain. "Individuals have different susceptibilities to disease, and each may be more vulnerable at one point than at another," says Kenneth K. Carroll, director of the Human Nutrition Center at the University of Western Ontario.

If your cholesterol count is normal, your blood pressure low, and your family tree free of cancer, heart disease, and diabetes, dietary change may seem like a low priority. Few people, however, are lucky enough to be free of risk factors for all the diseases that have been linked to diet. And even some people without those risk factors might be helped by changing what they eat.

Half of all heart attacks, for example, occur in people with "normal" blood-cholesterol levels. One theory holds that dietary fat and cholesterol may contribute directly to arterial deposits in these people, without ever showing up as elevated cholesterol in the blood. If so, then a low-fat, low-cholesterol diet would be prudent heart-disease prevention for anyone, not just those who are clearly at high risk.

The diet we've outlined offers global benefits. It provides a single protective umbrella that can lower the risk of a number of chronic diseases. Beyond disease prevention, it provides a recipe that can contribute to your overall fitness and health.

And, as we show in the following report, it offers a bounty of good-tasting food.

EATING RIGHT
IT'S EASIER
THAN YOU THINK

Moderate but consistent changes can improve your diet dramatically.

Misconceptions about dietary change seem to have deterred many Americans from taking steps to improve their diets. Consumers frequently tell researchers they don't want to give up the foods they like. Yet change need not mean sacrifice. "There's room in a healthy diet for what you love, in some amount, virtually every day," says Mary Abbott Hess, past president of the American Dietetic Association.

Choosing wisely

The menus [in this article], prepared with the help of an ADA representative, show how easily an "average" diet can be changed to follow our experts' recommendations for an "ideal" diet. And the list of foods on page 00 shows the wide range of foods you can eat to meet those goals.

Here are some additional tips for choosing foods to make more healthful meals:

■ Try low-fat products. Nearly 1000 food products introduced in 1990 were low-fat or fat-free. Food manufacturers have stripped the cholesterol from eggs and siphoned the fat from cheeses, cookies, salad dressing, and sour cream. If you can't find a substitute you like, stick with the real thing but use it sparingly. Since "light" or "low-fat" claims are often fanciful, you may want to calculate the percentage of calories from fat in some of the foods

you buy and compare different brands. Each gram of fat is nine calories; multiply the number of fat grams in a serving by nine and divide the result by the total calories.

■ Stay clear of deep-fried foods. Even the benefits of zucchini or mushrooms are compromised when they're breaded and fried.

■ Trim visible fat from meat before cooking and remove the skin from poultry. Bake, broil, or roast meats instead of frying them.

■ When you eat red meat, choose lean cuts. (They're more flavorful when cooked in a stir-fry or marinated in herbs mixed with tomato juice, vinegar, fat-free yogurt, or wine.) Most "light" hot dogs still get two-thirds or more of their calories from fat, and even extra-lean broiled hamburger gets 57 percent of its calories from fat.

■ Cook stews and soups a day early and chill. Then skim off fat.

■ Choose very flavorful ingredients so you can reduce the portions of fatty foods. Try extra-sharp cheddar on tacos, for example, or extra-virgin olive oil in salad dressing.

■ Opt for milk and yogurt more often than other dairy foods—they're richest in calcium.

■ If you're trying to limit your sodium intake, go easy on condiments such as soy sauce, steak sauce, or catsup, as well as pickles, olives, processed meats, and most cheeses and canned soups. Put canned tuna or canned vegetables in a colander and give them a two-minute shower to remove the sodium. Flavor foods with herbs, spices, or lemon juice, and cook with less salt.

■ Eat fruits and vegetables with their skins and peels intact for more fiber, and cook them minimally to preserve nutrients and flavor.

■ Keep cut raw vegetables in water in the refrigerator for snacks.

■ Add shredded carrots, tomatoes, or bean sprouts to sandwiches.

■ Put vegetables into casseroles, soups, salads, and pastas.

■ Add sliced fruits to cereals, frozen yogurts, plain yogurt, pancakes, and other foods.

■ Choose brown rice and whole-grain breads, cereals, and pastas for extra vitamins, minerals, and fiber.

A philosophy of food

The specific foods you serve should fit into an over-all plan for dietary change that is both workable and feasible. Here are some basic principles:

Balance your diet over the course of a week. If you aim to get 25 percent of your calories from fat, that doesn't mean every food or every meal has to meet that goal. Instead, try to meet dietary guidelines for fat, cholesterol, calcium, and the like over the course of several days. You need not, for example, deprive yourself of fried eggs for Sunday brunch if you see no more high-cholesterol foods for the week.

Don't keep a calculator by your plate. It's worthwhile to check food labels to keep a loose tally of what nutrients you're getting. But don't overdo it. If you eat the recommended number of servings and a variety of foods in each food group of the Food Guide Pyramid (see page 110), you'll get all the vitamins, minerals, and protein you need. If you select most foods from our "Choose Often" column, you'll also keep fat, cholesterol, and added sugars low.

Make room for your favorites. There's no need to feel deprived if your favorite foods are high in fat. Just keep portions small and limit other sources of fat.

Adopt a new eating style gradually. Think of a move toward low-fat, high-carbohydrate foods as a permanent change in eating style instead of a dieting regime that succeeds or fails. Experiment with new recipes and foods, with the understanding that you won't like them all. Sonja L. Connor, research associate professor at Oregon Health Sciences University, speaks of moving "from meat to beans in ten short years." Her point is to be easy on yourself if you find the transition difficult; it's likely that your tastes will gradually change so high-fat foods have less appeal.

MENU ALTERNATIVES

A more healthful diet doesn't have to leave you feeling hungry or deprived. Below, we've transformed two days' worth of standard American meals and snacks. The Typical meals, with familiar foods and reasonable portions, derive more than 40 percent of their calories from fat, an amount that's usual for many Americans. The Prudent meals substitute low-fat dressings, spreads, and dairy products, bring on fresh fruits and vegetables, and go for high-fiber grains. They are still familiar, filling, and tasty, and they meet the goals set by the Government's Dietary Guidelines for Americans. The Ideal meals make additional changes in the same direction, reaching the ideal levels of fat and carbohydrate advised by our experts. Here, fat is dramatically reduced, yet the essence of familiar American meals remains intact. For all meals, total calories are in a range appropriate to the average man; women would likely have smaller portions. Both days' menus provide close to or more than the U.S. RDA for all nutrients, with one exception: Typical meals on Day Two are slightly low in zinc and vitamin C.

DAY 1

Typical	Prudent	Ideal
BREAKFAST		
2 scrambled eggs in 1 tsp. butter 2 slices white toast with 1 tsp. butter, 1 tsp. jam 4 ounces orange juice 1 cup lowfat (2%) milk Coffee or tea	1 egg yolk, 2 whites scrambled in 1 tsp. soft margarine 2 slices whole-wheat toast with 1 tsp. soft margarine, 2 tsp. jam 8 ounces orange juice 1 cup lowfat (1%) milk Coffee or tea	3-egg-white Spanish omelet (tomato, peppers and onions) in 1 tsp. soft margarine 2 slices whole-grain toast with 1 tsp. soft margarine, 2 tsp. all-fruit preserves 1 cup strawberries 1 cup skim milk Coffee or tea
LUNCH		
Ham sandwich 3 ounces regular ham on white bread with 1 tbsp. mayonnaise, lettuce ⅓ cup potato salad 1 ounce tortilla chips	Ham sandwich 3 ounces extra-lean ham on whole-wheat bread, 1 tbsp. fat-free mayonnaise, lettuce, tomato ½ cup German potato salad 1 ounce pretzels	Turkey sandwich 2 ounces turkey breast on whole-grain bread, 1 tbsp. cranberry sauce, lettuce ½ cup three-bean salad and ½ cup carrot-raisin salad 1 ounce whole-wheat pretzels
SNACK		
1 ounce peanut brittle	4 fig bars	1 small bran muffin
DINNER		
4 ounces meat loaf with ¼ cup mushroom gravy Lettuce and tomato with 1 tbsp. regular blue-cheese dressing 1 biscuit ½ cup broccoli with 2 tbsp. cheese sauce ½ cup vanilla ice cream	3 ounces lean meat loaf with ¼ cup tomato sauce Mixed greens and tomato salad with 1 tbsp. low-calorie blue-cheese dressing 2 slices French bread with 1 tsp. soft margarine ½ cup steamed broccoli with 1 tsp. soft margarine ½ cup vanilla ice milk with 1 sliced fresh peach	1 cup spaghetti with 2 ounces extra-lean ground meat, ½ cup spaghetti sauce Mixed greens and tomato salad with 1 tbsp. fat-free blue-cheese dressing 1 whole-wheat roll with 1 tsp. soft margarine ½ cup broccoli with garlic sauteed in ½ tsp. olive oil ½ cup nonfat ice cream with 1 cup fresh fruit salad
LATE SNACK		
1 cup lowfat (2%) milk 2 small chocolate chip cookies	1 cup lowfat (1%) milk 6 vanilla wafers	1 cup skim milk 6 graham-cracker squares
TOTALS		
2239 calories 11 grams of fiber 777 milligrams of cholesterol	2211 calories 23 grams of fiber 353 milligrams of cholesterol	2230 calories 37 grams of fiber 116 milligrams of cholesterol

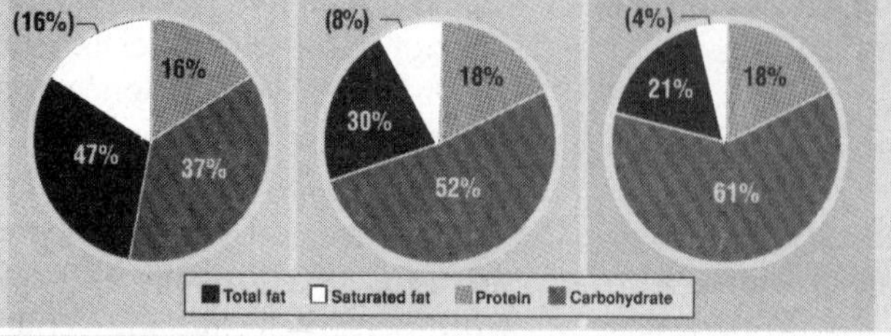
(16%)
16%
47%
37%
(8%)
18%
30%
52%
(4%)
21%
18%
61%
Total fat
Saturated fat
Protein
Carbohydrate

DAY 2

Typical	Prudent	Ideal
BREAKFAST		
1 cup corn flakes 4 ounces apple juice 1 cup lowfat (2%) milk Coffee or tea	1 cup wheat-flake cereal 1 banana 4 ounces orange juice 1 cup lowfat (1%) milk Coffee or tea	1 cup bran-flake cereal 1 cup blueberries 1 orange 1 cup skim milk Coffee or tea
MORNING SNACK		
1 glazed doughnut	1 small blueberry muffin; 1 tsp. margarine	1 bagel; 2 tsp. soft margarine; 1 tsp. jam
LUNCH		
Tuna sandwich 3 ounces oil-packed tuna, 2 tbsp. mayonnaise on white bread with lettuce ½ cup macaroni salad 1 ounce corn chips 1 slice apple pie	Tuna sandwich 2 ounces water-packed tuna, 2 tbsp. cholesterol-free mayonnaise on whole-wheat bread with lettuce, tomato ⅓ cup pasta salad 1 ounce tortilla chips 1 baked apple	Tuna sandwich 2 ounces water-packed tuna, 2 tbsp. light mayonnaise on thickly sliced whole-grain bread with lettuce, tomato ½ cup cucumber-onion salad and ½ cup tortellini-vegetable salad 1 ounce no-oil tortilla chips 1 apple
SNACK		
½ cup frozen yogurt	½ cup lowfat frozen yogurt	1 cup lowfat frozen yogurt with ½ cup fresh fruit salad
DINNER		
Baked ½ chicken breast and chicken drumstick with skin ½ cup french fries ½ cup canned green beans ½ cup chocolate pudding (2%) milk)	Baked ½ chicken breast and chicken drumstick without skin 1 cup mashed potatoes with lowfat (1%) milk, 1 tsp. soft margarine ½ cup steamed green beans with 1 tsp. soft margarine ½ cup chocolate pudding (1%) milk)	½ baked chicken breast without skin 1 baked potato with 2 tbsp. half-and-half sour cream topping 1 cup stir-fried vegetables with garlic in 1 tsp. oil ½ cup chocolate pudding (skim milk)
TOTALS		
2588 calories 9 grams of fiber 284 milligrams of cholesterol	2199 calories 20 grams of fiber 182 milligrams of cholesterol	2217 calories 36 grams of fiber 127 milligrams of cholesterol

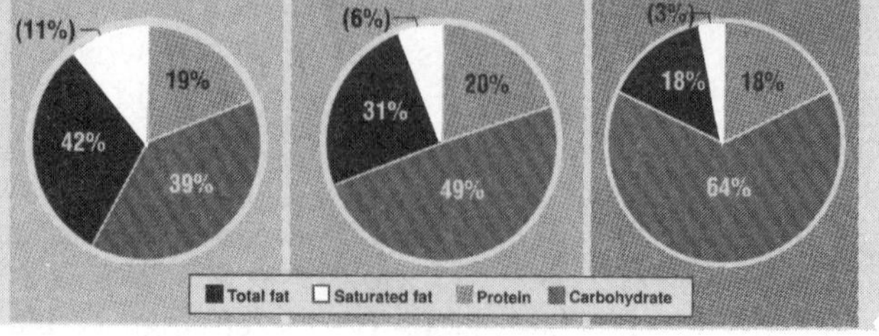
(11%)
19%
42%
39%
(6%)
20%
31%
49%
(3%)
18%
18%
64%
Total fat
Saturated fat
Protein
Carbohydrate

Consultant: Mindy Hermann, R.D., spokesperson, American Dietetic Association

To Salt OR Not to Salt –

Not a Simple Question

Mary Carole McMann

MARY CAROLE MCMANN, M.P.H., R.D./L.D., IS A FREELANCE WRITER LIVING IN HOUSTON, TX.

One might assume that there are good data to support recommendations for universal dietary change. In the case of salt restriction, this assumption is grossly mistaken.

SALT RESTRICTION TO REDUCE sodium is now a basic part of most dietary guidelines promulgated in the U.S., including those published in the Surgeon General's Report and by the American Heart Association and the National Research Council. Similar dietary guidelines have been published in many other countries. One might assume that there are good data to support recommendations for universal dietary change. In the case of salt restriction, this assumption is grossly mistaken.

The primary interest in sodium intake stems from its perceived role in high blood pressure — hypertension. Hypertension is both a disease and a risk factor for other serious diseases. It is one of three major risk factors for coronary heart disease. It is *the* major risk factor for stroke and is also a risk factor for kidney disease and congestive heart failure.

Beliefs Underlying Present Recommendations

The general recommendation to restrict sodium is based on several beliefs. The first involves people who actually are hypertensive. For these individuals it is assumed that sodium restriction is the best initial treatment. Furthermore, since many cases of hypertension go undiagnosed, general sodium reduction would benefit people who are unaware that they are hypertensive. It is generally thought that lowering blood pressure for these individuals reduces their risk of having a heart attack. The second belief focuses on healthy people. It assumes that sodium restriction may prevent them from developing hypertension. A third belief is that even if sodium restriction doesn't achieve the first two goals, it is a prudent measure that can't do any harm.

Undeniably there are studies that support these theories and highly respected, well-intentioned researchers who are convinced of their validity. However, there is a growing body of evidence challenging each of these beliefs.

Is Salt Reduction Good for All Hypertensive People?

Hypertension affects approximately 20 to 25 percent of the adult American population—about 50 million people. It is estimated that less than half of the hypertensive population is "salt sensitive," *i.e.*, can lower blood pressure by decreasing sodium intake, and the reduction must be drastic. Therefore, more than half the hypertensive people who try to reduce sodium will not benefit from this measure. In fact, those hypertensive individuals who are not salt sensitive can actually experience increased

From *Priorities*, Summer 1993, pp. 33-36. Reprinted with permission from *Priorities*, a publication of The American Council on Science and Health, Inc., New York, NY.

119

blood pressure in response to decreased sodium intake.

It is important that we learn to identify salt-sensitive people in the hypertensive population. Some studies have shown a higher prevalence of salt sensitivity in hypertensive individuals with a family history of hypertension; in those with higher initial blood pressures; and among obese, older patients and African-Americans. Other studies indicate that salt-sensitive individuals may have a higher heart rate or abnormalities in the mechanisms regulating calcium. Research is underway to detect factors associated with salt sensitivity that can help identify these individuals.

Almost all hypertension studies measure resting blood pressure. Broad rec-

More than half the hypertensive people who try to reduce sodium will not benefit from this measure.

ommendations based on these data may be invalid because these measurements do not represent blood pressure the majority of the time. One study investigated this problem by comparing the effect of high and of low salt intakes on both resting and ambulatory blood pressures in healthy and hypertensive individuals. Although hypertensive patients experienced a significant reduction of resting blood pressure while restricting sodium, their 24-hour ambulatory blood pressure readings were not significantly lower. Further analysis of round the clock blood pressure readings showed that there was a small, but significant lowering of blood pressure at night but no difference during the day. To what degree might the antihypertensive effect of sodium restriction have been overestimated in studies measuring only resting blood pressure?

Another argument for sodium restric-

tion in hypertensive patients is that it increases the efficacy of antihypertensive medications. Some, but not all, studies have shown sodium restriction to contribute to the effects of B-blockers and converting enzyme inhibitors; however, sodium restriction may actually increase blood pressure in people taking calcium channel blockers. Recent studies show that the addition of sodium restriction to diuretic therapy had little or no effect and may lead to dizziness, weakness, orthostatic hypotension and abnormally low concentrations of sodium and potassium in the blood.

Based on these uncertainties, it seems neither reasonable nor wise for physicians to prescribe sodium restriction as the first step in treating hypertensive patients. In addition, research has failed to prove that lowering blood pressure actually reduces the risk of heart attack.

Is Reducing Salt Good for the General Public?

Is recommending sodium restriction for everyone a reasonable public health measure? It has long been a basic tenet of medicine that people should only be treated for diseases that they actually have.

The rationale for recommending sodium restriction to the general public is based on epidemiological data showing the presence of both hypertension and a high sodium intake in the same populations. The inference from such studies is that a high sodium intake actually causes hypertension, but this has never been demonstrated. In fact, data from the Health and Nutrition Examination Survey I, obtained from more than 10,000 people who had no history of hypertension and had not changed their diet, showed just the opposite. Higher intakes of sodium, potassium and calcium were associated with a lower absolute risk of hypertension. Those people found to have hypertension had lower, not higher, sodium intakes.

Much has been said about the INTER-SALT study, which included more than 10,000 people from around the world.

Although the data showed a positive association between sodium intake and blood pressure in individual subjects within a center, the association disappeared when data across the centers were analyzed. In fact, the data indicated that other factors such as obesity, alcohol consumption and low intakes of potassium were more highly correlated with hypertension than was sodium intake.

Population studies can only suggest association. They can not prove cause and effect. For proof of a cause and effect relationship between sodium and hypertension, intervention studies in which blood pressures are observed during manipulation of sodium intake are necessary. In controlled studies, an increased sodium intake has not been shown to increase blood pressure in healthy people. The study of ambulatory blood pressure, mentioned previously, showed that sodium restriction had no effect on blood pressure in healthy people.

The possible effect of a high sodium intake on the risk of young people developing hypertension later in life is one area of concern prompting restriction guidelines. Research has shown that higher blood pressures in adolescents are closely related to hypertension in adults. Although certain individual young people have a hypotensive response to sodium restriction, the majority of data show that dietary salt intake has little effect on blood pressure even in children with elevated blood pressure at baseline. One seven-year study of children age 6 to 17 years showed associations between hypertension and both low calcium levels and a high sodium/potassium ratio but no association with sodium alone.

Is General Salt Reduction Harmless?

Finally, we examine the belief that sodium restriction is harmless. This unfounded belief is perhaps the most dangerous of all since it is the fallback position of those people who can't justify sweeping recommendations for the public in any other way. To weigh the possible benefits of universal sodium restriction against the potential risks,

It is not good public health practice to recommend general sodium restriction in the face of its effectiveness in only a limited number of hypertensive individuals and its possible adverse effects in those individuals who are not sodium sensitive.

the public needs to be aware of negative effects that may be associated with sodium restriction.

• Sodium restriction increases blood pressure in some hypertensive patients; it leads to an increased production of hormones that constrict blood vessels, thereby raising blood pressure.

• Sodium restriction results in increased plasma renin activity which, in turn, leads to stimulation of angiotensin II; since angiotensin II stimulates growth of the heart muscle, these reactions have been suggested as a pathogenic factor in cardiovascular damage.

• People who are not salt sensitive and who reduce their intake of sodium not only fail to lower blood pressure but also significantly increase their blood levels of total cholesterol, LDL-cholesterol (so-called "bad" cholesterol), uric acid and creatinine and tend to have lower blood insulin levels. Data from the Primary Prevention Trial in Goteborg, Sweden indicated that when antihypertensive therapy results in even a small increase in blood cholesterol levels, it has no effect on rates of coronary heart disease.

• A low salt intake significantly increases ambulatory heart rate — a risk factor for developing chronic heart disease.

• Salt restriction reduces the body's capacity to handle other stressful situations, such as sporadic physical activity, bleeding, diarrhea and/or vomiting and heat stress. This is of special concern in people who are ill, have diabetes or are elderly.

• A low-salt diet may lead to a reduction of other important nutrients, such as calcium, iron, magnesium and vitamin B_6.

• Unnecessary restriction of sodium intrudes on an individual's quality of life and often necessitates an increased expenditure for special foods.

• There is circumstantial evidence that a low-sodium diet may contribute to disturbed sleep patterns.

The Case for Calcium and Potassium

It is impossible to review current research on sodium and hypertension without becoming aware of the strong evidence for an association between this disease and low levels of calcium and/or potassium. For example, studies show that dietary salt loading may lead to elevated blood pressure by enhancing the excretion of calcium and potassium. It has been suggested that the salt sensitivity noted in African-Americans and elderly people with hypertension may actually be associated with a lower intake of calcium and potassium.

A study of 60,000 women, a subset of the Nurses Health Study, demonstrated that a calcium intake above 800 milligrams per day (Recommended Dietary Allowance for most adults) carried a reduced risk of developing hypertension when compared to an intake of less than 400 milligrams per day. Although hypertensive people with a low calcium intake may benefit from increasing their intake to 800 milligrams, there is no additional benefit from consuming more calcium from a supplement.

Dairy products provide about 80 percent of the calcium in the Western diet. African-Americans have a relatively high incidence of lactose (milk sugar) intolerance, a condition that limits the consumption of dairy products. Researchers have theorized that the connection between low calcium intake and hypertension may help explain the high incidence of hypertension in African-Americans. Some experts suggest that an adequate intake of calcium and potassium may actually protect people against salt sensitivity.

Faulty Public Policy

It is unfortunate that those who recognize the fallacy of a general recommendation for sodium restriction have not been as widely heard as those setting public policy. It is not good public health practice to recommend general sodium restriction in the face of its effectiveness in only a limited number of hypertensive individuals and its possible adverse effects in those individuals who are not sodium sensitive. When all of the known facts are considered, they clearly show that there is no justification for recommending salt restriction in the general population.

The new thinking about fats

As most people see it, fat is the nutritional villain, clogging the arteries and settling around the waist. Americans have one of the fattiest diets in the world: about 37% of our calories now come from fats, up from 32% at the start of the century. The largest portion of our fats comes from animal sources—especially meat and whole-milk dairy products—and is thus highly saturated and accompanied by cholesterol. Thanks to recent research, we now know that the fat scenario is more complicated than it once seemed. Are hydrogenated vegetable oils (found in margarines, for example) necessarily better for us than animal fats (such as butter)? Should we adopt a "Mediterranean diet" that is rich in olive oil? Here are answers to these and other questions.

What are fats? Why are they high in calories?

Technically called lipids, the fats in foods are mostly triglycerides, which consist of three fatty acids attached to a glycerol molecule. Fats are the most concentrated source of food energy, supplying nine calories per gram; carbohydrates and proteins have four calories per gram. High-fat foods are thus always high-calorie foods. And a high-fat diet may increase the chance of obesity, which in turn increases the risk of cardiovascular disease, diabetes, and other disorders.

What's the difference between saturated and unsaturated fats?

All fats are combinations of saturated and unsaturated fatty acids, which is why fats are described with terms such as "highly saturated." Fatty acids vary in length and in degree of saturation (that is, how many hydrogen atoms they carry), both of which help determine whether a fat is solid or liquid (oil) at room temperature.

Saturated fatty acids carry all the hydrogen atoms they can hold. Highly saturated fats come chiefly from animal sources and include butter, milk fat, and the fat in meats; two vegetable oils—coconut and palm kernel oils—are also highly saturated.

Unsaturated fatty acids do not have all the hydrogen atoms they can carry. If a pair of hydrogen atoms is missing, these fatty acids are called **monounsaturated** (olive, peanut, and canola oils are largely monounsaturated). If two pairs or more of hydrogen atoms are missing, the fatty acids are called **poly-**unsaturated (corn, safflower, and sesame oils are primarily polyunsaturated). Plants and fish are the important sources of unsaturated fats. These fats generally are liquid at room temperature.

Should I avoid all fat?

That would be very difficult—and undesirable. You need to consume some fat to stay healthy. For instance, it supplies "essential" fatty acids—so named because the body can't make them and must get them from foods—which are crucial for proper growth and development. Essential fatty acids are the raw materials for several hormonelike compounds, including prostaglandins, that help control vital bodily functions. However, you don't need to consume any *saturated* fatty acids; your body makes all it needs. Fat also aids in the absorption of the fat-soluble vitamins (A, D, E, and K) and helps maintain healthy skin and hair.

Are all saturated fats bad?

Highly saturated fats raise overall cholesterol levels in the blood, especially LDL ("bad") cholesterol. Yet even this seemingly clear-cut fact has been complicated by recent research that has examined the interactions of various fatty acids in the body. At least one saturated fatty acid, stearic acid (a major component of the fat in beef, pork, and the cocoa butter in chocolate), appears to have a neutral effect on blood cholesterol. However, this has little or no practical implication, since no one eats isolated stearic acid, except in laboratory studies. In any case, what may be true of stearic acid alone isn't true of sirloin steaks, burgers, pork chops, and other foods rich in stearic acid. These foods still have two strikes against them—they contain other saturated fatty acids (notably palmitic acid) that clearly raise cholesterol in the blood, and most are high in cholesterol.

Is cholesterol a fat?

No, though it is also classified as a lipid. Cholesterol is a vital part of all cell membranes and nerve fibers and serves as a building block for hormones. It is the cholesterol that circulates in the blood that is so often discussed and measured. That's because this cholesterol can accumulate in the walls of blood vessels, leading to atherosclerosis and possibly heart attack or stroke.

Comparing oils (one tablespoon)

All vegetable oils contain 120 calories and 13.5 grams of fat per tablespoon (butter and margarine have 100 calories and 11.5 grams per tablespoon; lard 115 calories and 13 grams of fat). Look for an oil that is low in saturated fatty acids and, preferably, high in monounsaturated fatty acids.

TYPE	UNSATURATED		SATURATED
	MONO (g)	POLY (g)	(g)
BEST			
Almond	10	2	1
Canola (rapeseed)	8	4	1
Olive	10	1	2
Peanut	6	5	2
GOOD			
Corn	3	8	2
Cottonseed	2	7	4
Safflower	2	10	1
Sesame	5	6	2
Soybean	3	8	2
Sunflower	3	9	1
Walnut	3	9	1
WORST			
Coconut	1	—	12
Palm	5	1	7
Palm kernel	2	—	11
Butter	3	1	7
Margarine, stick	5	4	2
Lard	6	2	5

Cholesterol is found only in foods from animal sources, such as meats, eggs, and dairy products, which are usually also rich in saturated fats. If it were simply a matter of the cholesterol from food going directly into our bloodstream, we would only have to worry about how much cholesterol we eat. But the liver usually synthesizes most of the cholesterol in the body—a process only partly regulated by the amount of cholesterol eaten. Surprisingly, the amount and type of fat you eat generally affects blood cholesterol levels much more than the cholesterol in the foods you eat. Thus limiting your cholesterol intake but not your consumption of saturated fats can result in high blood cholesterol.

What's wrong with safflower oil and other polyunsaturates?

Highly polyunsaturated vegetable oils—such as safflower, sunflower, and soybean—used to be considered the most healthful oils because they dramatically lower overall cholesterol levels, especially LDL. But in recent years nutritionists have focused on the possible negative effects of these oils. First of all, large amounts of highly polyunsaturated fats also lower HDL ("good") cholesterol, and scientists now believe that a *low* HDL level is an independent risk factor for heart disease (monounsaturates may not lower HDL as much). In addition, studies on animals have found that large amounts of highly polyunsaturated vegetable oils increase the risk of several types of cancer—but that's not necessarily true for humans. (For more on fat and cancer, see page 124.)

What are those hydrogenated fats in margarine?

Manufacturers hydrogenate—that is, add hydrogen atoms to—soybean, corn, and other liquid oils to make them more solid and stable. This gives margarines and some puddings a creamy consistency, for instance, and prolongs the shelf life of crackers, cookies, potato chips, and other foods that contain the semi-solid oils. Because they are less likely to turn rancid, hydrogenated oils are also often used to cook french fries in restaurants. Usually oils are only partially hydrogenated; totally hydrogenated oils are suitable for few foods. Depending on the degree of hydrogenation, these artificially saturated vegetable fats may be no better for you than comparably saturated animal fats.

Most important, hydrogenation transforms many of an oil's unsaturated fatty acids, making them more saturated and changing their structure in other subtle ways—they are thus called *trans* fatty acids. Scientists have been concerned that these trans fats may increase the risk of coronary artery disease and perhaps other health problems. While a diet high in regular unsaturated fat lowers total blood cholesterol, a diet high in trans fats lowers it much less—or may even raise it—by increasing LDL cholesterol. In addition, trans fats lower HDL cholesterol, the type that carries cholesterol out of the arteries. This may help explain why a study from Harvard published in March in *Lancet* found that women who ate lots of foods high in trans fatty acids (especially margarine) had a 50% higher risk of coronary artery disease than women who ate these fats rarely. Another study, reported in the *American Journal of Cardiology* in April, found that people with coronary artery disease have significantly elevated levels of trans fatty acids in their blood.

A few years back, the National Academy of Sciences concluded that there was little or no cause for concern about trans fats because they make up only a small amount of our fat intake. Critics claim, however, that in recent years Americans have been consuming two to three times as much trans fat as was previously estimated—especially since food makers, pressured to reduce the use of highly saturated tropical oils (such as palm and coconut), have generally replaced them with hydrogenated oils. The fact is, no one really knows how much trans fat we eat. For one thing, food manufacturers often change the types of oils they use and the degree of hydrogenation of the oils. In addition, nutrition labels don't specify how much trans fats are in foods.

So should I avoid margarine and go back to butter?

Butter, lard, and coconut oil contain more saturated fat than margarine, so they probably raise blood cholesterol more than margarine. Butter and lard also contain cholesterol, while margarine doesn't. Still, if your diet is otherwise low in fat, you needn't worry about occasionally eating small amounts of butter, margarine, or any high-fat food.

If, however, you eat lots of margarine and many processed foods that contain hydrogenated oils, try to cut back. In general, the more solid the vegetable oil, the more hydrogenated, and therefore the more trans fatty acids it has—that's why tub and liquid "squeeze" margarines are preferable to stick margarine. "Diet" margarines are even better, since they are very soft and contain more water and only half the fat of other margarines.

When possible, use liquid vegetable oil (except coconut or palm oil) in cooking rather than butter or margarine. You can even use a little olive oil on your bread instead of either spread.

Is olive oil the way to go, then?

Olive oil, as well as other highly monounsaturated oils such as canola and nut oils, may not only help lower overall blood cholesterol level and artery-damaging LDL cholesterol, but also maintain the level of heart-healthy HDL cholesterol. Monounsaturated fats may also result in less oxidation of LDL (this chemical process appears to trigger a chain of events that causes plaque to build up in artery walls and that subsequently leads to a heart attack). Though the evidence is weaker, some studies have also suggested that olive oil can help lower blood pressure and control blood sugar levels. Highly monounsaturated oils are especially good for cooking: when overheated, they develop fewer "free radicals"—chemical agents that may be dangerous to human cells—than polyunsaturated oils do.

The recent surge in popularity of olive oil can probably be traced to the Seven Countries Study begun in 1958, which found that Mediterranean peoples, such as the Italians and Greeks, whose chief dietary fat is olive oil, have relatively low cholesterol levels and low rates of coronary artery disease, despite a fat intake as high as ours. It is important to remember, however, that the "Mediterranean diet" typically contains much more fruit and vegetables and less meat than ours, and these Europeans are generally more active than we are.

Still, no responsible scientists recommend that Americans simply swallow olive or canola oil by the tablespoon. Like other oils, they are 100% fat and contain 120 calories per tablespoon, and thus may cause you to gain weight. The important part of the equation is to use olive oil to *replace* animal fats and highly polyunsaturated oils.

What's special about the fat in nuts?

Like olive oil, most nuts are high in monounsaturated fat, and several recent studies have suggested that nuts may offer beneficial effects. For instance, a study published in the *Journal of the American College of Nutrition* in 1992 found that people on a low-fat diet lowered their total and LDL cholesterol levels significantly when they started eating 3.5 ounces of almonds a day (the percentage of calories derived from fat in their diet rose from 28% to 37%). Another study, using walnuts instead of almonds and published in the *New England Journal of Medicine,* found similar results (the percentage of fat calories stayed the same—30%). And a study of Seventh Day Adventists suggested that those who ate nuts most often had the lowest risk of heart attack (see *Wellness Letter,* February 1993). These results are promising, but it is still too early to recommend a daily handful of nuts—which are very high in calories—as a way to ward off heart attacks.

How strong is the evidence that fat causes cancer?

The strongest evidence concerns the link between a high fat intake and colon cancer. For other kinds of cancer, fat's role remains controversial (the *Wellness Letter* discussed the debate about breast cancer and fat in March 1993). Nonetheless, a low-fat diet makes sense if you're concerned about cancer, particularly since it helps guard against becoming overweight or obese, which in itself may be a risk factor for certain cancers, as well as for diabetes and heart disease.

Many scientists have noted that, with a few exceptions, countries with a high national fat intake also have the highest cancer rates. Some studies have found that a diet high in fat—saturated or unsaturated—increases the risk of cancer of the colon and breast, and possibly of the ovary, uterus, and prostate. Most recently, a study presented to the American Cancer Society found that among nonsmoking women, the risk of an uncommon form of lung cancer increases dramatically along with saturated-fat intake.

The mechanism for the link between a high-fat diet and cancer has not been determined, but there are theories. A diet high in fat affects the secretion of some sex hormones, which might cause cancer in the reproductive organs. Moreover, high-fat diets increase the amount of bile acids in the colon, which may be converted there by bacteria into carcinogenic by-products.

What about the polyunsaturated fat in fish?

Fish contains a type of long-chain polyunsaturated fatty acids commonly called omega-3s, which make the blood's platelets less likely to form a clot, thus reducing the chances of an artery blockage and heart attack. Get your omega-3s from fish, not from supplements, since many questions remain about the safety, effectiveness, and proper dosage of fish oil in liquid or capsule form.

The bottom line

Eat less fat, period. Virtually all health organizations and government agencies recommend that Americans reduce their fat intake so that less than 30% of all calories consumed each day come from fats. That translates to less than 66 grams of fat in a 2,000-calorie daily diet. Some health professionals advocate that total fat consumption should drop to 25% or even 20%.

Eat less saturated fat. Less than 10% of your calories should come from saturated fat, such as that in cheese, butter, and meat.

Limit your polyunsaturated fats. Less than 10% of your calories should come from polyunsaturated fat, such as that in safflower oil, soybean oil, and sunflower oil. Especially limit your intake of hydrogenated vegetable oils, found in so many processed foods. For instance, instead of stick margarine, which contains lots of hydrogenated fat, choose a tub margarine, which doesn't. The softer the spread, usually the less hydrogenated.

Eat monounsaturated fats in place of other fats. Olive and canola oils are the best choices among vegetable oils because they are highest in monounsaturated fat and among the lowest in saturated fat: use them instead of butter or margarine, when possible. You can also choose a peanut butter sandwich *instead of* a hamburger. Since avocados are another source of monounsaturates, opt for guacamole instead of cheese dip. But, of course, even better choices would be fish instead of the fatty hamburger, and salsa instead of the cheese dip, since the goal is to cut down on all fats.

Snack Attack

A junk food lover's guide to those empty hours between meals

Patricia Long

Patricia Long is a contributing editor.

SITTING IN BAR 234, a windowless, fluorescent-lit room, it's difficult to tell day from night, lunchtime from dinnertime. But the place fairly well shouts snack. The walls are lined with 22 mechanical dispensers that disgorge everything from Care Free gum to Famous Amos cookies, from pickles to Lay's potato chips, from Ultra Slim-Fast to the latest vending triumph, French fries cooked with hot air.

A uniformed U.S. Army major walks in the door and heads toward a machine. He presses his face up against the glass and plunks in a few quarters. I sidle up.

"Fritos, eh?"

"Excuse me?"

"Fritos. Kinda high in fat and salt, aren't they?"

Maybe I shouldn't be so confrontational with a guy trained in combat techniques. But orders are orders, and mine are to explore the workaday snacking habits that cost Americans $13.4 billion a year. Find out why we shove $2.5 billion of that into vending machines, yet of our 60 favorite selections, only three of them aren't extremely heavy in sugar or fat—Snak-Ens party mix, Snyder's hard pretzels, and Fig Newtons (and they're numbers 12, 42, and 43 in the ranking). I'm after the answer to perhaps America's most intriguing dietary question: Is there some way for even the stuff in vending machines to improve our national diet, rather than ruin it?

Bar 234 is named for its location on the second floor at the junction of corridors three and four in the world's largest office building: the Pentagon, situated outside Washington, D.C. The Pentagon is a perfect test environment, because offices—along with schools and factories—are where the nation's snacking culture truly thrives. While a visitor could easily get lost in the nearly 18 miles of corridors and among the 23,000 employees, there's little hazard of starving. At almost every turn sits a vending machine. Les Barnett, the Pentagon's snack vendor, figures that between the machines in the halls, in Bar 234, and in one other snack bar, every week he sells about 5,000 candy bars, 2,900 packages of cookies, crackers, and nuts, and 7,000 bags of chips, pretzels, and pastries.

One of those bags of chips is now being torn open by the major, a polite man.

"I tend to snack if I'm edgy," he says. "I feel guilty only when I get on the scale in the morning and weigh too much. Then I skip my snack that day." He hesitates, figuring how to upgrade his image from a Fritos-only type. "Once in a while I get a granola bar."

I haven't the heart to point out that regular granola bars aren't much better than Fritos. They're loaded with sugar and get between 38 and 55 percent of their calories from fat. But otherwise the major has the right idea. When his weight rises, he cuts back on snacking for a while. That's one good thing about being in the military: Twice yearly mandatory weight checks keep most personnel from letting themselves go to pot.

An army lieutenant colonel whom I corner at the burrito machine confirms this. "Because we're military," he says, "we're theoretically healthier than the rest of the drone population." He pauses as the smell of buttered popcorn—more than half its calories from fat—wafts over us. He shakes his head. "Someone convinced someone in this building that popcorn consumed in industrial-size bags will not make you pudgy."

Here's a man, I think, who's not deceived by marketing, who understands that while plain air-popped popcorn boasts less than 10 percent of calories from fat, the microwave kind we're smelling is in the same fat league as fried chicken. I ask him what he snacks on.

"Diet Coke and doughnuts."

He notes my surprise. "Put it this way," he says, backpedaling. "Working in this building is like attending one continuous meeting. I don't get regular meal breaks, so I just have to lay my hands on whatever's not moving."

No matter how you figure it, combining a diet soda with a greasy doughnut is living by a weird credo: "Sugar is bad, fat isn't." True, sugar offers little more than calories, but it's not the demon fat is. Too much fat is linked to cancer, obesity, and heart disease. That's why we're advised to hold fat to under 30 percent of calories.

That's also why one look at the way we snack will tell you we're in big trouble.

AMERICANS ARE VERY concerned about nutrition. Just ask them. Fifty-eight percent of those surveyed by the Food Marketing Institute believe fat in food is a "serious health hazard." But how many are doing anything about it? According to one food industry survey, some 86 percent of adults admit to eating between meals. As for what they're eating—well, the overall top-selling snack food in America is potato chips. From vending machines it's the Snickers bar.

"Everybody says, 'Boy, we'd really like to see some healthier snacks in vending machines,'" says Tim Sanford, executive editor of the trade magazine *Vending Times.* "And that's exactly what they mean. They don't want to buy them, they just want to see them."

Consider what happened to Ruth Ward-Gross, vice president of Vendmark Inc. in Eagan, Minnesota. To celebrate "nutrition week" in a local health center, she replaced all the vending snacks with healthier ones such as raisins and trail mix, leaving only one exception—a slot

The Vending Machine Top 30

SOME WE GREW UP ON; others only recently hit the popularity chart. Either way, these classic snack foods aren't going to disappear from machines anytime soon, despite the fact that (or maybe *because*) most are heavy in fat and sugar. Still, say nutritionists, it's okay to eat them every once in a while, if you follow the advice on these pages.

In the meantime, see how your tastes match up with those of America's other snackers, and then take a look at the real price of your favorite vending machine pick.

	% of calories from fat	calories
1. **Snickers bar** (*2.07 oz*)	42	280
2. **M&M's peanut candies** (*1.74 oz*)	47	250
3. **Reese's peanut butter cups** (*1.6 oz*)	54	250
4. **M&M's plain chocolate candies** (*1.69 oz*)	39	230
5. **Butterfinger bar** (*2.1 oz*)	39	280
6. **Baby Ruth bar** (*2.1 oz*)	43	290
7. **Pay Day bar** (*1.85 oz*)	43	250
8. **3 Musketeers bar** (*2.13 oz*)	28	260
9. **Hershey's almond bar** (*1.45 oz*)	55	230
10. **Cheetos** (*1 oz*)	54	150
11. **Twix caramel cookie bar** (*2 oz*)	45	140
12. **Snak-Ens snack mix** (*1 oz*)	17	133
13. **Milky Way bar** (*2.15 oz*)	32	280
14. **Famous Amos Chocolate Chip cookies** (*1 oz or 3 cookies*)	36	150
15. **Act II Microwave Popcorn** (*3 cups popped*)	51	140
16. **Fritos corn chips** (*1 oz*)	60	150
17. **Almond Joy bar** (*1.76 oz*)	50	250
18. **Nestlé Crunch bar** (*1.55 oz*)	47	230
19. **Oreo cookies** (*1 oz or 3 cookies*)	36	150
20. **Lay's potato chips** (*1 oz*)	60	150
21. **Planters peanuts** (*1 oz*)	74	170
22. **Doritos Nacho Cheese tortilla chips** (*1 oz*)	45	140
23. **Kit Kat bar** (*1.4 oz*)	47	220
24. **Mr. Goodbar** (*1.65 oz*)	55	260
25. **Planters cheese peanut butter sandwiches** (*1.4 oz or 6 sandwiches*)	45	200
26. **Nature Valley Oats 'N Honey granola bar** (*.83 oz*)	36	120
27. **Milky Way Dark bar** (*1.76 oz*)	33	220
28. **Cheez-It crackers** (*.5 oz or 12 crackers*)	51	70
29. **Starburst Original Fruit Chews** (*2.07 oz*)	19	240
30. **M&M's peanut butter candies** (*1.63 oz*)	45	240

Excludes gum. Based on vendors' dollar purchases for the year ending June 1992. Ranking source: DEBS, Ann Arbor, Michigan. Vended samples vary in size.

full of Snickers. Within two days she got a call for more Snickers. "That's the reality," she says.

And we're ashamed about it. Fully one in three snackers confess to feelings of guilt, according to a 1990 survey. Of those, nearly half say they feel worse about snacking than they do about lying about their weight or age or letting the answering machine take a call when they're home. A third think it's worse than breaking a date, taking a phony sick day, or cheating on taxes.

"I'll see someone in front of a machine," says Barnett, the Pentagon's vendor, "and I'll ask if something's wrong. 'No, I'm just looking,' they'll say. They'll stand there, and you can almost hear them thinking, *I really should get something healthy, but I really want such-and-such. I had a late lunch, I'm having an early dinner, I'm too fat.* It just goes on and on."

But, really, is all this guilt warranted?

Not in theory. Studies on both animals and humans show that snacks—if complementary to regular meals—can help you feel more alert, lose weight, and lower your levels of "bad" cholesterol.

For one thing, standard mealtimes aren't always in synch with the body's rhythms. "After lunchtime your circadian performance rhythms are on a downswing," says Bonnie Spring, a psychologist at The Chicago Medical School. "Fatigue will peak around one to three in the afternoon." Reports Robin Kanarek, a psychologist at Tufts University in Medford, Massachusetts, "Somebody looking at a computer screen—at letters or numbers or whatever—does worse after lunch than before." British researcher Andrew Smith describes the feeling archly: "Lethargic, feeble, clumsy, and muzzy."

Kanarek's research confirms that a snack can reverse the letdown. In two experiments, she asked 18 men to either skip or eat a moderate lunch. Hours later some got no snack (actually, a diet soda), while others got a snack (in one, a chocolate bar, in the other, a yogurt). Then the men took tests measuring memory, math reasoning, reading speed, and attention span. It didn't matter much whether the men had lunched or not. Those eating calories at snacktime scored higher than those who didn't.

If we could manage it, eating tiny meals all day long—a meal pattern researchers refer to, not surprisingly, as nibbling—would actually cut more than our muzziness. For instance, our weight and our heart disease rates. Lab animals fed two large daily meals—known as gorging

No-Guilt Everyday Snacks

NUTRITIONISTS WHO understand human nature agree that a once-every-week-or-so splurge on your snack of illicit choice (*Oh, Lorna!*) can actually help you manage your cravings and diet. But how are you supposed to satisfy your desires the *other* days?

These 21 snacks are low in fat or high in nutritional value (some are both), not too caloric, and tasty to many. (In other words, tofu didn't make the list.)

ANYTIME

Low in fat and filled with vitamins, minerals, or fiber

	% of calories from fat	calories
Nonfat yogurt with fruit (*8 oz*)	0	100
Baby carrots (*3 oz*)	4	40
Fresh fruit (*pear*)	6	98
Bagel (*1*)	6	152
Raisin bran (*1.4-oz box*)	6	111
Fig bar (*1*)	15	60
Graham crackers (*.5 oz or 2 crackers*)	15	60
Instant oatmeal (*1-oz package*)	18	100

ONCE A DAY

Low to moderate in fat

	% of calories from fat	calories
Hard candy (*1 piece*)	0	22
Nonfat pudding (*4 oz*)	0	100
Rice cakes (*2*)	8	70
Pretzel twists (*10*)	8	229
Air-popped popcorn (*1 cup*)	9	31
Animal crackers (*.5 oz or 5 crackers*)	26	70
Gingersnaps (*.5 oz or 3 cookies*)	30	60
Saltines (*5*)	30	60
Whole wheat crackers (*.5 oz or 3 crackers*)	30	60

WHEN YOU'RE ACTIVE

Fatty, but high in vitamins and minerals

	% of calories from fat	calories
Trail mix (*1 oz*)	57	131
Roasted pumpkin seeds (*1 oz*)	73	148
Roasted peanuts (*1 oz*)	76	163
Sunflower seeds (*1 oz*)	82	176

All of the above items have no cholesterol or only moderate amounts; people on low-salt diets should always check labels for sodium content.

—experience large surges in insulin. Some studies show that because insulin converts glucose into body fat, big-meal eaters have more weight problems than the critters who eat the same amount, but spread out over the day.

Weight-conscious people especially should eat something every four or six hours, say diet experts. Anything less, and the body thinks it's starving so slows down its metabolism (not exactly what a weight-watcher wants). It also grows famished; the liver stores only about 340 calories' worth of fuel to maintain steady blood sugar levels. In other words, the I-didn't-eat-anything-all-day diet is bound to fail, explains Evelyn Tribole, a Beverly Hills, California, dietitian and author of *Eating on the Run*. "If you have a light meal at lunch and no snack, then work out and don't eat dinner until seven o'clock, you are too hungry to exercise any self-control."

Such big meals lead to higher levels of cholesterol. In one study, David Jenkins, a nutrition researcher at the University of Toronto, fed two groups of men identical food. One group polished it off as three meals, the other as 17 snacks. Sure enough, snackers experienced drops in "bad" cholesterol levels, lowering their risk of heart disease. Researchers believe the insulin surges that follow big meals prompt the liver to generate more of the cholesterol that helps cause heart disease.

But before you start nibbling, look at what happens when lab animals are given *unlimited* access to either wholesome Purina rat chow or an assortment of tasty chocolate cookies, peanut butter, and marshmallows. They turn up their little noses at the boring chow, gorge on the snacks, and grow very, very fat.

You don't need a research study to know humans do the same thing. Big lunch at noon, candy at two, potato chips at four, and so on into the evening. "The downside to nibbling in real life is that most people don't have any self-control," says Jenkins. "They gain weight."

SO WHAT'S A snack lover to do? Here's what the experts advise:

THINK OF SNACKS AS MINI-MEALS

The way nutritionists see it, we'd be healthier if we skipped candy, chips, cookies, and other typical snack foods altogether or ate them only occasionally. Instead, we'd snack on "meal-type" foods, such as fruit salad, instant oatmeal,

New and Improved

STROLL THE SNACK aisle of any grocery store these days and you might think you've blundered into the health-food section. Cookies are sweetened with fruit juice, while tortilla chips sport ingredients like beets, carrots, and flax seed.

If you eat any of the four C's—cookies, cakes, chips, chocolate bars—it can't hurt to see if you like the lighter alternatives. Though some still have loads of sugar or salt, all of the newcomers are a *lot* lower in fat.

CHIPS

Some chip makers now bake instead of fry. But a "baked-not-fried" claim isn't the same as "fat free." For taste, some companies spike their dough with shortening; others spray fat on after baking.

	% of calories from fat	calories
OLD-TECH		
Regular tortilla chips	47	142
Regular potato chips	62	158
NEW-TECH		
Guiltless Gourmet Baked Tortilla Chips	11	110
Childers Oven Toasted Potato Chips	0	98
Mr. Phipps Tater Crisps	30	120

COOKIES AND CAKES

Commercial bakers are replacing fat with fruit pectin or vegetable gums—xanthan gum, for example, or cellulose gel—which help keep the products moist.

	% of calories from fat	calories
OLD-TECH		
Regular blueberry muffin	34	210
Regular oatmeal raisin cookie	41	44
Regular granola bar	38	134
NEW-TECH		
Entenmann's Fat Free Blueberry Muffin	0	150
R.W. Frookie Oatmeal Raisin Fat Free Cookie	0	45
Health Valley Fat Free Granola Bar	0	140

CHOCOLATE BARS

Bars are now being made with two new ingredients. Caprenin, a manufactured fat, provides about half the calories per gram of most fats. Polydextrose, a lower-calorie bulking agent, replaces some of the candies' carbohydrates.

	% of calories from fat	calories
OLD-TECH		
Milky Way *(2.15 oz)*	32	280
Hershey's *(1.55 oz)*	54	240
NEW-TECH		
Milky Way II *(2.05 oz)*	24	190
Hershey's Reduced Calorie and Fat *(1.37 oz; in test marketing)*	30	150

strawberry yogurt, snack-size cans of tuna, and bagels.

At the very least, we should avoid having our snacks make matters worse. Deep inside the Pentagon I meet an air force senior airman whose regular meals are high in fat and cholesterol. For breakfast, he says, he eats ham and cheese omelettes, bacon, toast, juice, and vitamins; for lunch, pizza; and for dinner, fried chicken, mixed vegetables, and rice.

In between? He consumes two Cokes and two bags of Fritos.

While this man looks fit enough, there's no telling what's happening to his arteries. And it wouldn't take a visit to a health food store every afternoon for snacks to become his healthiest meals. Pretzels, gingersnaps, animal crackers, popcorn (unbuttered, that is), bread sticks, and hard candy are *far* less fatty than what he eats all day. Fresh fruit would be even better. Instead of the soda, he could drink fruit juice (not fruit punch or fruit ade, which are mostly sugar water). Instead of the Fritos, he could eat fig bars, graham crackers, or oatmeal raisin cookies, which all have fiber.

COMPENSATE FOR SNACKS IN YOUR WORKOUT OR NEXT MEAL

"If I want a candy bar," says a senior master sergeant in the air force, "I'll flip it over, look at the grams of fat, and figure out how many miles I have to run to work it off." By that measure, after eating a 250-calorie Reese's peanut butter cup he would run 2.5 miles. (In general, you burn about 100 calories for every mile you walk or run.) His other choice? At dinner he could skip the caloric equivalent of a Reese's: an order of French fries or a cup of ice cream.

Here's one way to handle this internal bargaining: Pretend you're carrying around a grocery bag filled with all your day's food—the perfect number of calories (for the average man and woman, 2,200 and 1,600 respectively). You can eat whenever and however much you want until the bag is empty, but that's all you get. If you use up your allotment with high-calorie candy bars and potato chips, you won't need a very big sack. Fill it with lower-calorie fruits, vegetables, whole grain cereals and crackers, and you'll get to eat a lot more before your hand scrapes bottom.

AVOID MINDLESS SPEED-EATING

Perhaps the sole advantage of vending machines is that they force you to consciously get out of your chair, walk to a machine, and pay money for a single item (provided you don't stock up on *several* candy bars).

Less measured eating styles invite disaster. An air force captain cheerfully pulls out the second drawer of his desk to reveal a stash of Brach's mints and Gummy Bears. He tells me he eats them throughout the day for an "energy high." I tell him he's a candidate for "eating amnesia," what happens when your hand goes to your mouth repeatedly without your brain kicking in.

It's a particular problem with itty-bitty snacks. On the Ritz Bits label, for example, a serving is listed as 22 pieces totaling 70 calories. Three calories per bit seems like nothing, and some out of control snackers will keep munching until the box is empty. That's almost as much food as the average woman needs in a day.

Eating too fast is another problem, because it takes 20 minutes from the start of eating before your body can tell your mind that it's had enough. "It's not like putting your hand on a hot stove, and you instantly know it's hot," says Captain Ellen Stoute, an army dietitian at Walter Reed Army Medical Center in Washington, D.C. "If our bodies worked that way, no one would overeat."

INDULGE YOUR DESIRES— NOW AND THEN

"When I go to a vending machine, I'm usually thinking candy bar," says a woman air force technical sergeant who is a confessed lover of Mars bars. "Sometimes I can even feel my craving."

It's a feeling deep inside all of us. A newborn given a sweetened solution in place of an unsweetened one, say taste researchers, drinks more eagerly—and also looks more contented. So it can be with adults, says Evelyn Tribole. "Don't necessarily swear off all your favorite foods, because deprivation can lead to an overeating backlash. Instead, sit down and savor them."

Sounds reasonable to me. Back in Bar 234, despite the lack of windows, I can tell from my stomach that the day's getting on. I face the machines. Yogurt? (It's got calcium for bones.) Pretzels? (They're low in fat.) Orange juice? (I could use the vitamin C.) The choices seem tortuous.

Then again, maybe not. Smiling, I drop in the coins, remember the part about indulging every once in a while, and press the button . . . for a Reese's.

Exercise and Weight Control

Are you physically fit? Surely you must have heard by now that exercising regularly yields substantial health benefits. Despite the fact that most Americans believe that exercise is important to maintaining good health, only about 1 in 10 Americans actually exercise on a regular basis. Why such a low percentage? Each year, millions of people begin exercise programs, but half of them quit within the first six months. A major reason for this high dropout rate is that many people approach exercise with unrealistic expectations, and in a manner guaranteed to make it boring, painful, and frustrating.

While it is true that exercise reduces the risk of coronary heart disease, it also yields several other health benefits if done at least three times a week in sessions of 20 to 30 minutes in duration, with an intensity level of 60 to 80 percent of one's maximal heart rate. The following benefits are typical of what can be achieved by exercising in accordance with these specifications: reduced blood pressure, improved blood cholesterol levels, improved cardiovascular function (increased energy and endurance), enhanced bone density, increased muscle mass (a trimmer physique), reduced musculoskeletal disorders, reduced stress (better sleep and enhanced sense of well-being), and perhaps even an enhancement in immunological function (increased resistance to infectious illnesses). Unfortunately, many of these benefits can take weeks or even months before they become apparent, and in the meantime, the exerciser must put up with a certain amount of discomfort or even pain as the body adjusts to the physical demands that this level of exercise entails. One solution to the high dropout rate is to begin exercising at a relatively light activity level to reverse the pattern of inactivity, and then to gradually increase activity level as fitness level improves. This approach minimizes the pain and discomfort that often accompany exercise and help to establish it as an integral part of the daily routine. While the health benefits associated with low levels of activity are not as great as with higher levels of activity, research now indicates that *any* increase in activity level will provide some protection against coronary heart disease. "Exercise Without Injury" discusses several common sports injuries and presents some helpful advice on preventing such injuries. "To Be Active or Not to Be Active" examines the top 10 documented health benefits associated with exercise. "From Here to Immunity," an article found in unit 7, discusses how exercise may enhance the functioning of the immune system. "Pressure Treatment: How Exercise Can Help You Control Your Blood Pressure," also in unit 7, discusses situations in which exercise can be an effective treatment for hypertensive individuals.

The fitness movement this country is experiencing began in the early 1970s in response to medical reports that linked Americans' sedentary lifestyle to the rising incidence of cardiovascular disease and obesity. The early advocates of this movement took up jogging and racquet sports as a way to trim off excess pounds and reduce their risk of coronary heart disease. As the movement grew, so did the diversity of the exercise programs being offered. Many people found that jogging was painful and boring, and the popularity of racquet sports diminished in the face of rising costs and competition for facilities. These factors, coupled with a broadening interest in physical fitness, prompted the exploration and development of numerous fitness programs. What type of exercise program is best? The answer to this question is simple—one that you enjoy and will stick with. Given the diversity of fitness programs, chances are good that you can find one that is right for you.

Of all the exercise programs, the one that has the lowest injury rate, lowest equipment cost, and broadest age range is walking. Millions of Americans each year discover that walking is a near-perfect form of exercise because they can do it wherever they are, whenever they want, and at whatever level of intensity they choose. Unlike many other popular fitness programs, walking is truly a lifetime fitness sport. "Walk Off Calories and Get Fit" explores the benefits of walking and provides a self-test for assessing your fitness level.

Researchers who have studied the physiological benefits of exercise have concluded that, in addition to promoting cardiovascular endurance, muscle strength, flexibility, and coordination, exercise can also improve a person's outlook on life. While few controlled studies have been conducted regarding the psychological benefits of exercise, numerous individuals have reported enhanced self-esteem, greater self-reliance, decreased anxiety, and relief from mild depression as a result of exercising regularly. For many, exercise has become a tool for building a new self-image.

Even though exercise is widely recognized as an effective means for shedding unwanted pounds of body fat, it still rates a distant second to dieting for weight control. The obsession that Americans have about their weight is evidenced by statistics indicating that 90 percent of Americans think they should lose weight. Many of these individuals are either on a diet or have tried to diet at some point in their lives. This obsession is not limited to obese individuals, but is shared by many with normal and even low body weight. Young women of normal body weight who feel they are fat are of particular concern because some of them become so obsessed with their body weight that they turn to starvation as a way to control it. This approach to weight control may result in a medical condition known as anorexia nervosa. Still others with distorted body images resort to vomiting and to purging their systems with laxatives in an attempt to control their weight. This condition is known as bulimia. Both anorexia and bulimia are serious eating disorders that may have deadly consequences. The article "Chemistry and Craving" discusses new research findings that link our eating behavior (desire for carbohydrates and fats) to neuropeptides produced by the brain. These findings certainly suggest that neuropeptides play a major role in eating disorders ranging from bulimia to obesity.

America's preoccupation with body weight has given rise to a billion-dollar industry. Unfortunately for most, the money spent on dieting has thinned their bank accounts more than their bodies, and the prognosis for keeping pounds off among those who do lose weight is grim. Current statistics indicate that approximately two-thirds of those who lose weight will gain back the pounds they lost, and sometimes more, within a few months or years. This yo-yo pattern of weight loss and gain is not only unhealthy, but often results in a lowering of self-esteem. Why do diets fail? One of the major reasons lies in the mind-set of the dieter. Many dieters do not fully understand the biological and behavioral aspects of weight loss, and as a result, they have unrealistic expectations regarding the process.

Numerous diets are on the market, and each one purports to be the ultimate weapon in the battle of the bulge. Unfortunately, many are not only worthless but may actually be hazardous to health. Amid all this hype and controversy, how should one decide which program to follow? Most experts agree that, for a program to be successful, it must include some form of daily exercise in addition to alterations in eating behavior. The exact contribution of exercise to weight control is yet another controversial topic. Current findings support the claim that exercise can improve the body composition of a dieter (the ratio of muscle mass to adipose tissue), and there is mounting evidence that daily exercise may lower the set point. Less convincing are claims that exercise suppresses the appetite and increases the basal metabolic rate. Beyond the physiological effects, exercise also seems to help dieters reduce their anxiety and increase their self-confidence.

The American preoccupation with weight is primarily due to social factors such as appearance and group acceptance, rather than to concerns regarding health. Traditionally, most health experts believed that a healthy weight was one that fell within the ideal range on the standard height-weight table developed by the Metropolitan Life Insurance Company in 1959. According to this table, millions of Americans were classified as overweight. Health researchers changed the focus of the medical community in the late 1980s with the publication of studies indicating that from a longevity perspective people who maintained or slightly increased their weight between the ages of 47 and 74 lived longer than those who demonstrated a significant weight change either up or down. Medical experts are not certain why a slight weight gain as one ages appears to confer health, but they suspect that those who demonstrate significant changes die sooner due to physiological changes brought on by the yo-yo effect. The U.S. government responded to these findings in 1990 by publishing a new set of dietary guidelines, including a new height-weight table that is much more lenient in terms of ideal weight ranges. It clearly suggests that putting on a few extra pounds as one grows older may be desirable. "Losing Weight: What Works, What Doesn't" takes a comprehensive look at the issues of weight control and provides current research findings.

As we strive to contain the high cost of health care, the role that preventative health practices play in the solution will continue to grow. We must all strive to find the time to engage in some form of exercise so that we may not only increase our resistance to various disease processes, but also enhance our capacity to enjoy all that life has to offer.

Looking Ahead: Challenge Questions

Explain why the concepts of balance and moderation are crucial to any discussion regarding physical fitness or weight control.

How important is regular exercise to optimal health?

Why should exercise be included in weight control programs?

What advice would you give someone regarding the prevention of sports injuries?

How does American society encourage or contribute to weight control problems? What changes would you suggest?

How do you feel about people who are overweight? Has weight control been a problem for you? If so, what have you done about it?

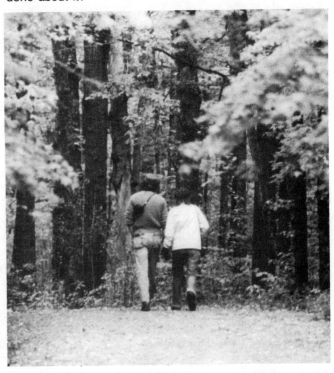

To Be Active Or Not To Be Active

That is the question for health-minded individuals in the '90s. A review of research on the health benefits of physical activity suggests that the choice is more important than we may have imagined.

LEN KRAVITZ, MA,

ROBERT ROBERGS, PHD

Len Kravitz, MA, is a doctoral student in health promotion and exercise science at the University of New Mexico and a regular contributing editor for IDEA Today. *He is the author of two books and the producer of four exercise videos, including his newest, "Phenomenal Abdominals."*

Robert Robergs, PhD, received his master's degree in exercise science and cardiac rehabilitation at Wake Forest University. He completed his doctorate in bioenergetics at Ball State University and is currently an assistant professor of exercise physiology and biochemistry at the Human Performance Laboratory, University of New Mexico.

It is commonly acknowledged in the scientific community and the fitness industry that physical activity and exercise exert a positive impact on many aspects of health. Recently, a host of health products, diet books, exercise videos and fitness clubs have emerged.

In addition, a more health-conscious community has developed growing markets for professional health services (e.g., exercise physiologists, personal trainers and health promotion professionals).

Though much has been made of the potential to look and feel better through exercise, it is likely that many people who come to you for instruction or information do not know specifically *how,* or to what degree, activity affects health. This research review offers an overview of the health benefits of physical activity and exercise so you will be equipped to educate your current and future clients.

Your mission to educate is becoming increasingly important. The U.S. Department of Health and Human Services (USDHHS) has defined its public health agenda for the 1990s with the release of *Healthy People 2000: National Health Promotion and Disease Prevention Objectives.* The three broad goals put forward in this report are (1) to increase the span of healthy life for Americans, (2) to reduce health disparities among Americans and (3) to achieve access to preventive services for all Americans. Physical activity and fitness are essential for meeting these goals.

The widespread need for effective promotion of physical fitness is well documented. Despite the merits of physical activity, 24 percent of the United States population over the age of 18 report no physical activity, with inactivity rates especially high in older age groups; and approximately one person in five (22 percent) reports physical activity for at least 30 minutes five or more times a week (USDHHS, 1991). According to a 1985 National Health Interview Survey, only 7.6 percent of persons in the United States exercised at the level recommended to attain cardiopulmonary benefits (Caspersen, Christenson & Pollard, 1986).

Health Benefits: The Top 10

Although research on health benefits continues to expand, conclusive studies now validate significant benefits of physical activity in these 10 broad categories:

1. coronary heart disease
2. hypertension
3. blood lipid and lipoprotein profile
4. cardiac function
5. bone mineral status
6. smoking risks
7. body composition and weight control
8. blood glucose regulation
9. musculoskeletal disorders
10. stress management and mental health

Health Benefit Area #1: Coronary Heart Disease

The incidence of coronary heart disease (CHD) has declined considerably over the last 25 years. According to the USDHHS (1988), deaths from CHD dropped 42 percent between 1964 and 1985. *Yet CHD is still the leading cause of death in the United States for both men and women.*

CHD is caused by a lack of blood supply to the heart muscle, resulting from a degenerative disorder known as atherosclerosis. This disorder involves a gradual buildup and deposition of fat and plaque on the inner lining of the coronary arteries. The annual costs associated with CHD range from $41.5 billion to $56 billion (Lenfant, 1992).

As a nation, our efforts to further decrease CHD need to be directed to *youth* as well as adults, because resounding evidence demonstrates that atherosclerosis begins in early childhood. As many as 60 percent of children in the United States exhibit by the age of 12 at least one modifiable adult risk factor for coronary heart disease (Berenson et al., 1980). Recent research suggests that physical activity in childhood is a determinant of physical activity as an adult (Powell & Dysinger, 1987).

People who are more active are less likely to develop CHD than their inactive counterparts. An analysis of the data from over 40 studies (referred to as a meta-analysis) by Berlin and Colditz (1990) indicated that CHD is 1.9 times more likely to develop in sedentary individuals than in physically active persons. This positive influence of exercise is independent of other CHD risk factors such as hypertension, smoking, obesity, diabetes or a family history of CHD. A number of studies have also indicated that when CHD does develop in physically active individuals, it occurs at a later age and tends to be less severe (Haskell et al., 1992).

In 1986, Dr. Ralph Paffenbarger presented the results of his landmark study of 16,936 Harvard University alumni men, who were followed over 16 years. Results of this famous study indicated that men who exercised and expended at least 2,000 calories per week *increased their life expectancy by one to two years* (Paffenbarger et al., 1986).

In 1989, the Cooper Institute for Aerobics Research in Dallas, Texas, published another landmark study involving more than 13,000 men and women over an eight-year period (Blair et al., 1989). Results of this study, which measured each participant's fitness level with a maximal treadmill test (Balke protocol), demonstrated that as fitness level increased, mortality decreased. The least fit men died at a rate almost 3.5 times higher than the most fit, while for women the ratio was 4.5 times higher.

The study divided participants into five categories based on their fitness levels, with the least fit (sedentary) in category 1 and the most fit (serious exercisers such as runners who logged 30 to 40 miles per week) in category 5. Most surprisingly, the moderately fit levels—those in categories 2 and 3—had almost one-third fewer deaths than those in category 1. There were additional, but minimal, gains for those persons in categories 4 and 5.

Health Benefit Area #2: Hypertension

Hypertension is abnormally high blood pressure. Often unrecognized, hypertension is a significant risk factor for cardiovascular and cerebrovascular disease. Hypertension is especially prevalent among African-Americans. If an individual's resting systolic blood pressure consistently exceeds 160 millimeters of mercury (mmHg), the risk of CHD is four times greater than normal. A consistent resting diastolic reading greater than 95 mmHg increases the normal CHD risk sixfold (Heyward, 1991).

The degree to which exercise can help a hypertensive person is currently unclear, due largely to methodological shortcomings in research designs. However, it is well established that *aerobic exercise can moderately lower systolic and diastolic blood pressure in normotensive and hypertensive individuals.*

Health Benefit Area #3: Blood Lipids and Lipoproteins

People who perform regular, vigorous endurance exercise have more high-density lipoproteins (HDLs) in their blood than do sedentary individuals (Haskell, 1984). This is especially true for the HDL2-C subfraction, which has been particularly associated with lowering the risk of CHD (Wood, 1987).

HDLs, manufactured in the liver, carry cholesterol from peripheral body tissues back to the liver, where the cholesterol is used to produce bile salts (which aid in the digestion of fat). HDLs are known as "good cholesterol" because they are associated with lowering the risk of artery disease by removing some cholesterol from artery walls. Positive, though modest, improvements in HDL concentrations can be realized very quickly after initiating an exercise program. The recent Helsinki Heart Study strongly demonstrated that raising HDL cholesterol levels lowered the risks of heart attack (Manninen et al., 1988). However, it is presently unclear how much exercise, at what intensity and for what period of time will optimally elevate HDL levels. Physical activity may also lower blood concentrations of the harmful cholesterols, known as low-density lipoprotein cholesterol (LDL-C) and very low density lipoprotein cholesterol (VLDL-C).

Exercise is also powerful in lowering blood triglyceride (fat) levels (Haskell, 1984). The body's triglyceride level tends to fall immediately after exercise and often remains low for several days. This change may be attributable to an increase in lipoprotein lipase (an enzyme), which facilitates the breakdown and assimilation of triglycerides in the body.

Another factor may be that production of insulin decreases with regular exercise, and this change may stimulate a decrease in the stimulus for triglyceride synthesis. Regular exercise helps prevent not only the development of insulin resistance by cells but also the increased insulin levels that often occur with advancing age.

In spite of lower insulin levels, physically active people have good blood sugar (glucose) tolerance as a result of cells that are able to respond more effectively to insulin.

Health Benefit Area #4: Cardiac Function

A number of processes closely linked to the efficiency of the cardiorespiratory system change with physical activity. Often a reduction in resting heart rate can be attributable to aerobic exercise. The heart's stroke volume (the amount of blood pumped per beat) increases at rest and during exercise as an adaptation to endurance training (McArdle, Katch & Katch, 1991). The volume of the left ventricular cavity, the pumping chamber of the heart, often adapts to cardiorespiratory training by increasing in size.

In addition, physically active individuals have larger coronary vessels than less fit persons. The most significant cardiovascular function change occurs when there is an increase in cardiac output, i.e., the amount of blood circulated by the heart each minute (cardiac output = heart rate x stroke volume). This functional change helps increase a person's physical work capacity.

Aerobic training will also improve the muscles' ability to extract oxygen from the blood, an ability referred to as the arteriovenous oxygen difference. This increased capacity to extract oxygen is believed to be due primarily to an increase in capillary density (Rowell, 1986). *The total effect of all these changes is a stronger, more efficient cardiovascular system.*

Several notable physiological changes also occur when the cardiorespiratory system is sufficiently overloaded. These adaptations include the following:

1. The trained muscle is more efficient at mobilizing and metabolizing fat. This is attributable to an increase of blood flow within the muscle and to greater activity of fat-mobilizing and fat-metabolizing enzymes.

2. The mitochondria, the subcellular structures responsible for the production of large amounts of ATP (the high-energy compounds from which our bodies derive energy) have a significantly greater capacity to generate ATP, due to an increase in their size and number.

3. The muscle's oxidative capacity increases in conjunction with an increase in glycogen (the form in which glucose is stored in the body), resulting in a greater capacity to oxidize carbohydrates.

Health Benefit Area #5: Bone Mineral Status

The prevention of osteoporosis in aging women has become a serious health issue. Approximately 1.2 million fractures occur each year as a result of this condition, including 227,000 hip fractures and 530,000 vertebral fractures (Johnson & Slemenda, 1987). Although exercise is recommended, along with calcium supplements and estrogen replacement therapy, information on the best form of exercise for preventing or reversing this bone degradation is still insufficient. Weight-bearing movements, such as low-impact activities, walking and jogging, increase the mechanical stress on the skeletal system and may reduce or reverse bone mineral loss in aging women (Smith & Gilligan, 1987).

Health Benefit Area #6: Smoking Risks

People who are physically active are less likely to smoke than their sedentary counterparts. In every category of smokers (i.e., nonsmokers; former smokers; light, moderate and heavy smokers), those who are physically active run a lower risk of developing CHD than sedentary people in the same category (Paffenbarger, 1987).

Health Benefit Area #7: Body Composition and Weight Control

Approximately 25 percent of the adult American population is obese. Obesity is a prominent problem in our society and a contributing risk factor in cardiovascular disease, hypertension and diabetes. Exercise offers both short-term and long-term benefits for obese individuals.

An immediate benefit of exercise is caloric expenditure. Studies on the increased metabolic demands of the body after an exercise bout have shown 1 to 25 percent increases in caloric expenditure that can last from one to 24 hours (Van Zant, 1992). Numerous factors—such as the type and intensity of exercise, the subject's fitness level and dietary intake prior to measurement—contribute to the range of increase in metabolic rate. However, recent data suggest that the bulk of the increased energy expenditure following an exercise bout occurs within the first hour of recovery (Brehm & Gutin, 1986; Gore & Withers, 1990).

Recent investigations seem to agree that one of the major benefits of exercise, as it relates to weight loss, is the positive impact exercise has on maintaining lean body mass while encouraging the loss of fat body weight (Hawk, 1989; Work, 1990).

Health Benefit Area #8: Blood Glucose Regulation

Regular physical activity can be beneficial in managing diabetes, particularly Type II, the noninsulin-dependent, or adult-onset, diabetes. Considerable deliberation continues regarding the best prescription of exercise within the total treatment program for diabetics. It does appear that a balance of regular physical activity, satisfactory medications and adherence to a proper diet will help diabetics keep their blood sugar under control.

Health Benefit Area #9: Musculoskeletal Disorders

Physical activity can reduce the potential for various musculoskeletal disorders such as osteoarthritis, bone fractures, connective tissue tears and low-back syndrome. Regular exercise that challenges the musculoskeletal system can increase bone mineral content (Smith & Gilligan, 1987). Physical activity programs designed to develop muscular strength and flexibility of the musculoskeletal system will improve structural weaknesses that can contribute to these disorders.

Health Benefit Area #10: Stress Management and Mental Health

Studies have shown that exercise brings about both short- and long-term psychological enhancement and mental well-being (Morgan & Goldston, 1987). A new position statement by the International Society of Sport Psychology (1992) has summarized a number of psychological benefits of physical activity, including the following:

• improvement in self-confidence and awareness
• relief of tension
• positive changes in mood
• relief of feelings of depression and anxiety
• increased mental well-being
• favorable influence on premenstrual tension
• increased alertness and clearer thinking
• increased energy
• the development of positive coping strategies in daily activities
• reduction in various stress indices
• increased enjoyment of exercise and social contacts

Individuals of all ages can realize these psychological benefits of physical activity.

Living the Benefits

The science documenting the positive changes caused by physical activity with respect to disease risk factors, several major chronic diseases and total health is dramatically clear. The last few years have seen a definite, and appropriate, shift in emphasis away from only vigorous exercise; now experts recognize that light to moderate levels of physical activity can also improve health. People should be encouraged to engage in activities that are pleasing to them, since personal satisfaction may increase adherence to physical activity. Now, more than ever, the involvement of exercise instructors, personal trainers and health promotion specialists with their clients, students and communities can play a significant role in achieving the goals for a healthy nation 2000.

References:

Berenson, Gerald S. et al. *Cardiovascular Risk Factors in Children: The Early Natural History of Atherosclerosis and Essential Hypertension.* New York: Oxford University Press, 1980.

Berlin, J. A. & Colditz, G. A. "A Meta-Analysis of Physical Activity in the Prevention of Coronary Heart Disease," *American Journal of Epidemiology,* 132, 4 (1990), 612-28.

Blair, S. N. et al. "Physical Fitness and All-Cause Mortality: A Prospective Study of Healthy Men and Women," *Journal of the American Medical Association,* 262, 17 (1989), 2395-401.

Brehm, B. A. & Gutin, B. "Recovery Energy Expenditure for Steady State Exercise in Runners and Nonexercisers," *Medicine and Science in Sports and Exercise,* 18, 2 (1986), 205-10.

Caspersen, C. J., Christenson, G. M. & Pollard, R. A. "Status of the 1990 Physical Fitness and Exercise Objectives—Evidence From NHIS 1985," *Public Health Reports,* 101, 6 (1986), 587-92.

Gore, C. J. & Withers, R. T. "Effect of Exercise Intensity and Duration on Postexercise Metabolism," *Journal of Applied Physiology,* 68, 6 (1990), 2362-8.

Haskell, W. L. "The Influence of Exercise on the Concentrations of Triglyceride and Cholesterol in Human Plasma," *Exercise Sport Science Reviews,* 12 (1984), 205-44.

Haskell, W. L. et al. "Cardiovascular Benefits and Assessment of Physical Activity and Physical Fitness in Adults," *Medicine and Science in Sports and Exercise,* 24, 6 (1992), S201-20.

Hawk, S. R. "Exercise and Weight Loss: The Uncertain Connection," *Health Education,* 20, 4 (1989), 11-15.

Heyward, V. H. *Advanced Fitness Assessment & Exercise Prescription,* 2nd ed. Champaign: Human Kinetics Publishers, 1991.

ISSP. "Physical Activity and Psychological Benefits: A Position Statement," *International Journal of Sport Psychology,* 23, 1 (1992), 86-91.

Johnson, C. C. & Slemenda, C. "Osteoporosis: An Overview," *The Physician and Sportsmedicine,* 15, 11 (1987), 65-8.

Lenfant, C. "Physical Activity and Cardiovascular Health: Special Emphasis on Women and Youth," *Medicine and Science in Sports and Exercise,* 24, 6 (1992), S191.

Manninen, V. et al. "Lipid Alterations and Decline in the Incidence of Coronary Heart Disease in the Helsinki Heart Study," *Journal of the American Medical Association,* 260, 5 (1988), 641-51.

McArdle, W. D., Katch, F. I. & Katch, V.L. *Exercise Physiology: Energy, Nutrition and Human Performance,* 3rd ed. Philadelphia: Lea & Febiger, 1991.

Morgan, W. P. & Goldston, S. E. (Ed.). *Exercise and Mental Health.* Washington: Hemisphere, 1987.

Paffenbarger, R. S. "A Round Table: The Health Benefits of Exercise," (part 1 of 2), *The Physician and Sportsmedicine,* 15, 10 (1987), 115-32.

Paffenbarger, R. S. et al. "Physical Activity, All-Cause Mortality and Longevity of College Alumni," *New England Journal of Medicine,* 314, 10 (1986), 605-13.

Powell, K. E. & Dysinger, W. "Childhood Participation in Organized School Sports and Physical Education as Precursors of Adult Physical Activity," *American Journal of Preventive Medicine,* 5 (1987), 276-81.

Rowell, L. B. *Human Circulation: Regulation During Physical Stress.* New York: Oxford University Press, 1986.

Smith, E. L. & Gilligan, C. "Effects of Inactivity and Exercise on Bone," *The Physician and Sportsmedicine,* 15, 11 (1987), 91-2, 95-6, 98-9, 102.

U.S. Department of Health and Human Services. *Healthy People 2000: National Health Promotion and Disease Prevention Objectives* (DHHS [PHS] Publication No. 91-50212). Washington, DC: U.S. Government Printing Office, 1991.

U.S. Department of Health and Human Services. *The Surgeon General's Report on Nutrition and Health* (DHHS [PHS] Publication No. 88-50210). Washington, DC: U.S. Government Printing Office, 1988.

Van Zant, R. S. "Influence of Diet and Exercise on Energy Expenditure—A Review," *International Journal of Sport Nutrition,* 2 (1992), 1-19.

Wood, P. D. "A Round Table: The Health Benefits of Exercise," (part 1 of 2), *The Physician and Sportsmedicine,* 15, 10 (1987), 115-32.

Work, J. A. "Exercise for the Overweight Patient," *The Physician and Sportsmedicine,* 18 (1990), 113, 116, 119-22.

Exercise without injury

From runner's ankle and biker's knee to tennis elbow and swimmer's shoulder, there's hardly a sport or exercise that doesn't have an injury associated with it. Despite these names, most exercise injuries aren't limited to a single activity; they actually fall into just two broad categories. An understanding of these basic types may help you avoid injury, minimize the damage when you are hurt, and help speed your recovery.

The "stress and strain" injuries that befall active people most commonly result from damage done to those parts of the body responsible for movement: bones and muscles; major joints like the knee and ankle; and tendons and ligaments. This article will not discuss the injuries that physicians refer to as "direct trauma," such as cuts, scrapes, bruises, and broken bones—which usually require first aid and, often, a doctor's care. By contrast, the injuries discussed below can often be managed without professional help.

Note: Don't let concern about injuries keep you from exercising. A number of studies show that the benefits of exercise far exceed the risk of injury.

How injuries occur

When you exercise, you intentionally use certain muscles to increase their strength and endurance. As your body adapts to these efforts (depending on their intensity), you are likely to experience minor aches, twinges, and soreness. For example, one type of discomfort, called ischemic pain, occurs when muscle tissue doesn't have enough oxygen to continue working. This is the ache you feel when you attempt to perform more sit-ups or lift more weight than you are accustomed to, and it disappears when you stop exerting yourself.

An injury occurs when an exercise or activity actually damages tissue. The two basic types of sports injuries are those occurring suddenly (acute) and those developing gradually (overuse).

Five factors that put you at risk

1. Overdoing it. Pushing yourself too hard, too long, or too often is probably the leading cause of sports injury. Studies show, for example, that working out more than four times a week in a high-impact activity like running or aerobic dance puts you at significantly higher risk. So does dramatically increasing your workload—whether it's the amount of weight you lift, the speed or distance you cycle, or the number of hours you play tennis.

2. Inadequate footwear and equipment. Wearing improper or worn-out shoes places added stress on your hips, knees, ankles, and feet—the sites of up to 90% of all sports injuries. Running shoes, for example, offer virtually no protection from the sideways motions typical of aerobic dance, basketball, and racquet sports. With frequent use, athletic shoes can also lose one-third or more of their shock-absorbing ability in a matter of months.

Poor equipment is another risk factor. Riding a bicycle that is too small or that has its seat set too low, for instance, puts undue stress on the knees; a tennis racquet with too large a grip can strain your forearm.

3. Poor conditioning. Being out-of-shape and having weakened, tight muscles increases your risk of injury when you exercise. Problems can also arise from favoring one sport; this is likely to strengthen certain muscles at the expense of others, leaving tendons and ligaments unbalanced and thus vulnerable. For example, shin splints—a common running injury that causes pain in the front of the lower leg—are often the result of an imbalance between the powerful muscles along the back of the lower leg and the relatively weaker ones in front. Varying your activities is one way to prevent this muscle imbalance. Another precaution is to strengthen the muscle groups you underuse, and stretch all muscles involved in your workout.

4. Improper technique and training. In most activities, stress can result from poor form, whether it's landing on the balls of your feet (instead of your heels) when jogging, using an awkward backhand in tennis, or constantly cycling in the highest gears. Training practices like running on hills or on hard or uneven surfaces also increase risk. It may pay to consult an expert—such as a teaching tennis pro or trainer—if you have recurrent injuries.

5. Ignoring aches and pains. Studies show that starting to exercise before an injury has healed may not only worsen it, but greatly increases the chance of re-injury. Learn to monitor your body for abnormal sensations, and to apply appropriate treatment as early as possible.

Strains and sprains

An acute injury usually results from a single, abrupt incident that produces sharp pain, often accompanied by swelling. Most common are strains and sprains, conditions that are especially a problem for eager weekend athletes who don't know the limitations of their unconditioned muscles and joints.

• **Strains,** or "muscle pulls," occur when muscles or their tendon attachments are stretched to the point where their fibers actually start to tear. This can happen when you lift a heavy weight or suddenly overextend a muscle—for instance, when swinging a golf club or stretching to catch a baseball. The most common sites for strains are the hamstring and quadriceps muscles in the thigh and the muscles in the groin and shoulder—all large muscles that are used for sudden powerful movements.

Mild strains are usually only a nuisance; the tears are microscopic and, with rest, repair themselves easily. More severe strains involve a greater degree of fiber destruction and produce not only sharp pain but also loss of power and movement.

Tip: Cold, fatigue, and immobilization reduce blood flow and lessen muscle elasticity, increasing the risk of strains. Best prevention: warm up, then stretch all the muscles involved in your upcoming activity. A full-body warm-up, such as jogging in place or stationary cycling for five to ten minutes, increases blood flow and raises the temperature of large muscle groups. Or warm up by slowly rehearsing the sport or exercise you're about to perform. A light sweat usually indicates that you've warmed up sufficiently.

• **Sprains** damage ligaments (the bands connecting bones) and joint capsules. They are most often the result of a sudden force, typically a twisting motion, that the surrounding muscles aren't strong enough to control. As a result, the ligaments, which usually wrap around a joint, get stretched or torn. Like strains, sprains can range from minor tears to complete ruptures. *But sprains tend to be more serious than strains:* not only do they often take longer to heal, but a torn ligament can throw bones out of alignment, causing damage to surrounding tissues. A ruptured ligament requires medical attention.

Because of its construction and the fact that it must support your entire body weight, the ankle is the most frequently sprained joint—in fact, a sprained ankle is probably the most common sports injury. The knee, too, is vulnerable because it must absorb twisting stresses every time the body rotates from the hips. Ankle and knee sprains are most likely to occur during activities involving sudden twists or stop-and-start movements, such as dancing, tennis, soccer, hiking on rough terrain, and downhill skiing.

Tip: Strong, flexible muscles help protect against sprains. To safeguard your ankles, stretch your calf muscles (see Wellness Letter, *January 1990, for an illustration). To protect your knees, strengthen your quadriceps—the muscle group along the front of the thigh—as follows: lie on your back, flex your foot, and do leg lifts (this can be done with light weights); sit and do knee extensions while wearing light ankle weights (skip this if you're recovering from a knee problem); or stand and hold onto a wall while doing partial knee bends (don't go more than one-quarter of the way down).*

Overuse injuries

Also known as chronic or stress injuries, overuse injuries are brought on gradually as a result of wear and tear from a repetitive activity such as cycling, running, or hitting a tennis ball. Though a weekend athlete can experience overuse soreness, it is far more of a problem for people who do the same exercise repeatedly and/or often. In one survey of athletes, overuse injuries outnumbered acute injuries in all activities except basketball and skiing. In two of the most popular activities, running and tennis, almost 80% of all injuries were of the overuse variety.

Whereas you can almost always pinpoint the incident that caused an acute injury, *an overuse injury may have no obvious cause.* For instance, you suddenly increase the intensity or duration of your normal workout and feel a dull, annoying pain. Over the next few days, the pain recurs intermittently, but isn't bad enough to stop you from exercising. In effect, you have pushed your body beyond its ability to absorb the force of exercise effectively. As a result, muscle tissue has gradually developed microscopic tears that can cause pain, tenderness, and swelling. Initially, an overuse injury may seem less serious than an acute one. But as time passes, you usually feel pain during and after exercise. If you ignore the damage, it can worsen—and you may suffer a strain or other acute injury at the site of the weakened tissue.

• **Tendinitis** is the problem behind many common overuse injuries. The suffix "-itis" means inflammation (characterized by pain, swelling, warmth, and redness). Tendons—the fibrous cords that anchor muscles to bones—are vulnerable because the force of muscle contractions is transmitted through them. People who exercise regularly are especially at risk because of the strong forces produced by their well-conditioned muscles. These increase tension on the tendons, which can then rub against bones, ligaments, and other tendons, causing irritation.

Tendinitis is deceptive: the pain can be severe when you start exercising, then diminish as you continue—only to return sharply once you've stopped. Perhaps the most common form of tendinitis is tennis elbow, which affects not only tennis players but also rowers, carpenters, gardeners, and anyone else

---

Myth: You can "run through" the pain

Fact: If you feel pain (beyond mild discomfort), stop exercising and rest.

It may seem that many professional athletes bounce right back after an injury. But they usually have the benefit of care by experts who diagnose and treat their injuries quickly. Moreover, they are usually in better condition than the rest of us and are highly motivated to recover. In contrast, recreational athletes and other active people often ignore the pain or delay treating it, and thus aggravate the problem—so that full recovery can take weeks or months.

The surest way to avoid such trouble is to treat any recurring ache or pain right away, even if you're able to continue exercising in spite of it.

6. EXERCISE AND WEIGHT CONTROL

who repeatedly bends his arm forcefully. In sports and activities that involve running and jumping, tendinitis is most likely to develop in the knee, foot, and the Achilles tendon at the back of the ankle. For cyclists, knees are most vulnerable. Shoulder tendinitis can develop from pitching a ball, swinging a golf club, or swimming.

Tip: Stretching and strengthening routines can help prevent tendinitis, but equipment and technique may be equally important. For example, an improperly executed backhand is often the cause of tennis elbow (see Wellness Letter, *July 1989), and running shoes with worn-down heels contribute to Achilles tendinitis (see* Wellness Letter, *September 1988, for advice on how to evaluate signs of uneven wear on the soles of your exercise shoes).*

• **Stress fractures** are microscopic breaks in bone, usually in the foot, shin, or thigh. Common among long-distance runners, aerobic dancers, and basketball players, the fractures are brought on by the repeated impact of running or jumping. Often the pain is mild at first, occurring during or right after exercising. Continuing to exercise makes it gradually worse, but for the first few weeks such fractures are usually too small to be detected, even by X-ray. Fortunately, they rarely break through the bone, so they don't require splints or casts to heal, only rest.

Tip: Prevent stress fractures by increasing the intensity of your workouts gradually, not dramatically. Try to minimize impact on your legs: run and jump on soft or resilient surfaces—grass, carpet, mats, or suspended wooden gym floors—rather than concrete. Wear well-cushioned exercise shoes.

Now you can lose up to 18 pounds a year without dieting. How? Simply by walking. Our step-by-step guide tells you everything you need to know about the hottest new way to lose weight and get in shape safely.

Walk off calories and get fit

By *the editors of* The Walking Magazine

Why walk? Because it's wonderful for your heart, for your muscle tone and for your figure. If you're always on the sidelines while your friends are on the track, walking is a great way to get fit without running. It's a diet without dieting because you can trim down gradually without ever cutting out a morsel. It even will help you sleep better.

Why is walking such a good figure enhancer? Because when you walk, you burn off calories. In fact, you can burn off as many calories walking a mile as you would jogging the same distance — the difference is that walking just takes longer. The amount you burn varies, depending on your weight and how fast and how far you walk. For example, a 120-lb woman who walks 3 miles per hour burns 189 calories in one hour or 232 calories if she walks at a pace of 4 miles per hour. The chart on this page shows what walking can do for you. The figures shown, however, are for women only. You can calculate your speed by using this easy formula: 20 to 21 average-size steps every 10 seconds equals 3 miles per hour; 24 steps every 10 seconds adds up to 3.5 miles per hour; 27 to 28 steps in 10 seconds means you're walking 4 miles per hour.

In addition to what it does for you, walking is terrific because of what it doesn't do to you. It doesn't burden your bones and joints with extraordinary strain, as jogging and aerobic dancing do. It's a lot safer. It's a relatively trauma-free activity. Studies show that walking generates a downward force of about 1.5 times your body weight. That's a lot less than the force you generate while running, which is about 3 times your body weight.

To avoid getting off on the wrong

Walk it off!

Weight in pounds	Calorie Burn-off per hour at		
	3.0	3.5	4.0
100	156	175	192
120	189	207	232
140	219	245	272
160	252	280	308
180	282	315	348
200	315	350	388

foot, you need to know your current fitness level before you begin. Are you in average shape? Below average? This is important to determine because it gives you a realistic place to start, and it will keep you from attempting to do too much too quickly. (If you're a man over 35 or a woman over 40, and are fairly inactive, check with your doctor before starting this or any other exercise program.)

The advantage of this test is that you don't need all the expensive paraphernalia (electrodes, heart-monitoring devices) that are usually required to obtain a reading with scientific accuracy. In fact, says James M. Rippe, M.D. director of the Exercise-Physiology Laboratory at the University of Massachusetts Medical Center, Worcester, where the test was developed, all you need is a wristwatch with a second hand and a flat road or track.

First, you need to know how to determine your heart rate (pulse). To practice, walk in place for 30 seconds. Then place your second and third fingers on the inside of your wrist to feel your pulse. You can also check your pulse by gently pressing on the side of your neck next to your Adam's apple and below the jaw. Count your pulse for 15 seconds. To get your heart rate per minute, multiply this number by 4.

Next, walk one mile at top speed on a flat surface. The best place to do this is on a track, but you can also walk on any road that has a mile measured out. Walk as fast as you can. Don't start and stop, and try to maintain an even pace. Take your pulse as soon as you stop, because once you quit walking your pulse begins to drop. Note how many minutes it took you to walk a mile.

Now consult the "What is Your Fitness Level?" chart in your age category. Find on the bottom line the time it took you to walk one mile and locate your heart rate on the left. From each of these points, draw a line across the chart, and note where they intersect. The point of intersection in the shaded area determines your condition. If you're 35, have a 15-minute time and a heart rate of 145, you're in above average condition.

Another way to get a general idea of your fitness level is to rank yourself according to the following

From *St. Raphael's Better Health*, November/December 1987, pp. 21, 23-26. First appeared in *The Walking Magazine*.
Reprinted by permission.

criteria.

- You have a sit-down job and do not engage in any regular aerobic activities: *poor or "low" condition.*
- You are sporadically involved in weekend golf, tennis, jogging, swimming or cycling: *average condition.*
- You have an active lifestyle, and you swim, jog or cycle three times each week for 30 to 60 minutes: *above average condition.*
- You exercise or participate in vigorous activity four times a week for 60 minutes: *excellent or "high" condition.*

Your tailor-made workout

This walking fitness program has three components: a warm-up, which consists of short walk plus some simple stretches, the walk itself and a cool-down. The warm-up gets your muscles and tendons limber, and helps you mentally prepare for exercise. The cool-down, the flip side of the warm-up, is just as important. It prevents stiffness from setting in and helps the muscles to clear themselves of waste products, such as lactic acid, which build up when you walk.

The warm-up. You can start your warm-up by building up to your walking pace over a quarter of a mile. After this short walk—5 to 10

Walking facts

- Walking on sand or dirt can boost your energy expenditure by as much as a third. It also exercises more of the muscles in the foot, expecially if you walk barefoot.
- Over 5 million Americans walk to work without relying on any other form of transportation, according to the U.S. Census Bureau.
- Even though you burn more calories in high heels than in flat shoes, high heels are poor walking shoes--bad for your feet, legs, and lower back.
- Skip elevators and escalators. Several work-site studies have found that people who simply began using staircases improved their overall fitness by 10 percent to 15 percent.
- A West Virginia study of women aged 50 to 63 found that a 6-month walking program (2 miles a day, 4 days a week) produced "significant improvements in the cardiovascular and muscular systems" comparable to those produced by an aerobic dance program.

- It's not surprising that you burn more calories when you walk uphill than on level ground. But did you know that walking down hill also uses more energy?
- If it's too hot or cold outdoors, try walking in your local shopping mall. Many malls now have walking programs sponsored by the American Heart Association.
- When walking at night, wear reflective clothing. This is an extremely important safety measure, particularly if you walk in heavily trafficked or dimly lit areas.
- Health walking can be an ideal exercise for pregnant women. The breathing and posture techniques associated with health walking helps keep pelvic and abdominal muscles in good condition—essential to easy delivery.
- Take the talk test as you walk. If you can't carry on a conversation without becoming breathless, you're going too fast.

minutes—do each of the following stretches three times to aid your performance and reduce the risk of strained muscles.

- For the hamstrings (the major muscle group in the back of the thigh): Stand with feet 6 inches apart. With knees straight (but not

What is your fitness level?

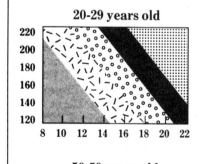

20-29 years old

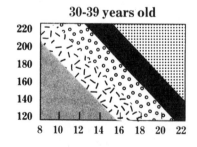

30-39 years old

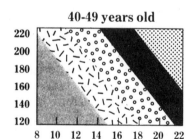

40-49 years old

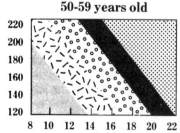

50-59 years old

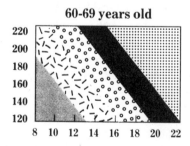

60-69 years old

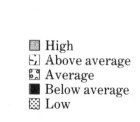

- High
- Above average
- Average
- Below average
- Low

■ Vertical numbers indicate heartbeats per minute. ■ Horizontal numbers indicate time in minutes.

Charts based on information from the Rockport Walking Institute, P.O. Box 480, Marlboro, MA 01752

locked), bend forward slowly and reach for the floor, arms dangling. Stretch as far as you can. Breathe deeply. Don't bounce. Hold for 20 seconds. Come up slowly. Repeat several times, stretching closer to the ground each time.

• for the calves and Achilles tendon: Stand at arm's length from a wall, place both hands on the wall, and move your left foot back one step. Keeping your heels on the floor, lean forward slowly, back straight, to the point where you feel you're stretching your left calf. Don't bounce. Breathe deeply and hold for 20 seconds. Relax. Switch feet and repeat.

The walk. Find the program that's right for you and stick with it for 4 weeks. *Poor or low condition.* Walk for 25 to 30 minutes at 3 miles per hour, five times a week. That's 1$\frac{1}{4}$ to 1$\frac{1}{2}$ miles.
Below average condition. Walk for 30 to 35 minutes at 3 miles per hour, five times a week. That's 1$\frac{1}{2}$ to 1$\frac{3}{4}$ miles.
Average condition. Walk for 35 to 40 minutes at 3 to 3.5 miles per hour, five times a week. That's 2 miles.
Above average condition. Walk for 40 to 45 minutes at 3.5 miles per hour, five times a week. That's about 2$\frac{1}{2}$ to 3 miles.

> *"Why walk? Because it's wonderful for your heart, for your muscle tone, and for your figure."*

Excellent or high. Walk for 45 to 50 minutes at 4 to 4.5 miles per hour, five times per week. That's 3 to 4 miles (Thirty to thirty-one steps every 10 seconds equals 4.5 miles per hour.)

As you feel more comfortable, gradually increase the distance you walk, adding no more than a quarter of a mile every two weeks. After about four weeks you may want to increase your pace so that your walking speed rises by approximately $\frac{1}{2}$ mile per hour. Experts say your cardiovascular system will benefit most if you get your heart rate up to what's called your target rate—that's 60 percent to 80 percent of your maximum heart rate. To determine your maximum heart rate, subtract your age from 220.
The cool-down. Cool down by gently slowing your pace over a quarter of a mile. If you feel stiffness in any area, repeat the warm-up stretches for those muscles.

Tips for walking
The appeal of walking is that you can do it almost anywhere and it requires no skills or major equipment. But no matter how much you walk, your technique probably could stand improvement. Some tips for your journey to health and fitness:
• Stand erect. This will improve the circulation of oxygen and blood in your body. Focus your eyes ahead of you and pull in your stomach.
• Swing your arms as you walk to help burn calories, aid oxygen distribution and promote balance. If you are in good condition, you may want to add $\frac{1}{2}$ lb. hand weights. They may increase calorie burn and improve upper-body fitness.
• Don't walk so fast that you find yourself huffing and puffing and straining. You should be able to carry on a normal conversation as you walk.
• Remember, warm up first and cool down later. If you find that you're too sore to repeat the same walk in 24 hours, you've done too much.

To subscribe to *Walking Magazine,* call toll free, 800-358-8888. And to receive a free copy of the kit, *Walking and Your Health,* send your name and address to: Raben Publishing, 711 Boylston St. Box 10 Boston, MA 02116.

LOSING WEIGHT

WHAT WORKS.
WHAT DOESN'T.

In the first large-scale survey of the major weight-loss programs, we found that no program is very effective. Here's why diets usually don't work, and how you can manage your weight more wisely.

Fifty million Americans are dieting at any given time, and these days, most of them are thoroughly confused. After decades in which medical authorities, the fashion industry, and most ordinary people agreed that the pursuit of thinness was an unmitigated good, the wisdom of dieting has come into question. Researchers have found that yo-yo dieting, the common cycle of repeatedly losing and regaining weight, may be as bad for you as weighing too much in the first place. Sobered by that research—and by the realization that many dieters become yo-yo dieters—members of a growing antidiet movement have urged people to throw away their calorie counters and eat whenever they're hungry.

Despite those developments, it is still possible and worthwhile for some people to lose weight. But a review of the scientific literature, interviews with experts in the field, and CU's own research show that a major shift in thinking about weight loss is in order. For the typical American dieter, the benefits of weight loss are no longer certain—and the difficulty of losing weight permanently has become all too clear.

Medical researchers have suspected for years that most diets end in failure; studies done at weight-loss clinics in medical centers showed that people almost always regained the weight they lost. But it was never clear whether people at those clinics had an unusually poor success rate because they were "hard cases" who needed special help.

Now CU has undertaken the first large-scale survey of people on ordinary diet programs and shown that they, too, usually fail at losing weight in the long term. We collected information from 95,000 readers who had done something to lose weight over the previous three years, including some 19,000 who had used a commerical diet program. . . . our survey showed that people do lose weight on these programs—but the great majority of them gain back most of that weight within two years.

Although different weight-loss programs use different diets and strategies, none have been able to overcome this basic pattern. The problem is that losing weight is much more than a matter of willpower: It's a process that pits the dieter against his or her own physiology.

Why people get fat

A small number of people have struggled with obesity since childhood and are massively overweight as adults. A greater number are not overweight when they enter adulthood, but become so as they gain 10, 20, or 30 pounds over the course of two or three decades. And about three-quarters of American adults are not overweight at all.

What makes for the difference? Primarily, it's the genes. An individual's body size, studies have conclusively shown, is genetically coded as surely as the shape of a nose. Inheritance overwhelms other factors in determining an individual's normal range of weight, which may be rela-

tively high for one person, low for another. While diet and exercise certainly play a role, they do so within limits set by heredity.

Over and over again, researchers have observed the human body's remarkable resistance to major weight change. Dr. Rudolph Leibel, an obesity researcher at Rockefeller University in New York City, describes how extremely obese people repeatedly enter the university's weight-loss clinic, lose dozens of pounds, go home, and return six months later having regained precisely the amount of weight they lost. Other clinicians have reported similar, if less dramatic, results.

What's less widely known is that the body resists major weight *gain* as much as it resists a major loss. In a classic study conducted in the 1960s by Dr. Ethan Allen Sims of the University of Vermont, a group of 20 prisoners of normal weight volunteered to gain as much weight as possible. Only by forcing themselves to overeat—some by thousands of extra calories a day—were the men able to add 20 percent to their weight and keep it on. Once the study ended, almost everyone returned quickly to his starting weight.

No one knows just how the body keeps weight within a fairly narrow range; researchers posit the existence of some sort of biochemical control system, but they haven't found it. Whatever the mechanism is, however, it allows weight to drift slowly upward as people get older. Two major changes take place with age. People tend to become less physi-

The first modern diet book
In 1863, the Englishman William Banting published his "Letter on Corpulence Addressed to the Public." His advice: Cut back on carbohydrates.

cally active. And, partly as a result of inactivity, people lose lean muscle mass, which burns calories more rapidly than fatty tissue.

No wonder, then, that the prime time for dieting is the mid-40s. "That's when people start to look fat or study a height-weight table and say to themselves, 'Gee, I've crossed over a line,'" says David Williamson, an epidemiologist who studies weight patterns for the Centers for Disease Control and Prevention.

Weight and health

Even if some people are genetically programmed to be fatter than others, their natural body size may not necessarily be a healthy one. Researchers are now struggling with a difficult question: At what point do the risks of overweight make the effort to lose weight worthwhile?

To begin to answer that question, scientists have used a measure called the body mass index, or BMI, which incorporates both height and weight to assess a person's level of fatness. You can find your own BMI by following the instructions on the opposite page. Scientists consider a BMI of 25 or less to be desirable for most people. A BMI between 25 and 30—mild or moderate overweight—carries a slightly increased risk of weight-related health problems such as high blood pressure, high blood cholesterol, heart disease, and Type II (adult-onset) diabetes. At a BMI of 30 or more—considered truly overweight—the risk of developing those conditions and others rises sharply.

There is little doubt that people with a *lifelong* BMI of 25 or less have the lowest risk of disease and premature death (except for cigarette smokers, who are both lean and suffer high rates of cancer, chronic lung disease, and cardiovascular disease). But the benefits of thinness may be greatest for people who have always been thin. Someone who starts out overweight and then slims down is still worse off than someone who never was overweight at all.

The people with the hardest decision to make about their weight are those who are mildly to moderately overweight, with a BMI between 25 and 30. If they have diabetes or cardiovascular risk factors, such as high blood cholesterol or high blood pressure, they may have a medical reason to try to reduce; if not, they may be relatively safe.

Age also affects the risk for this middle group. Americans' median weight rises steadily between the

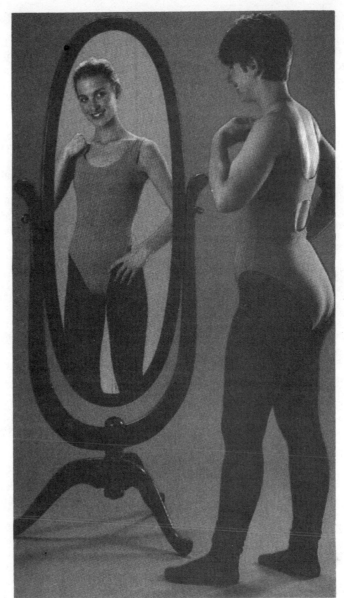

A clash of ideals The woman on the right—5-foot-4 and 130 pounds—has an ideal body type from a health standpoint. But many women her size long to attain a thinner ideal: the super-svelte body, shown in the mirror, that only a tiny fraction of the population can ever match.

ages of 20 and 55, and a number of studies indicate that isn't necessarily dangerous. The overall risk of moderate overweight apparently diminishes, or even disappears altogether, with advancing age. The reason is not entirely clear, and the data have been the subject of much debate. However, most researchers now accept the phenomenon as fact, as does the U.S. Government. Since 1990, the Government has published

weight guidelines for Americans that give different ranges for older and younger adults.

One other critical variable has emerged in the last several years: the waist-to-hip ratio, calculated as the measure of a person's waist at its smallest point divided by the circumference of the hips at their widest point. This ratio distinguishes "apples"—that is, people who carry excess weight above their waist—

from "pears," whose extra fat settles around the hips and buttocks. The higher the waist-to-hip ratio, the more apple-shaped the figure. Most men are apples, with the classic beer belly; most women are pears, although there is a significant minority of female apples.

The correlation between the waist-to-hip ratio and cardiovascular disease has been investigated in at least a half-dozen long-term studies, with consistent results: The higher the ratio, the greater the risk of disease, especially among people who are at least moderately overweight. Many scientists even believe that the waist-to-hip ratio predicts cardiovascular disease better than the degree of overweight. For men, the risk seems to rise above a waist-to-hip ratio of 0.95; for women, the cutoff point is 0.80. Paradoxically, surveys show that overweight men, most of whom are apples, are much less likely to try to lose weight than women, whose fat distribution is more benign.

Scientists think that abdominal fat does its damage because it is more metabolically active than below-the-waist fat. It's also associated with increased insulin resistance (a precursor to diabetes) and may be a cause of hypertension.

Why diets don't work

Even the most optimistic weight-control professionals admit that traditional dieting—cutting calories to lose weight—rarely works in the long term. Clinicians have tried everything to make diets more effective. They've devised ultra-low-calorie regimens that produce fast, large weight losses. They've brought patients in for months, even years, of behavior modification to help them deal with "impulse" eating and distract themselves from hunger pangs. The results are unvarying: When treatment stops, weight gain begins.

IS YOUR WEIGHT BAD FOR YOUR HEALTH?

While being overweight can raise the risk of disease, especially cardiovascular disease, your risk is only partially determined by the number you see on the scale. By completing this worksheet, you can get a fuller picture of how your weight is likely to affect your health. The approach used here is largely adapted from work by Dr. George Bray of the Pennington Biomedical Research Center at Louisiana State University and psychologist Thomas A. Wadden of Syracuse University. To begin, you need to calculate your body mass index (BMI) and your waist-to-hip ratio.

Finding your BMI

Using a calculator, you can calculate your BMI as follows: Multiply your weight in pounds by 700, divide by your height in inches, then divide by your height again.

BMI _____

Finding your waist-to-hip ratio

Using a tape measure, find the circumference of your waist at its narrowest point when your stomach is relaxed.

Waist: _____ in.

Next, measure the circumference of your hips at their widest (where your buttocks protrude the most).

Hips: _____ in.

Finally, divide your waist measurement by your hip measurement.

Waist/hip = _____ Waist-to-hip ratio

Determining your risk

Long-term studies show that the overall risk of developing heart disease is generally related to BMI as follows:

BMI of 25 or less—Risk is very low to low.
BMI between 25 and 30—Risk is low to moderate.
BMI of 30 or more—Risk is moderate to very high.

The BMI determines your likely range of risk. But where you fall within that range depends on the factors at right. The more items you have in the "High-Risk Factors" column, the higher your risk; the more you have in the "Low-Risk Factors" column, the lower your risk. Bear in mind that these factors give you only an approximation of your risk; your physician can give you more precise advice. (It's also possible for someone with a large number of high-risk factors to have a high risk of heart disease at any weight.)

HIGH-RISK FACTORS

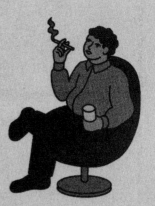

- Being male
- Under age 40 with BMI above 25
- Waist-to-hip ratio greater than 0.80 for women or 0.95 for men
- Sedentary life-style
- Smoking
- High blood pressure
- Blood cholesterol of more than 200 mg/dl
- HDL less than 35
- Heart disease or Type II (adult-onset) diabetes—personal or in family history

LOW-RISK FACTORS

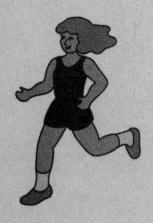

- Being female
- Waist-to-hip ratio of less than 0.80 for women or 0.95 for men
- Regular exercise
- Normal blood pressure
- Blood cholesterol of less than 200 mg/dl
- HDL more than 45
- No personal or family history of heart disease or diabetes

Scientists can't yet fully explain this nearly inevitable pattern, but the explanation may lie in our prehistoric roots. According to one hypothesis, humans evolved under the constant threat of famine. As a result, the human body is programmed by evolution to respond to caloric restriction as if starvation were at hand. After a few weeks on a low-calorie diet, the body goes on a sort of protective red alert. The basal metabolic rate—the speed at which the body burns calories when at rest—begins to decline. In addition, the body uses lean muscle mass as fuel in an effort to preserve fat, which is the major long-term source of energy. Both changes mean that the body burns fewer calories, making it more difficult to maintain a weight loss.

Finally, hunger—true, physiological hunger—increases. And, faced with hunger, "people are not able to keep up with the food restrictions required to maintain a lower weight," says David Schlundt, a psychologist at Vanderbilt University who specializes in obesity. Although the folklore of dieting says that hunger can be overcome by anyone with a decent amount of willpower, this basic biological drive is exceedingly difficult to ignore.

Most obesity researchers now believe that stringent dieting is actually a major trigger for binge eating. This connection was shown vividly in an experiment conducted during World War II by University of Minnesota physiologist Ancel Keys with a group of young, healthy men. Keys put the men on a balanced diet that provided about half their usual caloric intake—a regimen that he called "semistarvation" but that was remarkably similar to the diets prescribed by today's commercial weight-loss programs. When the men were released from the diet after six months, they went on massive eating binges, eating up to five meals and 5000 calories a day until they had returned to their normal weight. The lesson: "Going back to eating after a period of starvation is as natural as taking a breath," says Susan Wooley, a University of Cincinnati psychologist who specializes in obesity and eating disorders.

Is weight loss safe?

In addition to the high physical and emotional cost of dieting, new epidemiological evidence suggests that the practice may actually carry a greater health risk than staying overweight for some people.

For years everyone assumed that if overweight damaged a person's health, losing weight would improve it. That assumption seemed to be well-founded: Many studies have shown that as soon as dieters start to lose weight, their blood cholesterol levels and blood pressure drop and their insulin resistance declines.

Surprisingly, however, not a single long-term epidemiological study has ever proven that losing weight extends life. And over the past year, two important studies have provided evidence to the contrary.

One, headed by Elsie Pamuk of the Centers for Disease Control and Prevention, used the results of the First National Health and Nutrition Examination Survey, a Government survey of the health status of thousands of Americans. When they entered that study in the early 1970s, participants were given a complete checkup that, among other things, recorded what they weighed then and what was the most they had ever weighed. A decade later, the Government scientists tracked the participants to see who had died, and of what causes.

Recently, the CDC team analyzed the records of 5000 men and women who had been between the ages of 45 and 74 when they entered the Government study. The goal was to see whether those who had once been overweight but had lost weight lived longer than peers who had stayed fat. The team eliminated from the analysis anyone who had died within five years of starting the study, to make sure a pre-existing disease had not made them thin. They also adjusted their data to account for the effects of smoking, age, and gender.

The analysis did confirm one piece of conventional wisdom: Maintaining a stable adult weight and avoiding severe overweight is the best possible course. The data also supported the view that moderate overweight is not necessarily detrimental in middle age: Over the period of the study, men and women with a stable BMI between 25 and 30 had death rates as low as those with a stable BMI of 25 or less.

But when the CDC analysts looked at the effect of weight loss, what they found upset all their expectations:

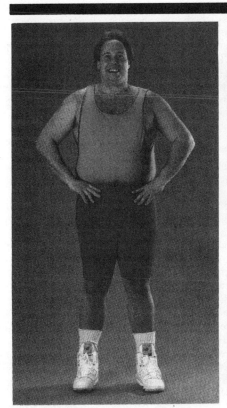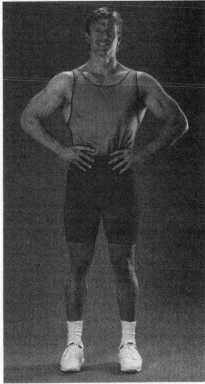

Same weight, different physique Weight is only one determinant of physical health. The man at left is 6 feet tall and weighs 240 pounds; the man at right is almost identical in height and weight, at 6-foot-1 and 230. But the man on the left is a classic "apple," with a high risk of heart disease, while the man on the right is muscular and at low risk.

Instead of improving health, losing weight seemed to do the opposite. Women who lost *any* amount of weight had a higher death rate than those who didn't; the more weight they lost, the higher their risk. Among the fattest group of men, who began with a BMI of 30 or above, those who had a moderate weight loss had a slightly lower than average death rate. But those who lost 15 percent or more had a higher death rate—unless, surprisingly, they were so fat that their weight loss still left them overweight.

The second study was even larger: It included 11,703 middle-aged and elderly Harvard alumni whose weight was recorded in the early 1960s and again in 1977. Like the CDC study, the Harvard study controlled for pre-existing disease.

In 1988, the researchers checked alumni records to see who had died. The men whose weight changed least between the 1960s and 1977 had the lowest death rates, whether the researchers looked at deaths from all causes, deaths from cancer, or, especially, deaths from cardiovascular disease. Any significant weight change, whether up *or* down, markedly increased the risk of dying from cardiovascular disease.

Researchers are hard-pressed to explain the findings of the CDC and Harvard studies. The most likely explanation, however, is that people whose weight changed the most over time were more likely to have had cycles of yo-yo dieting in between—especially if they were overweight. Since our culture stigmatizes fatness, anyone who has been overweight for more than a few years has very likely gone through at least one cycle of significant weight loss and regain. Of the 95,000 respondents to our diet survey, 40 percent had had two or more weight-loss cycles within the previous five years; in that survey, overweight people cycled more often than people of normal weight.

Other studies have suggested that repeatedly losing and gaining weight is hazardous to health. One recent analysis used data from the Framingham Heart Study, a long-term study of some 5000 residents of a Boston suburb that began in 1948. Compared with subjects whose weight remained the most stable, those whose weight fluctuated frequently or by many pounds had a 50 percent higher risk of heart disease.

Weighing your options

Studies like those will animate seminars at scientific meetings for years to come. But they're confusing to people who must decide right now what, if anything, to do about their weight.

For some groups, the decision is relatively clear-cut. People who are not already overweight should place top priority on avoiding weight gain through a combination of moderate eating habits and exercise. Most seriously overweight people—those with a BMI of 30 or more—should attempt to lose some weight; for them, the evidence favoring weight loss is greater than the evidence against it. Most adult-onset diabetics should also reduce, since blood-sugar control usually improves with even relatively small amounts of weight loss. Given the possibility that large losses and regains may be hazardous, however, the best strategy is to stay away from quick weight-loss diets and aim instead for slow, modest, but permanent weight loss using the approaches we'll describe below.

The choice for nondiabetic, moderately overweight adults is not so clear. They should do what they can to avoid gaining more weight. But it is not certain that losing weight in and of itself will reduce their risk—especially if they gain it back again.

Fortunately, there is an approach to losing weight through diet and exercise that doesn't involve low-calorie quick-weight-loss plans. It's safer than conventional dieting; it's more likely to be effective; and it can lessen the risk of cardiovascular disease dramatically, even if it doesn't result in a large weight loss.

The importance of exercise

Apart from the risk of developing shinsplints or being chased by a dog, there's almost nothing bad to be said about regular, moderate physical exercise. And a number of studies now show that exercise can be very effective in weight control.

In one recent study, Stanford University researchers put 71 moderately overweight men and women on a low-fat diet for a year, and another, matched group of 71 on a diet with the same kinds of foods—plus a three-day-a-week program of aerobic exercise. After a year, the diet-plus-exercise group had lost more weight overall and more pounds of fat, even though they actually ate more calories per day than the diet-only group. Other studies have shown that exercise can help people lose weight even if they don't change their regular diet at all.

The explanation lies in the nature of human metabolism. More than half the calories we take in are burned up by what's called basal metabolism—the energy expended just to stay alive. In addition to increasing the number of calories burned in activity, exercise increases the basal metabolic rate, so the body burns more calories even at rest. Studies have shown that the basal metabolic rate is closely linked to the amount of muscle on the body, which is built up through exercise.

For most people, exercise alone will be enough to prevent future weight gain; for many, it will enable them to lose weight effectively and safely. In addition, even if exercise doesn't help you lose pounds, it may help you become thinner. A pound of muscle takes up less space than a pound of fat. So as you build muscle and lose fat, you can lose inches even without actually losing any weight.

Exercise plays a critical role not only in burning fat, but in keeping weight off. That was shown dramatically in a study of 184 mildly overweight Massachusetts policemen and civil servants. All were put on a low-calorie diet, and half were also put through three 90-minute exercise sessions per week. After eight weeks, everyone had lost weight. But when the men were re-examined three years later, those who had never exercised—or who had stopped once the study ended—promptly regained all or most of the weight they had lost. In contrast, exercisers who kept at it maintained virtually all their initial weight loss.

The rationale for exercise goes well beyond becoming thinner. "A lot of the health benefits that people are seeking from weight loss can be achieved by exercise, even in the absence of any weight loss," says Steven Blair, director of epidemiology at the Institute for Aerobics Research in Dallas.

In 1970, scientists at that institute began keeping records on more than 13,000 then-healthy middle-aged men and women to determine the effects of physical fitness on cardiovascular risk. The results are now coming in: Exercise seems to protect against disease and death even in people whose risk factors would otherwise put them in danger. Physically fit men in the study who had high blood pressure, insulin resistance, a high BMI, or an unfavorable family history were less likely to die than unfit men with none of those risk factors. Overall, the fittest men in the study had a death rate less than one-third that of the least fit; for women, there was a five-fold differ-

Trading pounds for lung cancer? Smoking tends to make people thinner, and cigarette manufacturers once promoted their products as if they were diet aids. In 1928, the American Tobacco Company introduced the slogan, "Reach for a Lucky instead of a sweet."

ence. The rates for cardiovascular disease were even more dramatically affected by fitness.

This study has now been followed up by a number of others showing that, among people with almost any known cardiovascular risk factor, exercisers do better than nonexercisers. In addition, exercisers develop adult-onset diabetes about 40 percent less often than nonexercisers, according to a study of 21,000 male American doctors.

It may even be that lack of exercise, rather than excess body fat itself, is the true culprit behind many of the ill effects of obesity. Since inactivity often leads to weight gain, overweight may turn out to be more a result of an unhealthful life-style than a cause of ill health.

Despite the evident benefits of exercise, most people with a weight problem still choose dieting instead. One reason has been the exercise community's historic fixation on high-intensity aerobic exercise, with its intimidating target-heart-rate charts and elaborate workout schedules. Most people simply won't attempt such demanding, time-consuming regimens—especially not the sedentary, overweight people who have the greatest need to exercise.

But intense exercise may not be necessary. Blair's study at the Institute for Aerobics Research suggests that the chief benefits of exercise come when people go from a sedentary life-style to moderate activity—not when they move from moderate exercise to intense athletics. In that study, men in the moderate-fitness group had a death rate from all causes nearly 60 percent lower than that of the sedentary group. In contrast, the very fittest men had a death rate only 23 percent lower than that of the moderately fit group. (Moderate exercise was defined as the equivalent of 30 to 60 minutes a day of brisk walking, either in small spurts or all at once.)

Influenced by these findings, Blair has become a prominent advocate of what might be called opportunistic exercise, which is essentially the art of devising an activity plan that can mesh with any schedule, no matter how frenetic. Blair, like many fitness experts, recommends looking for exercise everywhere you can. Park at the far edge of the mall lot instead of next to the front door; get off a bus one stop early and walk the rest of the way; pace the floor while you're on the phone; use an old-fashioned reel-type mower instead of a gasoline-powered one; take the stairs instead of the elevator. Any kind of exercise, however mundane, has potential benefits.

Eat less fat, lose fat

In addition to exercise, changing the kinds of food you eat—even without changing the caloric content—can improve both weight and health. Despite the decades-old wisdom that a calorie is a calorie is a calorie, some recent studies have suggested that calories from fat follow a straighter trajectory to the hips or the belly than calories from other sources. The body can store fat very efficiently. But the body's ability to store carbohydrates is limited, so when people eat more than their bodies can use, the excess is burned.

For that reason, researchers have found that the composition of the diet may be more important than the number of calories in determining who gains and who loses weight. The percentage of fat in the diet was the single strongest predictor of subsequent weight gain, for example, among 294 adults monitored for three years by Memphis State University investigators. By contrast, the total calorie consumption they reported had only a weak relationship to weight gain for women, and none at all for men.

If a high-fat diet can add pounds, a low-fat diet may help take them off. Researchers at the University of Illinois at Chicago switched 18 women volunteers from a diet that derived 37 percent of calories from fat—roughly the fat content of the average American's diet—to a diet that was only 20 percent fat. Over the 20-week experiment, the women lost four to five pounds, even though they increased their caloric intake.

One way to reduce fat intake without feeling chronically hungry is to fill up on something else, namely fruits, vegetables, and whole grains. Those foods are all high in carbohydrates, and a diet rich in fruits and vegetables seems to lower the risk of cancer and cardiovascular disease.

Some high-fat foods are easier to give up than others, as scientists at Seattle's Fred Hutchinson Cancer Research Center found in a study of the relationship between dietary fat and breast cancer. They taught a large group of women simple ways to reduce their fat consumption, and tracked down some of the participants after a year to see if they'd kept up their low-fat habits. The easiest changes to sustain turned out to be those that were least noticeable from a sensory standpoint: switching to

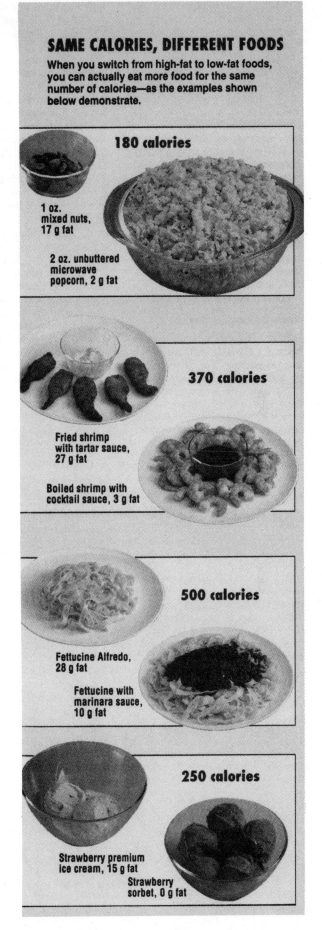

SAME CALORIES, DIFFERENT FOODS

When you switch from high-fat to low-fat foods, you can actually eat more food for the same number of calories—as the examples shown below demonstrate.

180 calories

1 oz. mixed nuts, 17 g fat

2 oz. unbuttered microwave popcorn, 2 g fat

370 calories

Fried shrimp with tartar sauce, 27 g fat

Boiled shrimp with cocktail sauce, 3 g fat

500 calories

Fettucine Alfredo, 28 g fat

Fettucine with marinara sauce, 10 g fat

250 calories

Strawberry premium ice cream, 15 g fat

Strawberry sorbet, 0 g fat

low-fat milk, mayonnaise, margarine, and salad dressing; trimming fat from meats and skin from chicken; having occasional vegetarian meals. Hardest to give up were the foods for which fat was an integral part of the food's appeal: pastries and ice cream, butter, hamburgers, lunch meats, and cheese.

Fortunately, the fat-reducing strategies that are easiest to follow can yield a significant decrease in total fat consumption. A group from Pennsylvania State University calculated the effect of such changes on an average woman's diet. They determined that by substituting skim milk for whole, switching to lower-fat meats and fish (such as skinless chicken and water-packed tuna), and using low-fat dressings and spreads, a woman could cut the fat in her diet from 37 percent of calories to 23 percent.

Your natural weight

Exercising and eating less fat are healthful changes that can benefit anyone, and may lead to weight loss as a bonus. But for many people,

especially those who have been overweight all their lives, even faithful adherence to healthful habits won't slim the body to the thin ideal our culture holds dear.

Janet Polivy, an obesity researcher at the University of Toronto, believes that people should learn to be comfortable with their "natural weight"—the body size and shape that results after a person adopts a healthful diet and gets a reasonable amount of exercise. Similarly, Kelly Brownell, a Yale University psychologist who has done extensive research on behavioral obesity treatments, speaks of a "reasonable weight" as an attainable goal. "It's the weight that individuals making reasonable changes in their diet and exercise patterns can seek and maintain over a period of time," he explains. Brownell suggests that people who want to lose weight should start by losing a moderate amount, 10 pounds or so, and should then see how comfortably they can maintain that lower weight before trying to lose a bit more, stabilizing again, and so on.

Accepting the goal of a "natural" or "reasonable" weight may involve giving up long-held fantasies of a slim, youthfully athletic body, and being content with the realities of a middle-aged shape instead. It means accepting a slower rate of weight loss, or none at all. For long-term dieters, many of whom have spent years monitoring everything they put into their mouths and suppressing hunger pangs, it also means learning anew how to eat normally—eating when hungry and stopping when full.

Nevertheless, we believe this moderate approach to weight control is the only one worth trying for most people. It makes sense whether you are trying to maintain your current weight, reverse middle-age spread, or deal with a weight problem that's plagued you all your life. If you change your eating and exercise patterns gradually, and maintain the changes over time, you will almost certainly look and feel better, have more energy, and reduce your risk of cardiovascular disease, whether or not you lose much weight.

Chemistry &Craving

NOT
THE SAME OLD
DIET STORY

HARA ESTROFF MARANO

some revolutions are waged with guns. Others are waged with words. But perhaps the major American revolt of the past two decades has been waged primarily with knife and fork. With butter banished, red meat in retreat, and humble grains advancing on our plates, we've toppled the old dietary regime on the grounds that you are what you eat.

Still, decisive victories in the battle of the bulge, the war on heart disease, and just plain healthy appetites elude us. And so we begin each year with solemn vows to tackle anew our waistlines and our arteries. But if a behavioral scientist in New York is right, a winning strategy can come only from a simple turn of the tables—we eat what we are.

In meticulous studies over the last 10 years, Sarah F. Leibowitz, Ph.D., of The Rockefeller University, has discovered that what we put in our mouths and when we do it is profoundly influenced by a brew of neurochemicals based in a specific part

of our brain. They not only guide our selection of morsels at breakfast, lunch, and dinner—and even the need for high tea—they are probably the power behind individual differences in appetite and weight gain. They appear to determine whether we are sitting ducks for the eating disorders that now afflict 30 percent of Americans.

Unless we take into account the physiological function of these brain chemicals in dictating natural patterns of food intake and metabolism, we will never get closer than annual avowals in regulating our eating behavior, whatever our reason for doing so. The only plausible way to control body weight is by working *with* the neurochemical systems that control appetite—and re-tuning them.

Leibowitz' studies point far beyond our forks. They challenge the deeply held belief that we are strictly self-determining individuals acting, at least at the table, by unfettered choice—whim, if the moon is right. Sooner or later, in

one context or another, we will have to overhaul our view of human behavior to acknowledge that there are a variety of physiological signals guiding what we now believe to be free will.

Leibowitz, however, has little taste for the philosophical soup. In classic meat-and-potatoes neuroscience, she has located the epicenter of eating behavior. It is a dense cluster of nerve cells, the neurochemicals they produce, and the receptors through which they act and are acted upon. They make up the paraventricular nucleus, deep in the brain's hypothalamus, a structure toward the base of the brain already known to control sexuality and reproduction.

A Matter of Energy

The neurons that affect eating are part of the body's elaborate mechanism for regulating energy balance, the power ensuring that we take in sufficient fuel, in the form of food, to meet internal and external energy demands to survive from day to day. This is

At the table, there are a variety of physiologic signals guiding what we now believe to be free will. Two brain chemicals—neuropeptide Y and galanin—control the appetite for carbohydrate-rich and fat-rich foods.

perhaps the body's most fundamental need.

Given so crucial a need, the location of the nerve cells of appetite in the hypothalamus is no accident of nature. They are the neurons next door to those that orchestrate sexual behavior. Leibowitz has found that we have clear-cut cycles of preference for high-carbohydrate and fat-rich foods, and they are closely linked to reproductive needs—that is, the ability of humans to survive from generation to generation. After all, the power to reproduce requires that we maintain a sufficient amount of body fat. The group of cells that tangle with sex and the cells that fancy our forks are in constant communication—like the sometimes overprotective mother she is, nature is constantly seeking reassurance that we have enough body fat for the survival of the species.

There are, in truth, many other brain areas that influence appetite. But from the lower brain stem up to the thalamus, which controls sensory processes such as taste, and on up to the forebrain and the cortex, where pleasure, affect, and cognitive aspects come into play, everything converges on the hypothalamus. The hypothalamus integrates all of the information affecting appetite. Its neurochemical signals coordinate our behavior with our physiology.

Through a daunting system of chemical and neural feedback, the brain monitors the energy needs of all body systems moment to moment. And it makes very emphatic suggestions to the stomach as to what we should ingest.

On the menu are the standard nutritional war-horses: carbohydrate for immediate fuel, fat for longer-term energy reserves—it is particularly essential for reproduction—and protein for growth and muscle maintenance. Directives from the brain to the belly are issued by way of neurochemical messengers and hormones. These directives, Leibowitz finds, have their own physiological logic, their own sets of rhythms, and are highly nutri-

> **Taste preferences for fat and carbohydrate, dictated by brain chemicals, show up early in life and reflect differences in genetic makeup.**

ent-specific. There's one thing we now know for sure—the stomach definitely has a brain.

A Taste for Carbo

In the dietary drama unfolding in Leibowitz' ground-floor laboratory, there are two star players. One is Neuropeptide Y (NPY), a neurochemical that dictates the taste for carbohydrate. Produced by neurons in the paraventricular nucleus (PVN), it literally turns on and off our desire for carbohydrate-rich foods.

In animal studies the researcher has conducted, the amount of Neuropeptide Y produced by cells in the PVN correlates directly, positively, with carbohydrate intake. The more Neuropeptide Y we produce, the more we eat carbohydrate.

"These Cells Tell Us To Eat"

"We can see these neurons and analyze the neuropeptides in them," says Leibowitz. "We know that these cells tell us to eat carbohydrate. In studies, we either give injections of a known amount of Neuropeptide Y, or measure the amount of Neuropeptide Y that's naturally there. Then we correlate it to what the animal ate in carbohydrate." Neuropeptide Y increases both the size and duration of carbohydrate-rich meals.

If production of Neuropeptide Y turns on the taste for carbohydrate, what sets production of Neuropeptide Y spinning? Probably signals from the burning of carbohydrates as fuel are the routine appetite stimulants. But Leibowitz has found that cortisol, a hormone produced by the body during stress, has a particular propensity to turn on the taste for carbohydrate by revving up production of Neuropeptide Y. High levels of Neuropeptide Y lead to weight gain by prompting overeating of carbohydrate.

Fat's Chance

The body also has a built-in appetite system for fat, the most concentrated form of energy, and it marches to a different neurochemical drumbeat, a neuropeptide called galanin, also

produced in the paraventricular nucleus of the hypothalamus. Galanin is the second star player in Leibowitz' studies.

These have shown that the amount of galanin an animal produces correlates positively with what the animal eats in fat. And that correlates with what the animal's body weight will become. The more galanin produced, the heavier the animal will become later on. To add insult to injury, galanin not only turns on the taste for fat, it affects other hormones in such a way as to ensure that fat consumed is turned into stored fat.

What turns on the taste for galanin? When the body burns stored fats as fuel, the resulting metabolic byproducts signal the paraventricular nucleus for more fat—a case of nature safeguarding our energy storage. But hormones also turn galanin production on. To be specific, the sexual hormone estrogen activates galanin.

"Estrogen just increases the production of galanin and it makes us want to eat. It makes us want to deposit fat," says Leibowitz. The influence of estrogen on our taste for fat "is important in the menstrual cycle and in the developmental cycle, when we hit puberty."

Of Time and the Nibbler

The two neurohormones of nibbling are not uniformly active throughout the day. Each has its own built-in cycle of activity.

Neuropeptide Y has its greatest effect on appetite at the start of the feeding cycle—morning, when we're just waking up. It starts up the entire feeding cycle. After overnight fasting, we have an immediate need for energy intake. Neuropeptide Y is also switched on after any environmentally imposed period of food deprivation—such as dieting. And by stress. "If you have lots of Neuropeptide Y in the system at breakfast," says Leibowitz, "you're going to be doing lots of eating."

Necessary as a quick-energy start is to get going, man cannot live by carbohydrate alone. After carbohydrate turns on our engines, the desire for this nutrient begins a slow decline over the rest of the daily cycle.

Around lunchtime, we begin looking for a little more sustenance. An afternoon of sustained energy expenditure stretches before us; we can afford to take in the other major nutrients—fat to refill our fat cells and protein to rebuild muscle. Both of these are converted more slowly to fuel. Our interest in protein rises gradually toward midday, holds its own at lunch, and keeps a more or less steady course during the rest of the day.

A Clockwork Orange

After lunch, the taste for fat begins rising, supported by increasing sensitivity to galanin and increasing galanin production; it peaks with our heaviest meal, at the end of the daily cycle. That's when the body is looking to store energy in anticipation of overnight fasting.

Take a late-afternoon coffee—or tea—break and you're virtually programmed to dive for energy-rich pastry, as appetite, spearheaded by the drive for fat, is gaining. We might, however, be better off appeasing the chemicals of consumption with a banana, or an orange.

Leibowitz believes that circadian cycles of neurochemical activity play a major role in eating problems. A late-afternoon fat snack, for example, could prime us neurochemically to consume more fat later into the night. Galanin activity late in the day gives fat consumed at dinner a head start, as it were, on our thighs.

Silent Signals

What drives us from a carbohydrate-rich breakfast to a more nutrient-mixed lunch? The carbohydrate we take in at breakfast has a direct impact on more widely distributed neurotransmitters such as serotonin. Active in many systems of the brain, including learning and memory, serotonin is believed to play a general role of modulator; it is essentially an inhibitor of activity.

Eating carbohydrate leads straightaway to synthesis of serotonin. Under normal conditions, rising levels of serotonin are the feedback signals to the paraventricular nucleus to shut off production of Neuropeptide Y and put a stop to the desire for carbohydrate.

Behind the Binge

Leibowitz now thinks that this serotonin signal is directly related to the bingeing behavior that is the *sine qua non* of bulimia. "Bulimics have a deficit in brain serotonin. The mechanism for stopping carbohydrate intake doesn't seem to be there."

Every meal, then, and the appetite for it, is differently regulated and presided over by a separate cocktail of neurochemicals. The neurochemically correct breakfast is a quick blast of carbohydrate right after awakening. Say, a glass of orange juice for speedy transport of sugar into the bloodstream to restore glycogen. Then a piece or two of toast, a more complex carbohydrate to deliver a more sustained supply of glucose over the morning.

For those who don't do it regularly, a breakfast of, say, eggs benedict—rich in protein and fat as well as carbohydrate—will send your neurochemicals spinning, throw off their normal rhythm of production, and affect many other neurotransmitters in the bargain. Ever wonder why you're just not sharp enough after an unusually rich breakfast?

The Big Switch

Not only are the neurochemicals of appetite active at different times over the course of a day, they are differently active over the course of development. Before puberty, Leibowitz finds, animals have no interest in eating fat. Children, too, have little appetite for fat, preferring carbohydrates for energy and protein for tissue growth. But that, like their bodies, changes.

In girls, the arrival of the first menstrual period is a milestone for appetite as well as for sexual maturation. It stimulates the first

desire for fat in foods. And that, says Leibowitz, is when a great deal of confusion sets in for anorexics.

"We hit puberty and that turns galanin on." The female hormone estrogen primes the neurochemical pump for galanin.

There are other sex-based differences in nutrient preference. In studies of animals, young females tend to have higher levels of Neuropeptide Y and favor carbohydrates. Their preference for carbohydrates peaks at puberty. Males favor protein to build large muscles.

When puberty strikes up the taste for fats, males are inclined to mix theirs with protein—that sizzling porterhouse steak. Women, their already high levels of Neuropeptide Y joined by galanin, are set to crave high-calorie sweets—chocolate cake, say, or ice cream. It's bread-and-butter nutritional knowledge that carbohydrate makes fat palatable in the first place.

This neurochemical combo particularly sets women up for late-afternoon snacking, possibly bingeing. Late afternoon may be the time when those who skip breakfast are particularly likely to pay for it, and there in turn with exaggerated increases in their Neuropeptide Y levels leading them into late-day gorging.

Patterns of Preference

When Leibowitz allows animals to choose what they eat, they show marked individual preferences for nutrients. These nutrient preferences, in turn, create specific differences in feeding patterns. In this animals are just like people, and fall into one of three general categories.

In about 50 percent of the population, carbohydrate is the nutrient of choice. Such people naturally choose a diet in which about 60 percent of calories are derived from carbohydrate, and up to 30 percent come from fat. They are neurochemically in line with what nutritionists today are recommending as a healthy diet. High-carbohydrate animals consume smaller and more frequent

Through a daunting system of chemical and neural feedback, the brain monitors the energy needs of all body systems moment to moment and makes very emphatic suggestions to the stomach as to what and how much we should eat.

meals, and they weigh significantly less, than other animals.

Some Like It Fat

A small number of people and animals are dedicated to protein. But 30 percent of us have a predilection for fat. And those who do take in 60 to 70 percent of their calories in straight fat, as opposed to the 30 percent considered appropriate to a lifestyle that's more sedentary than our ancestors'.

Not only is this not likely to sit well with arteries, but such preferences also correlate highly with body weight in animals. Those constituted to favor fat consume the most calories and weigh the most. And they seem to be particularly predisposed to food cravings late in the day.

Early Indicators

What is perhaps most intriguing in all of this to Leibowitz is that individual taste preferences first show themselves when animals are very young, notably at the time of weaning, even before their neurochemical profiles are fully elaborated. The same is true of people. "We know early in family life what we are going to become," she contends.

The New York researcher believes that by sampling infants' tastes, it will be possible to predict eating and weight-control problems long before they occur. And, of course, if we choose, do something to prevent them from ever occurring.

More than Metabolism

At the time of weaning—21 days in rat pups, 1½ to 2 years in human infants—taste preferences largely reflect differences in genetic makeup. And in those animals that prefer sucrose or fat—"you put it on an infant's tongue and watch how they react to it, whether they become active or not"—their appetite is strongly predictive of how much weight they will gain later on in life. And their neurochemical make-up.

"We believe there is strong appetitive component to pre-ordained weight gain," Leibowitz

says. "We think there's more to it than just metabolism. We are on the verge of linking that early taste with later eating behavior and weight gain."

The Wages of Stress

These ground-breaking studies of nutrient preferences show that inborn patterns are one way we can be set up for eating problems or weight gain we might prefer not to have. They also implicate another—stress. Stress potentially wreaks havoc with our eating patterns by altering us internally.

When we feel under stress, the body increases production of the hormone cortisol, from the adrenal gland. The purpose of this chemical messenger of alarm is to marshall forces of energy for immediate use—to prepare us, as it were, for fight or flight. It puts our whole system on alert, and makes us hyper-vigilant.

As it enters the bloodstream from the adrenal gland and circulates throughout the body, cortisol sees that carbohydrate, stored in muscles and liver as glycogen, is swiftly turned into glucose for fuel. If we are not burning up glucose, we have no energy. One reason cortisol is elevated in the morning is because the food deprivation of overnight fasting is a kind of stress to the body, destabilizing the system.

Cortisol, however, is also critical in the regulation of the neurochemicals that control eating behavior. "It up-regulates the neuropeptides when you don't want it to," says Leibowitz. Cortisol specifically stimulates production of Neuropeptide Y, which turns on the appetite—for more carbohydrate. "Stress is very much related to turning on Neuropeptide Y," reports Leibowitz. "It doesn't appear to increase galanin."

What's particularly tricky is that the effect of stress on eating is not uniform throughout the day. A bout of stress at the right time in the morning may keep Neuropeptide Y turned on all day. "We know that some people under stress get fat and others do

Skipping meals upsets the natural rhythm of neurochemicals, and that's important because the body works on routines. It affects your mood, your energy, even your sex life. And it turns your next meal into a high-carbohydrate binge.

not overeat. It depends on when the stress is occurring. Wouldn't it be nice to get your stress at a time when you are not so vulnerable?" Now if only she knew when that was.

Why We Overeat

What she does know is that if there is no muscular activity to use up the carbohydrate stress sets us up to eat, the carbohydrate is put directly into storage as fat. But wait—there are other consequences. It is an axiom of neuroscience that the same chemical messenger has different effects at different sites.

Through neurochemical cross talk in the hypothalamus, the increase in Neuropeptide Y activity affects the master switch for sexual and reproductive behavior in the cluster of cells next door. In this back-and-forth signaling between cell groups, high levels of Neuropeptide Y, hell-bent on carbohydrate intake, turn off the gonadal hormones, which are far more interested in fat. The upshot is a dampening of sexual interest and activity. This effect turns out to be critically important in anorexia.

Eating carbohydrate under stress, however, has something going for it. It chases away the stress-induced changes in neurochemistry. The hormonal alarm signals dissipate. "After we eat a carbohydrate-rich meal, the world actually seems better," explains Leibowitz. We feel less edgy. "That's why we overeat."

Dieting—Bad for the Brain

Many studies have shown that curbing body weight by food restriction—dieting—makes no sense metabolically; in fact it's counterproductive. Leibowitz finds it also makes no sense to the biochemistry of our brains, either. "All dieting does is disturb the system," she says emphatically. "It puts you in a psychological altered state. You're a different person. You respond differently."

Erratically skipping meals upsets the natural daily rhythm of neurochemicals; "that's important because the body works on routines. If you disturb the routine, you're going to be a different person at lunch than if you didn't skip breakfast." What's more, "the chemicals that regulate appetite also directly affect moods and state of mind, our physical energy, the quality of our sex lives," says Leibowitz.

Fasting—restricting, in the parlance of those who study eating behavior—is particularly counterproductive to appetite. It simply turns on the neurochemical switches. "It's got to come out somehow," says Leibowitz. It specifically drives up levels of Neuropeptide Y and cortisol. Then, when the next meal rolls around, it turns it into a high-carbohydrate binge. "Neuropeptide Y is truly the neurochemical of food deprivation." Fasting or dieting drives the body to seek more carbohydrate. Her studies show that animals that love carbohydrate have higher levels of Neuropeptide Y in the paraventricular nucleus.

The Way We Were

How, then to lose weight? Certainly not diet pills. One reason they don't work is that they don't even aspire to cope with the array of neurochemicals setting the table for appetite. Assuming such an approach to be possible or even desirable, it would, in fact, take assorted concoctions of

> We need to help people understand what they are, what their appetite is, and how to work with their body the way it is."

chemicals at different times of the day, since each meal is regulated differently.

Nevertheless, the way to control appetite and body weight, Leibowitz believes, is by working *with* the neurochemical systems—and re-tuning them. "We need to help people understand what they are and what their appetite is, and how to work with the body the way it is. Some people are more sensitive." This may be a far gentler approach than skipping lunch, but in the long run, it may be the only workable one, the only one that can possibly do away with the preoccupation with dieting that now consumes 50 to 70 percent of all women.

However deterministic biochemistry at first appears, that is not, within broad bounds, the case with behavior. We are not wholly slaves of neurochemistry. "Neurons are plastic. They change. We can therefore educate the neurons," explains Leibowitz. "You can say that God dictated this biochemical pattern. But we are here to mold ourselves and train ourselves."

The secret to modifying neurons is to introduce a very gradual shift in their sensitivity to the neurochemicals of appetite—to down-regulate them s-l-o-w-l-y.

Given the plasticity of neurons, early experience is heavily weighted in shaping the behavior of brain cells for life. Early exposure to a certain nutrient—say, a high-fat diet—will bias neurochemistry—It will up-regulate sensitivity to galanin and prompt production of greater amounts of it, aiding and abetting the appe-

tite for fat. "Your training, your habits, all have an effect," says Leibowitz. "We don't know how much is permanent and how much is reversible. It may be like the case with fat cells in the body; if you overeat when young and get fat cells, you may not be able to get rid of them." The bottom line is, we may be remarkably adaptable but not infinitely malleable.

Taste Texts for All?

The ideal, then, is to start the neurochemicals of appetite out on the right foot, "to modulate them before an eating disorder sets in, or any disturbance in dieting. It's got to be preventative. What you eat is going to affect production of these peptides." At some point in the future, it may be possible to determine the right calorie and nutrient mix even to dampen the genetically outlined production of the appetite hormones.

Leibowitz would bypass the dismal enterprise of dieting altogether with a taste test at age two. "We're aiming for the goal of trying to characterize people at a very early age, just as we can now do with animals. We can predict adult height at two years of age. We may also want to predict adult eating behavior and weight gain."

Then, with nutrition and planning and behavioral therapy she would set out to educate the appetite. "I'm not thinking drugs, but there could be drugs. If we could do this ahead of time, we could prevent the development of eating disorders," disorders that now affect, by her calculation, 30 percent of the population.

"The question is, can we find some specific dietary situation, different foods at different times, that might help us to reduce neuropeptide activity without depriving ourselves. The whole point is, we can't deprive ourselves. But if we know that what we eat and when we eat it affect the production of neuropeptides, we can modulate what we eat and work the appetite so that we can get a new routine in."

Gastronomy may never be the same again.

Current Killers

Over the past 30 years, Americans have witnessed remarkable scientific achievements in medical technology. Today not only are organ transplants a common occurrence, but human organs are even being replaced with artificial substitutes. While these medical marvels are a testament to America's technological sophistication, they have done little to prevent the ravages associated with cardiovascular disease and cancer—the leading killers in this country. The time has come for Americans to realize that they must rely less on medical technology and take a more active role in safeguarding their own health against these diseases.

Of all the diseases in America, cardiovascular disease is the nation's number one killer, and, within this category, coronary heart disease tops the list. Frequently, the first and only symptom of this disease is sudden death. While medical science has been unable to prevent this disease, epidemiological studies have revealed a number of risk factors that increase one's likelihood of developing it. These include hypertension, a high serum cholesterol level, diabetes, cigarette smoking, obesity, a sedentary lifestyle, a family history of heart disease, age, sex, and stress. Research further indicates that, as the number of risk factors increases, an individual's risk of developing premature coronary heart disease rises dramatically. While there is little doubt that the identification of these risk factors has helped the scientific community better understand coronary artery disease, there is some concern that the pharmaceutical industry has orchestrated the move to view hypertension and high cholesterol as diseases in themselves, thus serving as a marketing strategy for selling high-priced drugs. "The 'Diseasing' of Risk Factors" by Lynn Payer questions the motives of the pharmaceutical industry and suggests that financial considerations rather than medical concerns are the driving force behind the move to view hypertension and high cholesterol as diseases and not merely as risk factors.

The good news regarding coronary heart disease is that the majority of individuals may be able to prevent it by reducing their risk factors. There are lifestyle modifications that everyone can make to reduce the risk factors of coronary heart disease. "Pressure Treatment: How Exercise Can Help You Control Your Blood Pressure" by Kathleen Cahill discusses how exercise, excess body fat, and nutritional components such as salt and calcium can influence blood pressure.

While the link between high serum cholesterol levels and premature cardiovascular disease is irrefutable, the connection between dietary fat and elevated serum cholesterol is embroiled in controversy. The controversy is not whether dietary fat can raise the serum cholesterol level, but what percentage of the population is susceptible to this cholesterol-elevating effect. Over the past few years, A. E. Harper, professor of nutritional sciences and biochemistry at the University of Wisconsin, has been a vocal opponent of the National Research Council (NRC) recommendation concerning dietary fat. The NRC recommends that dietary fat should

constitute less than 30 percent of one's total caloric intake and that saturated fats should be replaced with monounsaturated and polyunsaturated fats whenever possible. Dr. Harper has argued that while this recommendation is valid for those individuals who test high for blood cholesterol, it is inappropriate and unnecessary for the majority of Americans. In the past, Dr. Harper has been criticized for this position, but new scientific findings provide strong evidence that he is correct. The medical community has been taken aback by the discovery that very low blood cholesterol levels, while reducing the risk of heart disease, increase the risk of dying from suicide, stroke, certain cancers, liver disease, and lung disease. Most striking is the finding that the mortality rate is the same for those with either high or low blood cholesterol levels. The article "Cholesterol: Put Knowledge Behind Your Numbers to Lower Your Confusion Level" provides a comprehensive look at cholesterol.

Cardiovascular disease may be America's number one killer, but cancer takes top billing in terms of the "fear factor." This fear of cancer stems from an awareness of the degenerative and disfiguring nature of this deadly disease. Today researchers are employing a variety of complex agents, such as monoclonal antibodies and interferon, in their attempts to fight it. Progress has been slow, however, and the results, while promising, suggest that a cure may be several years away. A very disturbing aspect of this country's battle against cancer is the fact that millions of dollars are spent each year trying to advance the treatment of cancer, but resources are not being provided for the technology that could be used to detect cancer in its early stages. A reallocation of funds would be appropriate, given the medical community's position that early detection and treatment are the key elements in the successful management of cancer.

Researchers have begun to examine dietary factors to determine if there are any positive links to the development of cancer. Medical experts now believe that dietary factors contribute to one-third of the 500,000 yearly cancer deaths in this country. Based on preliminary observations, some health experts believe that a reduction in dietary fat, coupled with an increase in dietary fiber, could help prevent colon cancer. While it is too early to make specific dietary recommendations concerning colon cancer, a high-fiber, low-fat diet is probably a good idea. Scientists have also been researching various foods, dietary supplements, and alcohol to determine what effect they may have on the development of cancer. It appears that some foods may actually reduce the risk of cancer. Of all the foods studied to date, the cruciferous vegetables, which include broccoli, cabbage, cauliflower, brussels sprouts, mustard, kale, and collard greens, seem to contain the most potent anticancer agents. "Eat to Beat Cancer" addresses the issue of diet and cancer by examining the evidence linking dietary factors to various forms of cancer.

In addition to diet, recent evidence also suggests that

exercise may lower the risk of certain types of cancer. As with dietary factors, the evidence supporting the protective influence of exercise is tentative. Preliminary findings suggest that while exercise appears to slow the growth of all malignancies, its protective influence appears greatest for colon cancer, breast, cervical, ovarian, and uterine cancer. It should also be noted that ovarian, breast, and uterine cancer appear to run in families; therefore, high-risk individuals should have themselves tested regularly for early warning signs. "From Here to Immunity" by Peter Jaret discusses recent scientific investigations demonstrating a possible link between moderate exercise and enhanced immune responses. He also discusses the physiological mechanisms that may account for this enhancement. "Your Health History" by Joanne Silberner discusses the importance of your family medical history as both a diagnostic tool and as a guide for making lifestyle decisions.

Of the three diseases discussed in this unit, AIDS has the potential to become the worst epidemic of this century. As medical researchers intensify their search for an effective AIDS vaccine, the disease continues to spread and infect countless innocent people. This disease has already been diagnosed in over 80,500 people. Of those diagnosed, half are already dead, and the rest are dying.

What is known about AIDS? Researchers have been able to identify the virus that causes AIDS. This virus, termed the HIV virus, has been found in both the blood and body fluids of infected persons, and case studies have documented that the disease can be transmitted through intimate sexual contact and the mixing of blood products. To date, there have been no documented cases of AIDS being spread through casual social contact, and most experts do not believe that the viral content of saliva is sufficient to spread the disease. Currently there is no vaccine available to protect a person from this dreaded disease, and there are no antiviral drugs available that can cure it. The only bright spots in this regard are the drugs AZT and DDI. Recent findings have revealed that while AZT has been shown to prolong the life of some AIDS patients, it is particularly effective in slowing the progress of this disease if taken prior to the appearance of symptoms. Unfortunately, researchers are also finding that the HIV virus in individuals receiving AZT for prolonged periods of time is capable of mutating to AZT-resistant strains. AZT may also produce side effects serious enough to preclude its use for certain individuals. These limitations have prompted the FDA to relax its testing and approval procedures for the drug DDI, so that it may also be used to treat AIDS patients. At this time, little is known regarding its therapeutic effectiveness or potential side effects. Until there is a safe and effective vaccine against AIDS, our best defense against this killer is education. "The Long Shot" by Mark Caldwell discusses why the world scientific community is pessimistic regarding its ability to devise an effective immunization or cure for AIDS in the near future. "Confront-

ing the AIDS Pandemic" discusses the current state of the pandemic, and speculates on how it will grow and the economic impact it will have on the world economy by the year 2000.

While coronary heart disease, cancer, and AIDS are all deadly diseases, many of the risk factors associated with each of them can be controlled through the lifestyle choices we make. This fact, coupled with our country's need to curb the high cost of health care, may be just what it takes to elevate the role of primary prevention to the forefront of health care, where it belongs.

Looking Ahead: Challenge Questions

Should doctors and other medical personnel be required to submit to AIDS testing? If so, how often should the testing be redone?

Do doctors have a right to know if their patients are infected with AIDS? If so, how should they secure this information?

What role can and should education play in combating the spread of AIDS?

What lifestyle changes could you make that would reduce your risk of developing cardiovascular disease, cancer, and AIDS?

What dietary advice would you give someone to reduce the risk of cancer?

Do you think that hypertension and high cholesterol should be treated as diseases?

To what extent should the government be involved in promoting preventative medicine?

Which chronic disease do you think you are most likely to contract based on your family history and lifestyle?

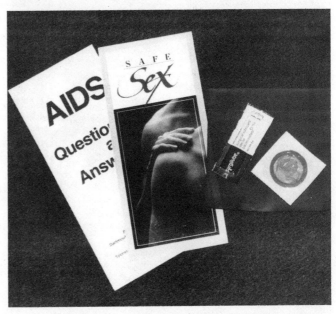

Your health history

Tracing your family's medical tree may well save your life

Try this quick test: If your grandparents are dead, can you say how old they were when they died and exactly what caused their deaths? If they're alive, do you know much about their health?

Recent advances in genetic technology have given scientists the tools to connect many diseases with the genes that cause

or trigger them. Just last month [December 1990], University of California researchers came close to locating the gene responsible for a type of breast cancer that strikes unusually early. Announcements of genes that lead to heart disease have become routine. It is just a matter of time before researchers unmask the genes that play a role in such common

illnesses as diabetes and high blood pressure, which tend to run in families.

Dig deep. Despite these advances, a genetic screening that lays out your health future is years away. A doctor can already hazard a good guess about your personal risk simply by checking your family history. But several genetics researchers claim doctors don't pay

---

THE LONGEVITY TEST

No test can predict with any certainty how long you will live. But a review of your health history, including heredity, can give you a fair sense of your life expectancy compared with that of the average American who lives into his or her 70s. The following longevity test is based on government studies and New York City cardiologist Elliott Howard's work with his patients. Your score may spur you to consider lifestyle changes—and add years to your life.

PERSONAL HISTORY
Choose all that apply.
- −2 No cancer or heart disease in parents who lived beyond age 75
- −1 No cancer or heart disease in one parent who lived beyond age 75
- +2 Coronary heart disease before age 50 in one or both parents
- +3 Coronary heart disease before age 40 in one or both parents
- +2 High blood pressure before age 50 in one parent
- +3 High blood pressure before age 50 in

both parents
- +1 Diabetes mellitus before age 60 in one or both parents
- +2 Cancer in a parent or sibling
- +2 Stroke before age 60 in one parent

Total:

WEIGHT
Your weight is:
- 0 Always at or near ideal weight
- +1 Now 10% over ideal weight
- +2 Now 20 to 29% over ideal weight
- +3 Now 30 to 39% over ideal weight
- +4 More than 40% over ideal weight

Total:

BLOOD PRESSURE
Your blood pressure is:
- −2 Below 121/71
- 0 121/71 to 140/85
- +2 141/86 to 170/100
- +4 171/101 to 190/110
- +6 Above 190/110

Total:

CHOLESTEROL
Your blood cholesterol level is:
- −2 150 to 170
- −1 171 to 190
- 0 191 to 210
- +1 211 to 240
- +2 241 to 280
- +3 281 to 320
- +4 Over 320

Your high-density lipopro-

tein (HDL) cholesterol level is:
- −2 66 to 80
- −1 51 to 65
- 0 41 to 50
- +1 31 to 40
- +2 25 to 30
- +3 Below 25

Total:

SMOKING
You don't smoke now. In the past, you:
- −1 Never did, or quit over 5 years ago
- 0 Quit 1 to 5 years ago
- +1 Quit within the past year

You now smoke:
- +1 Pipe or cigars
- +2 Less than a pack of cigarettes a day
- +3 A pack a day
- +4 1 to 1½ packs a day
- +5 2 packs a day
- +5 *And* drink alcohol 5 or more times a week
- +3 *And* take birth control pills

You have smoked:
- +3 For at least 10 years
- +5 For more than 20 years

Total:

ALCOHOL
You drink:
- −1 Never or rarely
- 0 No more than a 5-oz. glass of wine or a 12-oz. glass of beer or 1½-oz. of hard liquor, 5 times a week
- +1 Two glasses of alcohol a day
- +2 More than two glasses a day

Total:

EXERCISE
To keep fit, you:
- −2 Exercise vigorously more than 45 minutes 4 or 5 times a week
- −1 Exercise vigorously at least 30 minutes 3 times a week
- 0 Exercise moderately

enough attention to family history. And patients often don't know much about their family's health.

You can help your doctor, and yourself, by creating a medical family tree. Filling in the blanks could take some digging, but it is worthwhile. You may be able to fend off your genetic legacy. Keeping your cholesterol down, for example, could mitigate a tradition of heart disease. If a disease seems inevitable, as certain forms of cancer can be, frequent health checks can alert you to a problem while there's time to treat it.

The warning could save your life. Comedian Gilda Radner gritted her way through a year of pain, crushing fatigue and intestinal distress before doctors diagnosed the ovarian cancer that eventually killed her in 1989. Caught early, the survival rate for ovarian cancer is 85 percent; once the cancer spreads beyond the pelvis, chances drop to 15 to 20 percent. And Radner's cancer could have been caught early if she or her doctors had realized that her aunt, her first cousin and probably her grandmother had suffered from the disease. That lineup boosted her risk of ovarian

cancer from the usual 1 in 70 to 1 in 2.

Cancer geneticists think 5 to 10 percent of cancers are rooted in heredity, but only rarely, when the genes have been determined, do they know whether a particular breast or colon or reproductive tract tumor was predestined. In general, having one parent or sibling with cancer triples the risk that you will have it, estimates John Mulvihill, chief of human genetics at the University of Pittsburgh. Given many cases of one type of cancer in your family tree, most doctors would urge earlier and more frequent screening for that type—mammography for breast cancer, for example.

Cancer data. You can benefit from researchers' interest in "cancer families." In exchange for information on your family, several registries will provide instruction on ways to reduce your risk and let you know if any of your relatives have already volunteered information. The National High Risk Registry, at (800) 521-9356, deals with breast cancer. The Hereditary Cancer Institute at Creighton University School of Medicine in Omaha, at (402) 280-2942, covers all cancers, and the Gilda Radner Familial Ovarian

Cancer Registry, at (800) 682-7426, is for women worried about ovarian cancer.

Doctors can better estimate your own risk of cancer if they know when it struck your relatives. Henry Lynch, a cancer specialist who runs Creighton's Hereditary Cancer Institute, has found that in families with many cases of colon cancer, the condition hits at an average age of 44 years instead of the more typical 60 or 65; hereditary breast cancer comes on at an average age of 42 instead of 63.

Age is also a factor in families where heart disease is common. University of Utah researchers studied nearly 15,000 family trees and found that men under 40 with two siblings or parents who had a heart attack before age 55 had 12 times the risk of early heart disease as men of the same age with no such family history. Women in the same category had eight times the risk. Heart-disease data from a long-term study in Framingham, Mass., show that people whose parents or siblings had heart attacks before age 60 have twice the risk of early coronaries. Many can easily be identified by a blood test that reveals high cholesterol levels or low levels of high-density lipoprotein (HDL),

---

	at least 30 minutes 3 to 5 times a week	diets once or twice a year	

+1 Exercise moderately at least twice a week

+2 Exercise usually on weekends or less than twice a week

+3 Rarely or never exercise

Total:

....

DIET
Your eating habits include (choose all that apply):

+2 Using salt freely without tasting food first

+2 Eating cabbage, broccoli or cauliflower less than 3 times a week

+3 Eating high-fiber grains, such as whole-wheat bread, brown rice and bran cereal, less than once a day

+3 Eating fruits and vegetables less than 3 times a day

+1 Following fad crash

You eat beef, bacon or processed meats:

+3 5 to 6 times a week
+2 4 times a week
+1 2 times a week

You eat eggs:

+3 2 every day
+2 6 to 8 eggs a week
+1 4 to 6 eggs a week

You eat ice cream, cake or rich desserts

+2 Almost daily
+1 Several times a week

You eat butter, cream, cream cheese and cheese:

+3 Every day
+2 Almost daily
+1 2 to 3 times a week

Total:

....

STRESS
Describe your personality:

+1 Intense desire to get ahead
+2 Constant driving for success

+2 Easily frustrated, annoyed or irritated

+2 Angry and hostile if losing in competition

+3 Angry and hostile even if successful

+2 Don't express anger or feelings

+2 Frequent knots in stomach, poor sleep or headaches

+2 Hardly laugh, depressed often

+2 Constantly strive to please others rather than yourself

+2 Rarely discuss problems or feelings with others

−1 None of the above

Total:

....

MOTOR VEHICLE SAFETY
When you travel, you (choose all that apply):

−1 Usually use mass transit

0 Travel by car less than 200 miles per week

+1 Travel by car 200 to 400 miles per week

+2 Travel by car over 400 miles per week

+2 Rarely use a seat belt

+2 Often exceed the speed limit

+2 Ride a motorcycle

+4 Ride a motorcycle without a helmet

+4 Sometimes drink and drive or ride with a driver who has been drinking

+6 Often drink and drive or ride with a driver who has been drinking

Total:

....

INTERPRETING YOUR SCORE
Add the totals for all categories and find the result below.

−14 to 3
Low risk. Odds are you will live a long and healthful life if you continue to limit risks.

4 to 30
Moderate risk. You can ex-

pect to live a long life but risk ill health. Like most Americans, you can change a few habits and greatly reduce your risk of cancer, stroke, heart disease and motor vehicle accidents and perhaps add years to your life.

31 to 70
High risk. You are at considerable risk of developing a serious illness and shortened life. But you can improve your life expectancy by changing some of the habits that earned you scores of 2, 3, 4 or higher.

Over 70
Very high risk. Based on your lifestyle and personal history, you are at dangerous risk for serious illness and premature death unless you see a physician and eliminate as many risk factors as possible.

USN&WR—Adapted from "Health Risks" by Elliott J. Howard, M.D. ($19.95 hardback, $8.95 paper, Foundation for Study of Exercise, Stress and the Heart, 1986)

a protective form of cholesterol. Absence of heart disease in your family doesn't free you to be sedentary, smoke or eat a high-fat diet. "We live in a society where it's easy to overcome the best genes," says William Castelli, medical director of the Framingham Heart Study.

Everyday killers beyond cancer and heart disease have genetic links, too. The children of two parents with childhood diabetes—technically insulin-dependent type I diabetes—have up to a 20 percent chance of developing the condition, for example. That is more than 40 times the risk when both parents are free of diabetes. Doctors and parents can watch for the weight loss and increased thirst that herald the disease and begin treatment before a child could otherwise end up in the hospital. The risk relationship isn't as well established with adult, or non-insulin dependent-type II diabetes, but the genetic connection is well enough known so that anyone with a parent who had this type of diabetes should stay slim, since this can protect against diabetes.

A disease-ridden family tree is not always dangerous. Having several relatives with emphysema sounds ominous, but if they all smoked, that rather than genes is the likely culprit. And people who have lived past the age at which many family members died of a particular condition can generally relax.

Working out your family's health history may be as easy as checking the family Bible, but it might also demand real effort. Stigmas against cancer and mental illness sometimes shroud these conditions in euphemisms. And family lore may be none to reliable. "The story was that my Grandpa Jake died in his mid-40s of acute indigestion because of my grandmother's cooking," says Jeremy Nobel, a lecturer in health policy and management at the Harvard School of Public Health. When Nobel's father died of a heart attack at age 46, the family realized that the "intestinal distress" was more likely a heart attack. Nobel got the message. Now 36, he exercises regularly and eats prudently.

No history. The records of doctors who have treated members of your family can help fill in a health history, but reliability can be a problem here, too. Cancer specialist Lynch and his colleagues scanned the charts of patients who they knew had several relatives with cancer. Over 70 percent of the charts listed no such family history.

When the doctor's records (or the doctor) are no longer around, you might try the hospital where a relative died.

Hospitals generally release records to the next of kin who apply in writing. In some states, hospitals have to keep records for only five years, so you may have to go further. States retain death certificates permanently. While death certificates are not always accurate or precise—the exact cancer might not have been known—they may at least tell you that cancer was present. The local health department can steer you to the state agency that handles death records. These are in the public domain, so you don't have to be the next of kin to get them.

Perfect knowledge doesn't equal perfect health, of course. Fifteen years ago, genealogist Dorothy Payne of Arlington, Va., discovered that not only her father but her grandmother and great grandfather had died of emphysema—and her father had been the only smoker among them. She heavily lobbied her sons not to smoke, but couldn't break her own habit. "I come from the generation that says do as I say, not as I do," explains Payne, 58. Once you know what medical history your parents have bequeathed you, the next step is in your hand. You can't chop down the tree, but you can plant your own.

Joanne Silberner

Cholesterol

Put knowledge behind your numbers to lower your confusion level

"My doctor just gave me the results of my cholesterol test. He said, 'Your good cholesterol is low—that's bad, and your bad cholesterol is high—that's bad too. You need to raise your good and lower your bad—that would be good.' "

Confusing? You bet it is.

Chances are you know your cholesterol level is important and that it shouldn't be too high. But beyond that you may be unsure exactly how cholesterol fits into the cardiovascular disease puzzle.

Maybe you're too concerned about your cholesterol. Maybe you're not concerned enough.

In the following pages, we answer common questions, such as:
■ What exactly is cholesterol?
■ How can cholesterol be both good and bad?

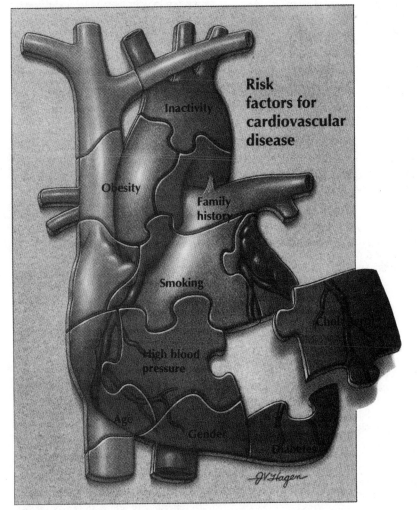

This puzzle includes nine major risk factors for cardiovascular disease, the nation's No. 1 killer. Cholesterol is among the most complex and important of all risk factors.

■ What does cholesterol do in your body?
■ What is an elevated cholesterol level?
■ When should you be concerned?
■ What can you do about your concerns?

Why all the fuss about cholesterol?

Your blood cholesterol is important. Heart and blood vessel (cardiovascular) disease is the No. 1 killer of Americans, and study after study points to elevated cholesterol as a major contributor to the problem.

In general:
■ The higher your cholesterol level, the greater your risk of cardiovascular disease.
■ The higher your cholesterol level, the greater your chances of dying of cardiovascular disease.
■ You can lower your risk of cardiovascular disease by lowering your cholesterol level.

Cholesterol and cardiovascular disease

The good news . . . Deaths from cardiovascular disease continue to fall. This encouraging trend is due to improved treatment and modification of cardiovascular disease risk factors, including cholesterol.

In 1980, heart attacks accounted for 163 deaths per 100,000 people. By 1990, this number had dropped to 112 people per 100,000.

The numbers for stroke are improving, too. In 1980, strokes claimed 41 people per 100,000. By 1990 this figure was down to 28.

The bad news . . . Far too many people still die from cardiovascular disease. The American Heart Association reports that cardiovascular disease still kills almost 1 million Americans each year. This is more than all cancer deaths combined.

Many of these deaths occur because of narrowed or blocked arteries (ath-

From *Medical Essay,* supplement to *Mayo Clinic Health Letter,* June 1993, pp. 1-8. © 1993 by Mayo Foundation for Medical Education and Research, Rochester, MN 55905. Reprinted by permission.

erosclerosis). Cholesterol plays a significant role in this largely preventable condition.

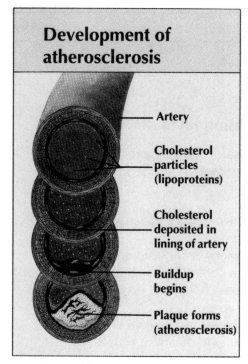

Development of atherosclerosis

- Artery
- Cholesterol particles (lipoproteins)
- Cholesterol deposited in lining of artery
- Buildup begins
- Plaque forms (atherosclerosis)

A high number of cholesterol particles (lipoproteins) in your blood increases your risk for a buildup of cholesterol within the wall of your artery. Eventually, bumps called plaques may form, narrowing or even blocking your artery.

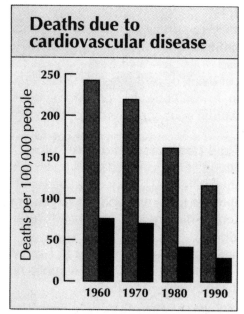

Deaths due to cardiovascular disease

Deaths per 100,000 people (y-axis: 0, 50, 100, 150, 200, 250; x-axis: 1960, 1970, 1980, 1990)

Deaths from heart attacks (gray bars) and stroke (black bars) are declining. This encouraging trend is due to improved treatment and modification of cardiovascular disease risk factors, including cholesterol.

(Sources: National Center for Health Statistics and American Heart Association.)

Atherosclerosis (ATH-ro-scler-OH-sis) is a silent, painless process in which cholesterol-containing fatty deposits accumulate in the walls of your arteries. These accumulations occur as bumps called plaques. (See illustration.)

As plaque builds up, the interior of your artery narrows. This reduces the flow of blood. If reduced flow occurs in your coronary (heart) arteries, it can lead to a type of chest pain called angina pectoris.

As a plaque enlarges, the inner lining of your artery becomes roughened. A tear or rupture in the plaque may cause a blood clot to form. Such a clot can block the flow of blood or break free and plug an artery downstream.

If the flow of blood to a part of your heart is stopped, you'll have a heart attack. If blood flow to a part of your brain stops, you'll have a stroke.

Many factors influence the clogging of arteries. Cholesterol is important in the process, but it's not the only piece of the puzzle.

What is cholesterol?

Cholesterol is a waxy, fat-like substance (lipid). Although it's often discussed as if it were a poison, you can't live without it. Cholesterol is essential to your body's cell membranes, to the insulation of your nerves and to the production of certain hormones. It's used by your liver to make bile acids, which help digest your food.

The confusion that clouds cholesterol is partly due to the way some people use the word. "Cholesterol" is often a catch-all term for both the cholesterol you eat and the cholesterol in your blood.

■ *Your dietary cholesterol*—Cholesterol exists in your food as a dietary lipid. You'll find cholesterol only in animal products, such as meat and dairy foods.

■ *Your blood cholesterol*—Cholesterol also exists in a different way as a natural component of your blood lipids.

The cholesterol in your blood comes both from your liver and from the foods you eat. Your liver makes about 80 percent of your blood cholesterol. Only about 20 percent comes from your diet.

The amount of fat and cholesterol you eat may influence all levels of your blood lipids, including your blood cholesterol levels.

Blood cholesterol—the good, the bad and the ugly

To be carried in your blood, your body coats cholesterol with proteins called apoproteins (AP-oh-PRO-teens). Once

coated, they form a package called lipoproteins (LIP-oh-PRO-teens).

Lipoproteins carry both cholesterol and triglycerides (another blood lipid) in your blood.

Some of your lipoproteins are called low-density lipoproteins (LDLs). They contain lots of cholesterol. Others are called high-density lipoproteins (HDLs). They contain mostly protein.

A third type of lipoprotein is called a very-low-density lipoprotein (VLDL). This type contains cholesterol, triglycerides and protein.

Some people call LDL "bad cholesterol" and HDL "good cholesterol." Here's why:

Cholesterol serves as a building material in cells throughout your body. LDL particles, which carry cholesterol, attach themselves to receptors on cell surfaces and are then received into your cells.

If there are too many LDL particles in your blood, if your liver cells (LDL receptors) do not receive LDL particles normally, or, if there are too few LDL receptors in your liver, your body's cells become saturated with cholesterol from the LDL particles. Cholesterol is then deposited in your artery walls.

At this point your high-density lipoproteins (HDLs) play their "good" role. They actually pick up cholesterol deposited in your artery walls and transport it to your liver for disposal.

The situation can turn ugly if too much cholesterol from LDL particles remains deposited in your artery walls. Your arteries will develop plaques and begin to narrow. This is atherosclerosis.

This is why a high HDL level relative to an LDL level is good. It can help protect you from developing atherosclerosis.

What's to blame?

Why do some people have high cholesterol? High levels result from genetic makeup or lifestyle choices, or both. Your genes can give you cells that don't remove LDL cholesterol from your blood efficiently, or a liver that produces too much cholesterol as VLDL particles, or too few HDL particles.

Lifestyle choices such as smoking, diet and inactivity can also cause or contribute to high cholesterol levels, leaving you at risk for atherosclerosis.

The cholesterol test

The only way to find out if your blood lipids are in a desirable range is to have them tested. The test is done by taking a blood sample after you have fasted overnight. You should have this test every three to five years—more often if you have a problem with your cholesterol level.

How much fat is that?

Limit fat to "30 percent of daily calories." Good advice. But what does it really mean?

This table converts this recommended guideline into the actual amount of fat you should limit yourself to daily.

If you eat . . .	Allow yourself this much fat daily . . .
1,400 calories	47 grams
1,600 calories	53 grams
1,800 calories	60 grams
2,000 calories	67 grams
2,200 calories	73 grams
2,400 calories	80 grams
2,600 calories	87 grams
2,800 calories	93 grams

Note: 1,400 calories is the minimum you should eat if you're trying to lose weight. 1,600 calories is about right for many inactive women and some older adults. 2,200 calories is about right for many sedentary men, most children, teenage girls and active women. 2,800 is about right for teenage boys, many active men and some very active women.

Calorie allowances are based on recommendations of the National Academy of Sciences and on calorie intakes reported by people in national food consumption surveys.

The test should measure your total cholesterol, HDL cholesterol and triglycerides. (Total cholesterol is made up of your LDL, HDL and other blood cholesterol particles.)

Some laboratories measure LDL directly, as part of the blood test. However, if your triglycerides are normal, your doctor can calculate your LDL level using the following formula:

$$\text{Total cholesterol} - (HDL + \frac{\text{triglycerides}}{5}) = LDL$$

In addition to your LDL level, your doctor might calculate the ratios between your LDL and HDL cholesterol, or between your total cholesterol and HDL.

Today, physicians pay more attention to your HDL number. Studies show that even with a desirable total cholesterol level, if you have a low HDL level, you may be at risk for cardiovascular disease.

It's critical to realize that numbers in the table on this page are only guidelines. If your numbers stray from the desirable ranges, your physician will counsel you.

Remember this too: Each number takes on greater meaning when you look at it in relation to the other numbers on your test and in relation to your other cardiovascular disease risk factors.

Other cardiovascular risk factors— the remaining puzzle pieces

To make the picture of your cardiovascular health more complete, you must consider your other risk factors for cardiovascular disease. (See illustration.) Each risk factor may influence your lipid levels.

The more risk factors you have, in combination with undesirable lipid levels, the greater your risk of developing cardiovascular disease. If you have several risk factors, their effects don't simply add up, they amplify each other.

For example, if you have high total cholesterol and you smoke, you're at much greater risk than a nonsmoker with the same cholesterol level.

However, you can make this amplifying effect work for you. Eating a diet low in fat, combined with exercise, can help you lose weight. At the same time, you can reduce your risk of high blood pressure, heart attack and stroke.

Risk factors for cardiovascular disease are divided into those you can change and those you can't. Consider

---

Your blood test: What do those numbers mean?

Your lipid levels can tell your doctor whether you're a candidate for cardiovascular disease. As you compare your numbers with these, remember: Numbers alone don't tell the whole story. Rely on your physician to interpret your test results.

Test	Your level (in mg/dl)*		
	Desirable	*Borderline*	*Undesirable*
Total cholesterol	Below 200	200-240	Above 240
HDL cholesterol	Above 45	35-45	Below 35
Triglycerides	Below 200	200-400	Above 400
LDL cholesterol	Below 130	130-160	Above 160
Cholesterol/HDL	Below 4.5	4.5-5.5	Above 5.5
LDL/HDL	Below 3	3-5	Above 5

* For people without known heart disease

Note: The numbers in this table represent a compilation of informed medical opinions from a variety of sources.

how each risk factor affects your blood cholesterol and triglycerides.

Here are factors you can change:

■ *Smoking*—Smoking cigarettes damages the walls of your blood vessels, making them prone to accumulate fatty deposits. Smoking may also lower your HDL by as much as 15 percent. If you stop smoking, your HDL may return to its higher level.

■ *High blood pressure*—By damaging the walls of your arteries, high blood pressure can accelerate the development of atherosclerosis. Some medications for high blood pressure increase LDL and triglyceride levels and decrease HDL levels. Other medications don't.

■ *Inactivity*—Lack of physical exercise is associated with a decrease in HDL. Aerobic exercise is one way to increase your HDL. Aerobic activity is any exercise that requires continuous movement of your arms and legs and increases your breathing. Even 30 to 45 minutes of brisk walking every other day helps protect your cardiovascular system.

■ *Obesity*—Excess weight increases your triglycerides. It also lowers your HDL and increases your VLDL cholesterol. Losing just five or 10 pounds can improve your triglyceride and cholesterol levels.

■ *Diabetes*—Diabetes can increase triglycerides and decrease HDL in many people. Diabetes accelerates the development of atherosclerosis which, in turn, increases the risk for heart attack, stroke and reduced circulation to your feet.

If you have diabetes, have your total cholesterol, triglycerides and HDL tested at least annually. Keep your weight and blood sugar under control. Still, complications may develop. Diabetes is not a risk factor you can always change. (See *Mayo Clinic Health Letter* Medical Essay on diabetes, June 1992.)

These are risk factors you can't change:

■ *Age*—As you age, your level of LDL cholesterol usually increases. Researchers aren't sure why. The increase could be caused by aging or by an increase in your body fat.

■ *Gender*—Until age 45, men generally have higher total cholesterol levels than women. Also, up to about this age, women tend to have higher HDL levels. However, after menopause, women's total cholesterol rises and the protective HDL drops.

Caution: Don't think of cardiovascular disease as mainly a man's disease. Cardiovascular disease is also the No. 1 killer of women, claiming almost 500,000 women each year. Cancer kills fewer than 220,000 women. Women get cardiovascular disease as often as men; it just happens later in life.

■ *Family history*—If members of your family have undesirable lipid levels and cardiovascular problems, your risks for these problems are increased.

Your first lines of defense against high cholesterol

Diet and exercise are your first lines of defense against undesirable lipid levels. Changes in your diet, along with exercise, can reduce your blood cholesterol level by up to 15 percent. However, some people have genetically determined lipid problems (especially LDL) that don't respond to diet and require medication.

Making diet changes to improve your blood cholesterol levels involves three steps:

■ *Reduce your weight by reducing your total fat*—Limit all types of fat, saturated, polyunsaturated and monounsaturated, to no more than 30 percent of your total daily calories. Because all foods with fats contain a combination of these fats, it's important to reduce total fat.

Don't assume each food you eat must have less than 30 percent of its calories from fat. Use the guideline as a daily average. By balancing occasional high-fat foods with low-fat choices, your fat intake should average 30 percent of your daily calories.

■ *Reduce saturated fat*—No more than one-third of the fat you eat should be saturated. Major sources of saturated fat are butter, cheese, whole milk, cream, meat, poultry, chocolate, coconut, palm and palm kernel oil, lard and solid shortenings.

■ *Reduce dietary cholesterol*—Your daily limit for dietary cholesterol is 300 milligrams. A good way to accomplish this goal is to avoid dairy products made with whole milk and cream, and organ meats such as liver and tongue.

These limits on fat and cholesterol can also help you lose weight, which can improve your blood lipid levels. . . .

Exercise enhances the benefits of diet

A low-fat, low-cholesterol diet can improve your VLDL cholesterol level. If you also exercise and lose excess weight, you may see even greater improvements in your triglyceride and cholesterol levels.

Exercise helps you lose excess weight and reduces your chances of gaining weight as you get older.

For these benefits, set up your program using these guidelines and your doctor's advice:

■ *Choose aerobic activity*—Get involved in brisk walking, jogging, bicycling or cross-country skiing.

■ *Build up time and frequency*—Gradually work up to exercising for 30 to 45 minutes at least three times a week. If you're severely overweight or have been inactive for many years, take several months to gradually work up to this level. The higher the level of your activity, the greater your rate of weight loss.

■ *Keep it up*—Schedule a regular time for exercise. Make exercise fun. If it's not enjoyable you'll have difficulty exercising regularly, year in and year out.

Find a friend, or join an exercise group, to keep you motivated and committed to exercise. Or take up an activity that keeps you active.

Unless you stay with your program, you may not be able to keep off the pounds exercise helped you lose. Staying active also may prevent a gain in weight that often accompanies age. This, in turn, may help maintain lower levels of blood fats.

When are medications necessary?

Often changes in diet, exercise and smoking habits will improve your VLDL cholesterol and triglyceride levels. But if you've carried out these important lifestyle changes and your total cholesterol, especially your LDL level, remains high, your doctor may recommend a medication.

Before recommending a medication, your doctor will use careful judgment and weigh many variables—your changeable risk factors, your age, your current health, and the drug's side effects. If you need a medication to lower your cholesterol, chances are you will need it for many years.

Your LDL cholesterol level is usually the deciding factor. If you have no risk factors for cardiovascular disease, an LDL level over 190 generally requires medication. With two or more risk factors, an LDL level over 160 may require medication.

And remember . . .

The issue of cholesterol and cardiovascular health is important, but by no means simple. Just knowing your total cholesterol level is not enough. Understanding how your other blood fat levels and your cardiovascular disease risk factors influence this number is essential.

Only with this knowledge can cholesterol assume its proper place in the cardiovascular disease puzzle.

The "Diseasing" of Risk Factors

Lynn Payer

Lynn Payer has written for the Medical Tribune *and edited* The New York Times Good Health Magazine. Disease Mongers *is her third book on medical topics.*

When epidemiologists started studying the characteristics that make people more prone to heart attack and stroke, they started identifying "risk factors" such as high blood pressure, high cholesterol, smoking and diabetes. Identifying such risk factors was useful, because it helped scientists understand something about how heart attacks and strokes developed and how they might be prevented.

The two risk factors that were the most susceptible to being modified by drug therapy—high blood pressure and high cholesterol—soon came to be labeled "diseases" in themselves.

But the two risk factors that were the most susceptible to being modified by drug therapy—high blood pressure and high cholesterol—soon came to be labeled "diseases" in themselves. From this labeling grew a whole infrastructure of national committees, specialists and specialized centers—and the pharmaceutical companies that marketed drugs for high blood pressure and cholesterol—all having a stake in emphasizing their importance. There were several dramatic consequences to this:

- Risk factors have come to be seen as bad in themselves, even in situations where they are of very little risk to the people who have them.
- People assume that by treating the risk factors, they are preventing the disease for which the factors predict risk, which doesn't always prove to be the case.
- When there is no clear dividing line between who is normal and who is "high," the line is frequently drawn in such a way that the maximum number of people are labeled "at risk" and are therefore candidates for medical intervention.

As a consequence, many people are worrying about risk factors, spending money for testing for them, and even dying of the treatment for them, when these factors might better have been ignored, or at least kept in perspective.

Risk Factors Are Promoted as Diseases in Themselves

Consider the white woman who has high blood pressure (up to a diastolic pressure of 100) but doesn't smoke, has a normal cholesterol level and is not obese or diabetic. Her risk of having a heart attack or stroke is slightly higher than that of an otherwise comparable white woman without high blood pressure, but her absolute risk of having either a heart attack or a stroke is very low. While it probably wouldn't hurt for such a woman to adopt some kind of regular exercise plan, drug treatment is another matter; in fact, in the largest trial yet for the drug treatment of mild hypertension, women in this category who were treated with antihypertension drugs actually had a higher death rate than those treated with a placebo! There is little evidence that such women benefit from taking drugs for their high blood pressure, and since high blood pressure usually produces no symptoms, drug treatment cannot be justified by the fact that it makes them feel better since it may actually make them feel worse.

Yet such women are usually treated with drugs in the United States, and in fact some hypertension specialists believe they are among the most treated, simply because they tend to be compliant patients. Because high blood pressure is more common in women (even though it is associated with such a low risk), some disease-mongers call high blood pressure a greater problem for women than for men, thereby totally dissociating the

From *Priorities*, Winter 1993, pp. 27-29. Excerpted from *Disease-Mongers: How Doctors, Drug Companies and Insurers Are Making You Feel Sick*, by Lynn Payer. © 1992 by Lynn Payer. Reprinted with permission from John Wiley & Sons, Inc.

risk factor from the risk that originally defined it!

A similar situation pertains to women with high cholesterol as their sole risk factor. While it might be better if these women's cholesterol were lower, their absolute risk of having a heart attack is still not very high. Like most labels, high cholesterol has vastly different meanings depending on who has it. While a man who smokes heavily, is obese, doesn't exercise and has high blood pressure and a cholesterol level of 300 and a slender, nonsmoking woman whose cholesterol is 220 may both speak about their "high cholesterol," this "disease" implies a vastly different risk for each. The man's risk of heart attack is high, and treatment may lower it significantly, resulting in a net benefit for him. The woman's risk is low, and there is a high probability that the treatment will be worse than the disease.

Treating Risk Factors Doesn't Always Reduce Risk

It was logical for the medical profession to assume that if high blood pressure and high cholesterol increased the risk of stroke and heart attacks, lowering both would reduce the risks. This worked for stroke, particularly for people with very high blood pressure.

But when the rate of heart attacks in the treated group was studied, observers were disappointed: bringing blood pressure down to normal didn't seem to cut the risk of heart attacks very much. In fact, the use of some types of blood pressure medications in some patients actually raised the death rate: a 1991 study performed at the Joslin Clinic in Boston showed that diabetics who also had high blood pressure had a higher death rate if given diuretic drugs for their high blood pressure than if their hypertension went untreated. Nobody knows quite how this happens, but diuretics tend to raise cholesterol, thus raising one risk factor in the process of lowering

another. Another study published in 1991 showed that people taking any type of medication for hypertension increased their risk of becoming diabetic.

These findings caused some of the more thoughtful players in the hypertension field to rethink their assumptions, and they began to emphasize that the total risk should be evaluated, not the individual risk factors, If treating one risk factor had an adverse effect on the others, they concluded quite logically, they should then proceed with caution.

We can all start taking risk factors with a bit more skepticism. the proverbial grain of salt may be bad for your blood pressure, it's definitely good seasoning to take with your medical information.

A similar dilemma haunted those looking carefully at the evidence that drug treatment of cholesterol was doing any good. High cholesterol, like high blood pressure, does increase the risk of having a heart attack. But when people whose cholesterol was very high were treated with cholesterol-lowering drugs and their survival was compared with people being given a placebo, two things became apparent. First, the drugs did seem to cut down on deaths from heart attack, although the magnitude of the reduction was quite mild. Second, in study after study there was no difference in the total mortality, because the deaths from heart disease in the group receiving placebo were always balanced by an increased death rate from something else—accidents, suicides, or cancer—in the groups receiving the cholesterol-lowering drugs. Some studies, in fact, have shown more deaths in people treated for

their cholesterol than in those not treated.

Despite the fact that treating large numbers of people with expensive drugs and restrictive diets yielded such modest results, the National Institutes of Health (NIH) launched a National Cholesterol Education Program to get all Americans to know their cholesterol level and presumably to try to lower it—even though the NIH's own advisory council opposed such an emphasis in the face of such slight evidence.

Dietary Therapy

Some people might argue that while perhaps the cholesterol-lowering drugs shouldn't be promoted, there's certainly no harm in trying to control cholesterol with diet. Most people agree that the American diet is high in fat, and we would probably be better off with less of it. Some people find that cutting down on fats has no negative effect on their quality of life.

But even here the health benefits are probably going to be very modest. W. C. Taylor and his associates from Boston, Massachusetts, developed a model that assumes cholesterol reduction is effective and safe in reducing the risk for death from coronary heart disease (CHD). For persons aged 20 to 60 years at low risk, they calculated a gain in life expectancy of three days to three months from a life-long program of cholesterol reduction. For persons at high risk, the calculated gain ranged from 18 days to 12 months. This was an average—some people's lives would be prolonged more, some not at all.

For many people, cutting down on fats in their diet does affect the quality of life. "Many healthy, hungry men are worried, frustrated and unhappy eating oat bran and rice bran, following diets without eggs, milk, butter or red meats and gorging on fish or the latest cholesterol-lowering fad food because they, their families or even their physicians are convinced that immortality is ensured by unrealistically low serum cholesterol levels," wrote Dr. Hal B. Richerson, of the University of Iowa College of Medicine, in a letter to the *New England Journal of Medicine.* It's interesting that Sir Richard Doll, an English epidemiologist credited with first showing the relationship of smoking to lung cancer, of radiation to cancer and many other correlations, once said that he considered one of his greatest accomplishments was showing that people didn't have to go on bland diets for gastric ulcers. That finding, he said, "contributed to saving millions of people from having miserable diets imposed on them." Thomas N. James, M.D., a past president of the American Heart Association, was quoted in an article in *The New York Times* as saying, "One of the saddest things is to see patients who are in their 70s or 80s

and who are terrified by what they are eating. One of the first things they want to know is what their cholesterol level is." Citing the fact that some elderly were even malnourished because they were afraid to eat their favorite foods, Dr. James said, "The obsession of the elderly with diet and cholesterol is a national tragedy."

What can be done? It's useful to look at what's happening in other countries. In Canada, for example, a working group strongly supported a general public health campaign to encourage community-wide changes in diet and lifestyle. It did not, however recommend the universal screening of the adult population, and, as reported in the *New England Journal of*

Medicine, cutoff points for intervention were set higher than those adopted in the U.S. on the grounds that "mass medicalization was not a sensible approach to a community-wide problem."

On a personal level, we can all start taking risk factors with a bit more skepticism. Avoiding mass screening programs is one way, since the results are likely to be inaccurate. Coupling risk factors to the diseases for which they predict risk is another: if your doctor says your blood pressure is high, try to pin him or her down on what your overall risk of heart attack or stroke is, and decrease your risk. While the proverbial grain of salt may be bad for your blood pressure, it's definitely good seasoning to take with your medical information.

Pressure Treatment

How exercise can help you control your blood pressure.

Kathleen M. Cahill

KATHLEEN M. CAHILL, *former senior editor of* Walking, *is a freelance writer based in Needham, Mass.*

High blood pressure, also known as hypertension, is a condition with virtually no symptoms. It creates no pain and interferes little, if at all, with one's lifestyle. It is troublesome only for what it represents: a possible heart attack or stroke sometime in the future. Too often, the condition goes untreated until it's too late. The good news is that consistent aerobic exercise—e.g., walking three to five times a week for at least 30 minutes—can be a form of treatment.

Until recently, doctors recommended exercise only because it helped hypertensive patients lose weight. But now there's proof that exercise, even without weight loss, can help control blood pressure. This is important news, particularly for those with mild hypertension, the group that can benefit most from exercise. People in this group, with blood pressure readings just above 140/90 mm Hg (the top number represents "systolic" pressure, and the bottom one "diastolic"), are often unaware that even borderline hypertension can cause serious heart damage. "Mild elevations of blood pressure are not as innocuous as we used to think," notes Dr. Stevo Julius, chief of the division of hypertension at the University of Michigan.

Many people with mildly elevated blood pressure ignore the problem and the need to take medication for a condition that causes them no apparent symptoms. "I've had mild hypertension most of my life," reports Gerald Lawson, a 56-year-old plumbing and heating contractor from Durham, N.C. "The doctor did flips when he saw my blood pressure reading back in high school. But I've never taken medication for it. I don't like to go to doctors, and I never take medication for anything if I can help it."

For other people, hypertension crops up later in life. "I never had a problem until I was 56," says nurse Patricia Porcelli, also of Durham. "I gained about 30 pounds and was under a lot of stress due to illnesses in my family. My blood pressure went up to around 155/90." Porcelli knew she needed to take steps. "I have a family history of heart disease," she says. "My sister had a stroke at 41, and my mother had a heart attack in her early 60's."

Although Lawson and Porcelli didn't know each other at the time, they had a lot in common. Both had mild hypertension and were slightly overweight. Neither had participated in exercise or sports. And both responded to a newspaper advertisement from a Duke University researcher seeking sedentary people with mild hypertension to participate in a study to determine whether aerobic exercise like walking could reduce mild hypertension. The two joined the experiment, and were chosen to be in the group that would walk, jog, bike, and do other aerobic exercises three times a week for four months. Lead researcher and psychologist James Blumenthal says he conducted the study because "We know that people with high blood pressure are at increased risk of stroke and heart disease, and that the standard medications may have side effects. They compromise the quality of a person's life, and that means that people don't take their medications." Blumenthal reasoned that a non-drug alternative such as exercise would be a boon to some people.

Both Lawson and Porcelli successfully lowered their blood pressure to a safe level during the four months they were exercising. That was three years ago. After reducing his blood pressure from 160/90 to 142/80 by walking, jogging, and biking for the study, Lawson went on to lose 27 pounds, whittling his weight down from 182 to 155. The 5-foot-8-inch amateur pilot now runs in races, including a marathon last year, "to keep motivated." His blood pressure has dropped even lower, to 138/80. "I was never an athletic person," Lawson says. "But now, I feel much more in touch with my body, and I've gained a sense of well-being."

For Porcelli, the Duke experiment reduced her blood pressure from a high of 155/90 to 130/80, and it has stayed there ever since. Porcelli keeps up her exercise with water aerobics, which she says has improved her sense of physical well-being. "I have a lot more stamina; I'm more energetic, not tired. My circulation is better, and I'm less prone to swollen ankles at night."

Among others who have demonstrated that exercise can be a potent tool for lowering blood pressure is John J. Duncan, Ph.D., associate director of the Department of Exercise Physiology at the Cooper Institute for Aerobic Research in Dallas. "When we've looked at the effect of exercise on the mildly hypertensive group, we've found that exercise can not only lower their blood pressure readings but keep them under control, below 90 [diastolic] in most cases," says Duncan. Although researchers are trying to isolate the effect of exercise to determine its ability to lower blood pressure independent of such factors as weight loss and diet, other lifestyle changes may be equally or even more important. Losing

 From *Walking Magazine*, June 1992, pp. 17-18.

weight is a major one. For anyone who is overweight, exercise and diet is a sound approach to treatment, says Edward Roccella, coordinator for the National High Blood Pressure Education Program. "Anyone who is overweight may be able to reduce his or her blood pressure simply by losing pounds."

Nutrition is another factor. Salt has long been linked with a higher rate of hypertension, Roccella says. "We consume 3 to 20 times the amount of salt we need." Although some experts believe that salt's role in reducing blood pressure has been overemphasized, Roccella notes that the evidence for the link remains strong.

Other minerals, such as calcium and potassium, may also play a role in hypertension. Some doctors recommend that hypertensive patients increase their intake of calcium, but Roccella reports that the relationship between blood pressure and calcium intake is far from fully documented. He does, however, support the recommended daily dietary allowance of 800 milligrams of calcium, the equivalent of nearly 3 cups of milk a day.

"The calcium factor is controversial. We see some evidence to support a higher intake," says Dr. Meir Stampfer, associate professor of epidemiology at the Harvard School of Public Health. "People with the lowest intakes of calcium appear to have a higher risk of hypertension." But he cautions that the need for calcium is "not nearly as important as losing weight. If you want to lose some points on your blood pressure, the first thing to do is lose pounds. Calcium, at best, will have a modest effect."

Heavy alcohol consumption also affects blood pressure, Stampfer adds. At a moderate level (two drinks a day), alcohol has no effect. But heavy drinking may increase

---

How's Your Blood Pressure?

Blood pressure is the force created by the heart as it pushes blood into the arteries and through the circulatory system. Normally, the small blood vessels, or arterioles, contract or expand as the blood surges through them. If the arterioles remain constricted, they create the condition of high blood pressure, also known as hypertension.

A blood-pressure reading has two parts. The first, known as systolic pressure, is the pressure of the blood flow during heartbeats. The second number, diastolic, is the pressure between beats. Blood pressure is measured in millimeters of mercury, which is abbreviated mm Hg. A reading of 120/80 mm Hg is considered normal. High blood pressure in adults is defined as a systolic pressure equal to or greater than 140 mm Hg and/or a diastolic pressure equal to or greater than 90 mm Hg. The diastolic portion is sometimes further classified as mild (90 to 104 mm Hg), moderate (105 to 114 mm Hg), or severe (115 mm Hg or higher).

---

blood pressure. For people who drink heavily, reducing alcohol consumption is extremely important.

Beyond exercise, weight control, and nutrition, gender may be a factor in hypertension. Most studies of blood pressure have been done on men, not women, points out the Cooper Clinic's John Dun-

can. "And women may respond differently than men to virtually any kind of treatment," he says.

There is some evidence that women respond better than men to exercise as a means of lowering blood pressure. "In one study, women had a 15-millimeter reduction in systolic pressure, and a 10- to 12-millimeter reduction in diastolic pressure, compared with only 12 to 15 in systolic pressure, and 8 to 10 in diastolic pressure in men. Exercise training—like walking programs—could potentially be more effective in women than men," Duncan concludes.

Current recommendations for treating hypertension do not differ for men and women, leading some experts to warn that women are being treated without adequate data on how they respond to medications, diet, and exercise. The possible side effects of medication are a particular concern.

There is a confusing variety of drugs prescribed for hypertensive patients. One group of drugs, called *diuretics*, works by eliminating excess fluids and salt, thereby reducing blood volume and pressure. *Beta blockers* reduce the heart rate and the heart's output of blood. *Sympathetic nerve inhibitors* are still another class of drugs. These inhibit the nerves that constrict the blood vessels. *Vasodilators* can cause the muscle in the walls of a blood vessel to relax, allowing the artery to dilate. *Angiotensin converting enzymes* (ACE inhibitors) interfere with the body's production of angiotensin, a chemical that causes the arteries to constrict.

Anyone with hypertension should not hesitate to take medication if the doctor prescribes it. But for those people who have borderline or mild hypertension with no other complications, lifestyle changes such as diet and exercise may be just the ticket.

FROM HERE TO IMMUNITY

Don't feel under the weather this winter: Keep your body's defenses primed with a daily dose of walking.

Peter Jaret

Peter Jaret writes on health issues for magazines such as National Geographic *and* Health, *where he is a contributing editor.*

It wasn't long before Verlene Roark began to feel better. "I had more energy. My breathing was better. I felt stronger," Roark recalls. After years of inactivity, Roark was participating in a study of the health effects of regular walking at Appalachian State University in Boone, N.C. Five days a week she and 15 other women walked 2 miles. Roark enjoyed the companionship that the exercise program offered. She was also glad to feel her energy returning. But it wasn't until the 12-week study was almost over, as winter set in amidst the fir trees of Boone, that she became aware of another side effect: "Save for a little case of the sniffles," Roark says, "I wasn't sick one day."

A healthier heart, stronger muscles, a leaner physique: Most of us know the value of regular exercise. But now there's growing evidence that moderate exercise—even a brisk daily walk around the neighborhood—can boost the body's immune system, making walkers far less susceptible to not only the misery of cold and flu season but also more serious illnesses, including cancer.

YOUR CENTERS FOR DISEASE CONTROL

To understand how a walk in the park might keep the next wave of flu at bay, it is helpful to take a close look at the human immune system. Scientists say they are only beginning to understand this remarkably complex network that defends us against viruses, bacteria, and myriad other microscopic dangers. But they do know that the overall force is both enormous—hundreds of millions of cells circulate through our bloodstreams—and highly specialized.

The first line of defense comes from cells called macrophages. Spotting a virus, bacteria, or other foreign cell, macrophages engulf and consume the invader, literally digesting it. Macrophages (the name means big "eaters") also alert other immune cells, called helper T cells, to the presence of an intruder in the area. These helper T cells then recruit killer T cells, which immediately begin to multiply and swarm around the site of an infection. Killer T cells lock onto the invader and blast open its cell wall. At the same time, helper T cells send chemical signals to B cells, which begin to produce chemical weapons called antibodies. Specifically shaped to grab onto the surface of a foreign cell, antibodies may simply slow the intruders down long enough for killer T cells to target them, or they may set in motion a chemical process that also destroys the invader's cell wall. Killer T and B cells are also highly specialized. For example, one set of killer T cells is genetically programmed to attack only one kind of flu virus; another is programmed to knock off just one type of cold-causing virus.

Scientists have recently identified another type of immune defender, a kind of James Bond of disease control called the natural killer cell, which appears to be far more versatile. Able to recognize and destroy a wide range of viruses and cancer cells, natural killer cells roam the body, constantly rooting out potential threats before the symptoms of illness or infection can appear.

HOW DOES WALKING FIT IN?

One clue that exercise may influence immunity was discovered in 1989 by David Nieman, Ph.D., a professor of exercise science at Appalachian State and a leading expert on exercise and immunity. Nieman (who later directed Roark's study) recruited 50 women in their 30s and 40s. One group continued to do what they'd always done—a minimum of physical activity. The others walked for 45 minutes a day, five days a week. Both groups were asked to keep a diary of how they felt during the 15-week study. When Nieman studied the results, he realized that the walkers reported half as many days with cold or flu

   From *Walking Magazine*, November/December 1993, pp. 43-44, 46-47, 77. © 1993 by Walking Inc. Reprinted by permission.

symptoms as the non-walkers. It was possible, of course, that the walkers simply tended to ignore their symptoms. But when Nieman studied blood samples for signs of immune activity, he found that antibody levels climbed steadily among the walkers during the 15-week experiment. Nieman also charted a steady increase in the activity of natural killer cells.

"Moderate exercise such as walking seems to prime the body's immune system, preparing it to fight disease-causing organisms," says Nieman. "The changes are much like those that occur when the body begins to fight an infection. But exercise seems to prepare the body in advance—increasing the odds that the immune system will be able to head off a respiratory infection, for example, before we feel the first sniffle."

Why this happens is still a mystery, but there are theories. Some researchers have suggested that hormones produced during physical activity may act as signals that trigger immune cells to multiply. Beta-endorphins, for instance, the substances that have been linked to "exercisers' high," seem to boost immune-cell activity in laboratory experiments. Moderate exercise also raises levels of epinephrine and norepinephrine in the bloodstream—both of which put immune cells on "active alert," making their response to an invasion quicker.

But not all researchers are convinced that hormones are the answer. They point to the fact that at higher levels of exertion, the body releases a stress-related hormone, called cortisal, which may actually dampen immunity.

"Moderate exercise such as walking seems to prime the body's immune system, preparing it to fight disease-causing organisms," says Nieman.

Nieman suspects that regular walking works its wonders in a very practical and straightforward way. "To spot invading bacteria and viruses, immune cells must constantly circulate through the bloodstream, just the way cops patrol the streets on the lookout for trouble," he explains. "Physical activity increases heart rate and speeds up blood flow, which in turn speeds the circulation of immune cells through the body. Increased blood flow may even jog immune cells out of the lymph nodes, where they tend to gather, and into the bloodstream. That's crucial. The more immune cells you've got out there on the beat, the more likely they are to bump into the bad guys and arrest them."

Exercise may bolster immunity in yet another way. The increased blood circulation and the simple friction of muscles working together raise core body temperature—mimicking a fever. There's good evidence that the elevated temperature of a fever is itself an immune defense, slowing down viruses and bacteria and making them easier targets for antibodies and other immune cells. For example, when animals have been prevented from running fevers, they often die of runaway bacterial infections. Exercise physiologists speculate that the temporary rise in core body temperature during moderate physical activity may be enough to help the body sweep away bad bugs.

HARD NEWS FOR THE HARD-CORE

If a little bout of exercise is good for you, will a strenuous workout be even better? Here, researchers have uncovered a seeming paradox. While moderate exercise seems to boost immunity, a hard-core workout may actually weaken the body's defenses.

Nieman first began to suspect that strenuous exercise might be detrimental when he heard long-distance runners complain about coming down with colds and flus after competing in races. Nieman polled more than 2,300 athletes in training for the 1987 Los Angeles Marathon to find out if those complaints were widespread. Runners who trained 60 miles a week, Nieman found, were twice as likely to come down with colds or flu as those who trained fewer than 20 miles a week. Athletes who eventually competed in the marathon were six times more likely to get sick during the week after competition than equally trained athletes who sat out the race.

Their strenuous exercise regimens appeared to be making these athletes more susceptible to illness. To test his suspicions, Nieman asked 10 veteran marathoners to come into the exercise laboratory and run at their fastest pace for three hours. Blood samples taken before and after their bout of exhausting exercise clinched it. The effectiveness of the runners' natural killer cells had dropped by as much as 30%—and stayed low for as long as six hours after exercise. More recently, researchers discovered that heavy exercise can weaken other parts of the immune system as well—slowing the production of antibodies, for instance, and dampening the activity of killer T cells. While these slumps in immune activity are temporary, researchers are convinced they're enough to make competitive athletes more susceptible to disease.

Why does brisk walking bolster immunity and hard running weaken it? Some experts believe the answer may lie in a delicate balance of hormones. During moderate exercise, the hormone epinephrine, which increases immune function, begins to surge into the bloodstream. But when exercise intensity climbs above about 75% or 80% of aerobic capacity, cortisol spills into the bloodstream. Produced in response to stress—whether it's the strain of a demanding job, an unhappy relationship, or a bruising workout—cortisol is a potent immune suppressor.

Overdoing it on the workout floor may also pose other hazards. Researchers at the University of Oxford recently found that strenuous exercise may rob immune cells of the energy they need to function at their peak. The amino acid glutamine, which is produced, stored, and released by muscle tissue, is an important fuel for immune cells. But when athletes overtrain, the British scientists discovered, glutamine levels drop. Starved of the fuel they need for peak performance, immune cells may be impaired.

CAN YOU WALK AWAY FROM CANCER?

The benefits of regular walking may be even more profound—it may protect you against serious threats to your health, including cancer. In an analysis of 5,400 women, Rose Frisch, Ph.D., a Harvard professor of population sciences, found that sedentary women were almost twice as likely to develop breast cancer. In addition, inactive women were two and a half times as likely to develop reproductive-tract cancers than women who remained physically active during their lives. Other studies suggest that regular physical activity may offer protection against colon cancer.

Our bodies are continuously exposed to cancer-causing substances. By speeding up metabolism, regular exercise may simply flush these carcinogenic chemicals out of the system faster, thus reducing their potential for harm. But Mark Davis, Ph.D., associate professor of exercise science at the University of South Carolina at Columbia, has shown that physical activity also increases the activity of two critically important immune cells: macrophages and natural killers. The effect on macrophages may be especially important, Davis believes, since these cells function as the first line of defense against infection and cancer. By increasing the vigilance of macrophages, regular exercise may enable the immune system to destroy troublesome invaders before they have a chance to multiply.

It will take years of research to know whether moderate exercise is enough to prevent cancer. But there's already reason to think it might. Researchers typically test anti-cancer drugs by exposing a group of animals to cancer cells. Then half of them receive doses of an experimental drug while scientists check for results. Laurie Hoffman-Goetz, Ph.D., professor of health studies at the University of Waterloo in Ontario, recently conducted a similar study. Instead of testing an experimental drug, however, she tested the effects of moderate exercise—with encouraging results. Animals trained to run for 8 to 12 weeks and then exposed to lung cancer cells were significantly less likely to develop tumors than the sedentary animals.

In another experiment, animals exposed to cancer cells and then trained to run weren't protected against tumors. An immune system already geared up by exercise, Hoffman-Goetz suspects, may be necessary to sweep away cancer cells the moment they appear. Thus, making exercise a regular habit may be crucial.

Exercise may also turn out to be beneficial in the treatment of other serious diseases. After a small group of men infected with the HIV virus participated in a 10-week program of regular exercise, researchers at the University of Miami measured improvements in their immune cell functions. The changes were remarkably similar to the effects of AZT, the leading AIDS drug. However, no one knows whether these small changes will have any effect on the overall course of the disease.

Immunologists have long known that the immune system typically declines with age, putting older people at greater risk of serious infections. But Nieman has found evidence that this is not always the case. When he compared a group of sedentary elderly women in their 70s and 80s with a dozen exceptionally active women in the same age group—women who had engaged in regular physical activities such as competitive walking for at least the previous 11 years—the results suggested that declining immunity may not be inevitable. "By virtually every measure, the immune systems of the active elderly women looked exactly like those we'd expect to see in a woman in her early 30s," says Nieman. Natural killer cells, in fact, were sometimes even more active in the elderly athletes than in sedentary women half their age. A robust immune system, Nieman concludes, is the payoff for a long-term commitment to regular exercise.

Back in Boone, N.C., Roark is still striding around the track every chance she gets. She's convinced that walking a couple of miles five days a week has helped ward off colds—and perhaps even more dangerous infections. "I plan to go on walking for as long as I'm able," says Roark. "I don't think I've ever been healthier."

EAT TO BEAT CANCER

Mounting evidence points to a diet-cancer link

Kathleen Cahill Allison

Kathleen Cahill Allison is a health writer in Needham, Mass.

By now the message should have sounded loud and clear: Eat lots of fresh fruit and vegetables to reduce your risk of cancer. Researchers estimate that approximately one-third of all cancers are related to diet, most commonly those of the colon, rectum, stomach, breast and prostate. But as the results from hundreds of scientific studies pour in, this simple message is getting blurred. Unlike heart disease, which demands a lowfat diet immediately upon diagnosis, there doesn't seem to be one hard and fast rule from the kitchen for fighting cancer.

Just recently, the results of a study from Harvard Medical School linking low intakes of vitamin A to a higher risk of breast cancer made headlines across the country. Reporters quoted researchers who said that women could lower their risk of this deadly disease by eating more carrots, cantaloupes and sweet potatoes. But does eating these orange foods cancel out the negative effects of fatty foods and alcohol reported in earlier breast cancer studies?

Adding to the confusion are reports that link different types of cancers with different types of foods. The same fruits and vegetables now associated with preventing breast cancer have been reported in the past to prevent lung cancer but have shown mixed success at staving off colon cancer. Yet other reports find that quite different vegetables—broccoli and brussels sprouts, for instance—*do* lower colon cancer risk.

"Most people don't realize how great an influence the foods they eat have on their chances of getting certain types of cancer," says Dr. Peter Greenwald, director of cancer prevention research at the National Cancer Institute (NCI). That's a daunting thought, especially when you try to translate baffling scientific information into a grocery list.

Certain substances in food, such as fat and nitrite preservatives, may even promote cancer. At the same time, fiber, vi-

tamins C and E, folic acid, beta-carotene (which the body converts to vitamin A) and other substances are believed to play protective roles. The obvious questions: Which foods and how much of them should we eat or avoid to prevent cancer? Unfortunately, there are no easy answers.

That's because we're looking for a simple solution to a complicated problem, explains Dr. Paul Saltman, a professor of biology at the University of California at San Diego. "Cancer isn't one disease," he says. "It's many diseases with a common root of uncontrolled cell growth. Even though we understand cancers, we're only just beginning to understand their connection to diet."

There is compelling evidence that colon, prostate and possibly breast cancer are more prevalent among people who consume high-fat diets. And the problem is not just the total amount of fat: A number of studies have indicated that the *type* of fat consumed, most notably the saturated fat in animal products, affects the degree of cancer risk.

Colon cancer, taken together with closely related rectal cancer, is the most common form of cancer in the U.S. A study of more than 49,000 men published last year by the Harvard School of Public Health showed that those who ate a high-fat, low-fiber diet quadrupled their risk of developing precancerous colon polyps. Another Harvard-based study of almost 89,000 nurses found that those whose diets were high in red meat and animal fat were more likely to develop colon cancer than those who ate more poultry and seafood.

Prostate cancer, which afflicts approximately one in every 100 American men over age 65, has also been linked to fatty foods. A University of California at Loma Linda study of 6,700 men found that those who ate cheese, eggs, meat or poultry three or more times a week and drank more than two glasses of milk a day were more than three times as likely to die of prostate cancer. It's not clear, however, whether a high-fat diet contributed to the disease or to reduced survival rates after diagnosis.

7. CURRENT KILLERS

The breast cancer picture is even murkier. In Mediterranean countries, where the primary source of fat is the relatively benign olive oil, a monounsaturated fat, the rate of breast cancer is quite low. In the U.S. and parts of Europe, where the diet is high in total and saturated fat from dairy products and meat, breast cancer rates are correspondingly high. On the basis of these observations and laboratory studies, researchers have long believed that fat is related to the risk of breast cancer.

Yet despite the evidence, the link between fat and breast cancer was called into question by the same Harvard nurse study that linked fat to colon cancer. "Based on our findings," says Dr. Walter Willett, a professor of epidemiology and nutrition, who headed the study, "there is little evidence that a high-fat diet, per se, causes breast cancer."

Because some tumors depend on the female hormone estrogen for growth, many researchers now believe that it is the true culprit in breast cancer. According to Harvard coinvestigator Graham Colditz, an associate professor of medicine, obesity and a high percentage of body fat in postmenopausal women have been correlated with high estrogen levels and a concurrently high risk of breast cancer. "Postmenopausal women still have detectable levels of estrogen in their blood," he explains. "And while these women have lower levels than those of premenopausal women, obese postmenopausal women have higher levels than their lean peers."

Estrogen may also be the missing link in the suspected relationship between alcohol and breast cancer. Over the past decade, studies have shown a strong correlation between moderate alcohol use and breast cancer, but until recently, scientists couldn't explain *how* alcohol affected the disease. Earlier this year, an NCI study of 34 women indicated that two drinks a day can raise estrogen levels up to 32%. Researchers speculated that an alcohol-induced estrogen increase could explain the connection between drinking and an increased risk of breast cancer.

Food is a complex mixture of many chemical substances. Earlier diet and cancer research focused on the relationship of some of these substances to disease. But over the past decade, the scientific focus has switched to the relationship between food substances and good health. As a result, we know now that fighting cancer with food isn't just a matter of avoiding potential cancer-causing substances, it's also a matter of including in your diet those foods that might offer protection.

Fiber, specifically *insoluble* fiber from foods such as wheat bran and whole grain cereals, has long been thought to reduce the risk of cancers of the digestive tract, particularly colon cancer. Fiber helps waste matter move quickly, theoretically limiting contact between potential carcinogens and the lining of the colon. Beyond fiber's mechanical role in clearing the colon, recent studies indicate that vitamins, minerals and other substances found in high-fiber vegetables and grains may also protect against colon and other types of cancer.

A deficiency of the B vitamin folic acid may put women at higher risk for developing cervical cancer. Researchers at the University of Alabama at Birmingham found that women with high blood levels of folic acid had significantly lower rates of a precancerous condition known as cervical dysplasia. Folic acid may also play a role in preventing the development of precancerous polyps in the colon and the rectum, according to results from Harvard Medical School's Health Professionals Study and further reports from its nurse study. An analysis of dietary information supplied by study participants reveals that men and women with diets high in folic acid had the lowest occurrence of colon or rectal polyps.

Vitamins C and E and beta-carotene are now commonly referred to as antioxidant nutrients. Scientists believe that antioxidants offset a normal body process known as oxidation

A PRACTICAL GUIDE TO PROTECTIVE FOODS

Although no food has been shown to prevent any disease absolutely, many foods contain natural substances that experts believe may help prevent some cancers. Foods that contain significant amounts of these substances are listed below.

BENEFICIAL SUBSTANCE	ASSOCIATED CANCERS	FOOD SOURCES
Fiber (insoluble)	Colon, gastro-intestinal, rectal	Wheat bran, whole wheat and other whole grain cereals and bread products; raw and lightly cooked fruits and vegetables
Antioxidants (vitamins C and E and beta-carotene)	Breast, cervical, gastrointestinal, lung, stomach, prostate	Vitamin C: citrus fruits, dark-green leafy vegetables, kiwi, strawberries, tomatoes, sweet and hot peppers, parsley; vitamin E: vegetable oils, wheat germ, soy products, avocados and nuts; beta-carotene: deep-yellow and orange vegetables and fruit (sweet potatoes, winter squash, pumpkins, cantaloupe, mangoes)
Folic acid	Cervical, colon, rectal	Whole wheat products, wheat germ, dried beans, dark-green leafy vegetables, beets, asparagus, broccoli, winter squash, bean sprouts, sunflower seeds, cantaloupe, citrus fruit
Nonnutritive phytochemicals (including indoles and isothiocyanates)	Breast, colon, gastrointestinal, lung, prostate, stomach	Cabbage, broccoli, brussels sprouts, cauliflower, greens, horseradish, garlic, licorice root, soybeans

that results in the formation of altered molecules called free radicals. Free radicals, which steal electrons from other molecules, can cause irreversible damage to a cell's membrane and its DNA. Scientists believe that over time this cell damage may lead to the formation of cancer cells.

The body naturally produces antioxidants that protect cells from free-radical attack. Antioxidants in certain foods also fight free radicals in a variety of ways:

▶Vitamin E defends fatty cell membranes by blocking free radicals before they attack.

▶Vitamin C neutralizes free radicals in the watery areas within and between body cells.

▶Beta-carotene functions in fatty areas of the cell, in much the same way vitamin E does.

Vitamin antioxidants are just one group of phytochemicals—chemical compounds synthesized by plants—drawing researchers' attention. "There are many substances in everyday foods that may prevent different types of cancer," says Dr. Herbert Pierson, former director of the Designer Foods Program at the NCI. Pierson's work at the NCI and currently as a consultant to private industry has focused on isolating a variety of nonnutritive phytochemicals found in foods such as garlic and cruciferous vegetables. Although these substances have no known nutritional value, they appear to have anticarcinogenic and other disease-fighting properties.

Garlic, for one, is a "chemical puzzle," says Pierson, who has been trying for years to tease apart its various protective substances. "Raw garlic contains substances that have been shown to kill a variety of microorganisms. When those same substances are cooked in boiling water—in soup, for example—they create sulfide compounds shown to be protective against colon cancer in animals." Pierson believes that garlic has great preventive powers for gastrointestinal cancers.

Cruciferous vegetables—broccoli, cabbage and brussels sprouts—contain a substance called sulforaphen that may help protect cells against cancer-causing substances. According to Pierson and other researchers, sulforaphen and its chemical cousins have been linked to lower rates of stomach, colon and breast cancers in lab animals. In addition, Pierson is investigating a group of food substances known as indoles. Also found in cruciferous vegetables, indoles activate an enzyme that lowers estrogen levels. Meanwhile, research funded by the NCI is looking at chemical compounds in licorice root, flaxseed, citrus fruit juice, soybeans and root vegetables that may lend anticarcinogenic properties to these foods.

There is as yet no hard evidence that any of these substances protect against cancer when taken as supplements. Since the human body is self-regulating, overloading on supplements may even turn off its own natural production of antioxidants. And no one is really sure if there are risks involved in long-term use of certain supplements, such as the currently popular vitamin E.

Most health authorities recommend getting antioxidants and other cancer-fighting substances from a well-balanced diet, rather than by taking supplements. But as evidence mounts in favor of the protective value of various substances isolated from foods, more and more researchers say it won't be long before specific recommendations for supplements will be made. "No one argues with the fact that you need to eat a varied, balanced diet," says Dr. Jeffrey Blumberg, a professor of nutrition at Tufts University School of Nutrition. "But now it seems clear that there's also a rational role for using supplements as protection against cancer and other diseases, particularly since

CAN EXERCISE WARD OFF CANCER?

Just in case you need another reason to head to the gym, there's a growing body of evidence that regular moderate exercise lowers the risk of colon cancer, as well as cancers of the breast, uterus, ovaries, cervix and vagina.

Researchers questioned 17,000 male Harvard University alumni about their exercise habits in 1962 or 1966, and then again in 1977. Those who reported at both interviews that they typically burned at least 1,000 calories a week through exercise (equal to walking 10 miles or playing two hours of tennis) had a colon cancer risk half that of those who didn't work out. Experts theorize that exercise speeds the transit of wastes through the intestines, moving along food-borne carcinogens that might otherwise linger in the colon. But since the disease can take years to develop, consistency is key: The men who reported exercising at only one interview did not benefit.

Working out over the long haul may also reduce the body's exposure to estrogen, which is thought to play a role in breast cancer and reproductive-tract cancers. (The hormone seems to stimulate cell division, which increases the chance of a harmful mutation.) Since one-third of a woman's estrogen before menopause is produced by body fat, leaner, fitter women tend to make less of it.

In a study at the Harvard School of Public Health, 5,400 women who had graduated from college between 1925 and 1981 were asked about their diet, their health and their reproductive and exercise histories. Half the subjects were nonathletes; the other half had been college athletes, and 75% of this group reported that they had continued to exercise. After eliminating factors such as smoking and family history of cancer, "We found that the former athletes had a significantly lower rate of breast cancer and cancers of the reproductive system," says Dr. Rose Frisch, an associate professor of population sciences emerita, who headed the research.

Exercise may also help fight other forms of cancer because of its ability to boost the performance of two types of immune system cells—natural killer (NK) cells and macrophages. According to Dr. J. Mark Davis, an associate professor of exercise science at the University of South Carolina in Columbia, mice put through both moderate and exhaustive treadmill exercise showed improvement in macrophage assault on breast tumor cells. And in a study at the University of Waterloo in Ontario, mice made to exercise for nine weeks had enhanced NK-cell ability to kill lung tumor cells. Moreover, their heightened immunity was sustained once they stopped.

Animal data can't be directly applied to people, of course. Although intense treadmill running seems to enhance the immunity of laboratory animals, studies show that humans who exercise too intensely may be *more* susceptible to certain infections. Still, Frisch believes that active people do have a greater ability to fight cancer. "With the exception of skin cancer, the athletes had markedly less of *all* types of cancer—including nonreproductive-tract cancers—than sedentary subjects," she says.

Although NK cells and macrophages seem to nip cancers in the bud, Davis emphasizes that once a tumor takes hold, working out won't help the immune system get rid of it. (It may, however, prevent malignant cells from spreading.) Moreover, the jury is still out on exactly how much exercise is needed to lower cancer risk. The best advice? Work up a sweat for 20 to 30 minutes, three times a week—and keep at it.
—*Michele Wolf*

over 90% of the population doesn't even meet their RDA [recommended dietary allowance] for most nutrients."

Dr. Mark Kestin, a nutritional epidemiologist at the Fred Hutchinson Cancer Research Center in Seattle, also believes supplements can be used preventively in some circumstances. "If I were a smoker, I would think about taking beta-carotene because of its possible protective effect against lung cancer." But, he adds, "I still believe you should get your nutrients from food. We don't know enough yet to give specific advice on supplements."

Blumberg says it's better simply to quit smoking than to depend on beta-carotene. "Smokers have 20 times more chance of getting lung cancer than nonsmokers, and beta-carotene cuts that risk in half. But that means smokers who take beta-carotene are still 10 times more likely to get lung cancer than nonsmokers." For Blumberg, taking supplements can be likened to wearing seat belts: "They provide protection against injury, but they don't give you license to drive recklessly."

As researchers continue to probe the mysteries of food chemistry, one message is now clear: Supplements aren't substitutes for a healthful diet. For now, the guidelines established by the NCI provide the most sensible framework for a diet that reduces the risk of cancer:

►REDUCE DIETARY FAT TO 30% OR LESS OF TOTAL CALORIES. Choose leaner cuts of beef, pork and lamb. Substitute chicken, turkey, fish and shellfish for some of the red meat in your diet. Eat reduced-fat, lowfat and fat-free dairy products, salad dressings and snacks.

►INCREASE FIBER TO BETWEEN 20 GRAMS AND 30 GRAMS DAILY. Eat a variety of whole grain cereals and breads. Legumes such as pinto beans, black beans, chickpeas, lentils and kidney beans are all low fat sources of fiber.

►EAT A VARIETY OF FRUITS AND VEGETABLES EVERY DAY. Eat at least five servings of different fruits and vegetables each day, including those high in beta-carotene and vitamin C. Cantaloupe, papaya, broccoli and tomatoes are good sources of both vitamins.

Most types of fresh produce also contain significant amounts of fiber.

►LIMIT THE AMOUNT OF SALT-CURED AND SMOKED FOODS IN YOUR DIET. These include pickles, olives and sodium nitrite—preserved foods such as bacon or salami. Nitrites combine with amino acids in the stomach to produce carcinogenic substances called nitrosamines. Also limit smoked foods and animal foods charred by

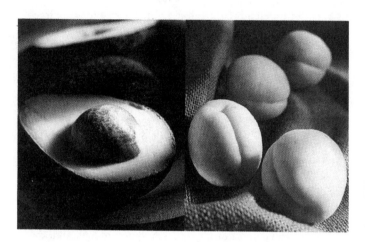

grilling or broiling: Mutagens formed from high-temperature burning of muscle protein have been linked to a variety of cancers in animals.

►AVOID OBESITY. Follow a suitable diet and exercise regimen to maintain the ideal weight for your height, age and body type (see "Can Exercise Ward Off Cancer?").

►DRINK ALCOHOL IN MODERATION, IF AT ALL. Besides its recent link with breast cancer, alcohol has been associated with cancers of the esophagus and throat. When combined with cigarette smoking, alcohol use is also thought to increase the risk of mouth, throat and liver cancers.

ANALYSIS

Confronting the AIDS Pandemic

**Daniel J. M. Tarantola
and Jonathan M. Mann**

Daniel J. M. Tarantola, M.D., is a lecturer in international health at the Harvard School of Public Health. Jonathan M. Mann, M.D., is director of the International AIDS Center of the Harvard AIDS Institute.

In 1986, the world undertook to mobilize against the AIDS pandemic in an effort that continued to grow until the beginning of this decade, when it began to stall. Today, the global HIV/AIDS pandemic is spinning out of control—its broad course has yet to be influenced in any substantial way by policies and programs mounted against it.

In 1991–1992, the Harvard-based Global AIDS Policy Coalition undertook a review of the state of the AIDS pandemic. The findings of this review, which appear in our new book *AIDS in the World* (Harvard University Press, December 1992), raise the alarm and call for an urgent revival of the response to AIDS.

The magnitude of the pandemic has increased over 100-fold since AIDS was discovered in 1981. From an estimated 100,000 people infected with HIV world-

wide in 1981, it is estimated that by early 1992, at least 12.9 million people around the world (7.1 million men, 4.7 million women, and 1.1 million children) had been infected with HIV. Of these, about one in five (2.6 million) have thus far developed AIDS, and nearly 2.5 million have died.

The spread of HIV has not been stopped in any community or country. In the United States, at least 40,000 to 80,000 new HIV infections were anticipated during 1992; in 1991, more than 75,000 new HIV infections occurred in Europe. In just five years, the cumulative number of HIV-infected Africans has tripled, from 2.5 million to over 7.5 million today. HIV is spreading to new communities and countries around the world—in some areas with great rapidity. An explosion of HIV has recently occurred in Southeast Asia, particularly in Thailand, Burma, and India, where, within only a few years, over one million people may have already been infected with HIV. HIV/AIDS is now reported from areas that, so far, had been left relatively untouched, such as Paraguay, Greenland, and the

Pacific island nations of Fiji, Papua New Guinea, and Samoa. The global implications are clear: During the next decade, HIV will likely reach most communities around the world; geographic boundaries cannot protect against HIV. The question today is not *if* HIV will come, but only *when*.

INCREASED COMPLEXITY

The pandemic becomes more complex as it matures. Globally it is composed of thousands of separate and linked community epidemics. Every large metropolitan area affected—Miami, New York, Bangkok, London, Amsterdam, Sydney, Rio de Janeiro—contains several subepidemics of HIV going on at the same time. The impact on women is increasing dramatically, as heterosexual transmission accounts for almost 71 percent of HIV infections. Worldwide, the proportion of HIV infected who are women is rising rapidly, from 25 percent in 1990 to 40 percent by early 1992. The epidemic also evolves over time: In Brazil, the proportion of HIV infections linked with injection

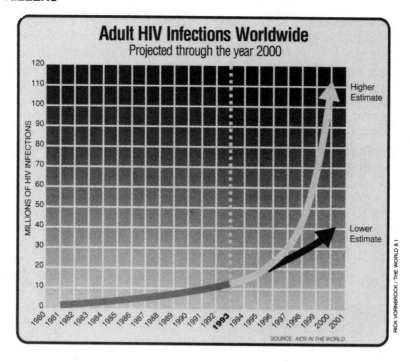

Adult HIV Infections Worldwide
Projected through the year 2000

SOURCE: AIDS IN THE WORLD.

RICK VORNBROCK / THE WORLD & I

drug use has increased over tenfold since the early 1980s; in the Caribbean, heterosexual transmission has now replaced homosexual transmission as the major mode of HIV spread.

The pandemic's major impacts are yet to come. During the period 1992–95 alone, the number of people developing AIDS—3.8 million—will exceed the total number who developed the disease during the pandemic's history prior to 1992. The number of children orphaned by AIDS will more than double in the next three years: from approximately 1.8 million today to 3.7 million by 1995. The pandemic has not peaked in any country—no community or country can claim "victory" against HIV/AIDS. By 1995, an *additional* 5.7 million adults will become infected with HIV. Thus, from 1992 to 1995, the total number of HIV-infected adults will increase by 50 percent. During the same period, the number of children infected with HIV will more than double, from 1.1 million to an estimated 2.3 million.

By the year 2000, the Global AIDS Policy Coalition has projected that between 38 million and 110 million adults—and over 10 million children—will become HIV infected. The largest proportion of HIV infections will be in Asia (42 percent), surpassing sub-Saharan Africa (31 percent), Latin America (8 percent), and the Caribbean (6 percent). By the end of this decade, 24 million adults and several million children may have developed AIDS—or up to 10 times as many as today.

Only a few years ago, tuberculosis was considered a stable problem that was endemic mostly in the developing world. If it was also prevalent in certain socioeconomic groups in industrialized countries, there was a common belief that the situation was largely under control. This general sense of complacency, denounced by many who had been fighting the disease, led to a decline in resources allocated to surveillance, prevention, and treatment services. When HIV came on the scene, it found a vulnerable population.

There is a dangerous synergy between HIV and tuberculosis that makes the combined effects of both worse than their separate effects added together. HIV makes individuals and communities more vulnerable to tuberculosis; it increases the rate of reactivation of tuberculosis infection, shortens the delay between TB infection and disease, and reduces the accuracy of diagnostic methods. Recent outbreaks of multiple-drug resistant tuberculosis have occurred in New York City and in Miami, especially in hospitals and prisons. Combining its projections with estimates made by the World Health Organization, *AIDS in the World* estimates that, by early 1992, there were more than 4.6 million people with both TB and HIV infection worldwide, 81 percent of them in Africa.

TAKING STOCK

Confronting the growing pandemic are national AIDS programs. These actions may involve governmental institutions and agencies, nongovernmental organizations, and the private sector.

> **Geographic boundaries cannot protect against HIV. The question today is not *if* HIV will come, but only *when*.**

Almost invariably overseen by ministries of health, they are generally implemented through government agencies and health services.

The success of a national AIDS program involves the extent to which it helps curb the course of the HIV epidemic and provides quality care to those already affected. On this basis, no program in the world can yet claim success.

Of the 38 countries surveyed by the Global AIDS Policy Coalition, 24 reported having conducted an evaluation since the inception of their national program. In general, the evaluation findings can be summarized as follows:

• Once created, programs become operational rapidly.

• They were successful in raising public awareness on AIDS issues although they did not always prevent (and at times they even generated) misperceptions among certain communities.

• They raised appropriate human rights issues and in some instances managed to prevent violations of these rights.

• They exchanged information—and in some cases made funds and skills available—at the international level.

Industrialized countries were generally able to secure the financial, human, and technological resources required to increase drastically the safety of blood and blood products, and establish diagnostic and treatment schemes reaching most (but not all) people in need. The same could not be said, however, about developing countries, which are constrained by lack of resources, weak infrastructures, and multiple developmental or even survival issues.

Common criticisms of these programs are their lack of focus and priority setting, their weak management, their lack of inte-

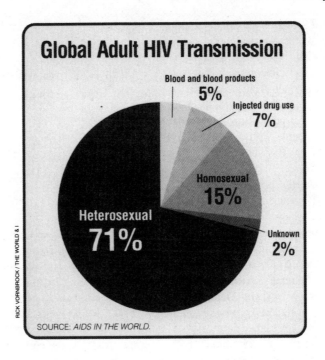

Global Adult HIV Transmission

Blood and blood products **5%**

Injected drug use **7%**

Homosexual **15%**

Unknown **2%**

Heterosexual **71%**

RICK VORNBROCK / THE WORLD & I

SOURCE: *AIDS IN THE WORLD.*

gration with existing disease prevention and control services, and their inability to actively involve other health programs, sectors, and nongovernmental organizations. Denial persists about the pandemic's impact upon women; prevention and research efforts worldwide still inadequately involve them.

In its report, the Global AIDS Policy Coalition suggests indexes that can be applied at the national or regional levels. Similar indexes are being developed for the assessment of community vulnerability.

THE COST OF AIDS

AIDS policies and programs used to be guided by two motives misperceived by many as antagonistic: a human rights/humanitarian approach and a public health perspective. The economic argument was seldom raised because it was not politically advantageous to make the cost of AIDS a major public issue. It did not conform to the humanitarian agenda (cost is secondary to human rights) nor to the public health perspective (the population must be protected). But with

the rising number of people and communities affected by the pandemic, the cost of prevention and care and the general economic impact of AIDS have become critical issues.

The economic perspective considers the impact of AIDS in a decade that began in a worldwide recession. It can be argued that the impact of HIV/AIDS on young, productive adults and their children will jeopardize the national development of many countries. In July 1992, a study conducted by an American team estimated the economic impact of the pandemic by feeding epidemiological projection data into a computer model of the global marketplace. It concluded that by the year 2000, the pandemic could drain between $356 billion and $514 billion from the world's economy, and developing countries are expected to be the hardest hit.

The Global AIDS Policy Coalition estimated that money spent on AIDS in a one-year period during 1990–91 was in the range of $1.4–$1.5 billion for prevention, approximately $3.5 billion for adult AIDS care alone, and $1.6 billion for research, for an adjusted total of $7.1 to $7.6 billion (including costs for treating those persons with HIV before AIDS occurs). Interestingly, about 95 percent was spent in industrialized countries that have less than 25 percent of the world's population, 18 percent of the people with AIDS, and 15 percent of HIV infections worldwide.

For HIV prevention activities in 1991, about $2.70 was spent *per person* in North America and $1.18 in Europe. In the developing world, spending on prevention amounted to only $0.07 per person in sub-Saharan Africa and $0.03 per person in Latin America. Of the $5.6 billion spent on AIDS research since the discovery of AIDS in 1981, $5.45 billion, or 97 percent, has been spent in industrialized countries. The United States is the biggest contributor to global AIDS research spending, with $4.8 billion, or 86 percent of the world total. Domestic and international research have led to a considerable advancement of knowledge. Research funds benefited from annual increases in the late 1980s, but resources supporting this research are reaching a plateau.

**The United States
is the biggest contributor to
global AIDS research spending,
with 86 percent
of the world total.**

For AIDS care, 89 percent of world spending in 1990 was used to help less than 30 percent of the world's people with AIDS—those living in North America and Europe. And yet, the cost of medical care for each person with AIDS—roughly equivalent to annual per capita income in developing countries—is overwhelming individuals and households everywhere. Inequities in treatment and prevention are growing. The cost of one year's treatment with AZT is about $2,500, while per capita income in all developing countries averages $700—in sub-Saharan Africa the

figure is $470—or less than one-fifth the cost of AZT for one year. Individual studies have indicated that the annual cost of care for an adult with AIDS varied in 1990–91 from $32,000 in the United States to $22,000 in western Europe, $2,000 in Latin America, and a mere $393 in sub-Saharan Africa.

These figures translate into the harsh reality of length of survival and quality of life of people with AIDS. The need for AIDS care and the inequity in access to quality services will continue to grow: The number of AIDS treatment years for adults alone will increase from an estimated 433,000 in 1992 to 619,000 in

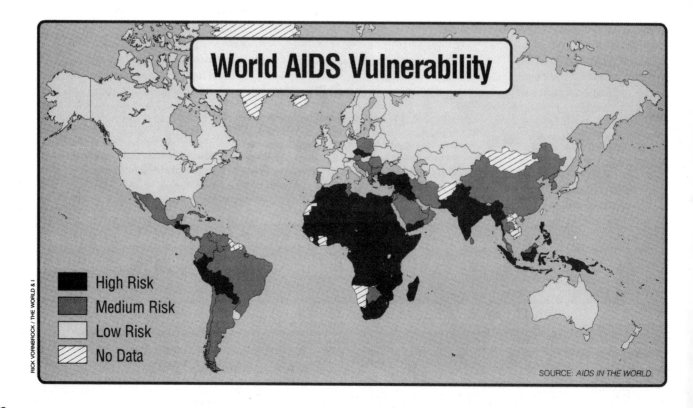

World AIDS Vulnerability

- ■ High Risk
- ▨ Medium Risk
- □ Low Risk
- ▨ No Data

RICK VORNBROCK / THE WORLD & I

SOURCE: *AIDS IN THE WORLD.*

1995; almost 60 percent of these will be in Africa and 26 percent in the industrialized world. Built into these estimates, however, is the average duration of survival of an adult with AIDS, which in Africa is estimated at about one year after diagnosis, less than half of the survival duration of an adult with AIDS in the industrialized world.

Despite the introduction of HIV diagnostic tests over seven years ago, unscreened blood is currently responsible for at least 5 percent of global HIV infections. Most sub-Saharan African countries still cannot afford a safe blood supply. And even if an AIDS vaccine became available today, its impact on the world would be limited by inequities in access to it.

NEED FOR A GLOBAL VISION

Where efforts have been made to provide a coordinated response to the growing crisis, there are clear signs of positive individual responses. But where programs are confronted with weak national commitment, declining resources, and a growing sense of complacency, national AIDS programs are in jeopardy and, together with them, the people they are intended to serve. Many governments, constrained by their lack of resources, continue to avoid the reality of the pandemic: More people become infected because they do not have sufficient access to information and services; more individuals require care that they cannot afford; more families and communities are affected by the impact of a pandemic that has only begun.

Industrialized nations are turning away from coordinated efforts, showing a growing preference to work independently, on a bilateral basis, with chosen developing countries. Fragmentation of efforts by industrialized countries has led to competition among donors in some countries. It is clear that as the pandemic continues to worsen, AIDS programs will be forced to struggle with insufficient funds.

Global efforts have failed to motivate low-prevalence countries to act before the epidemic reaches them in force. India, Burma, and the Sudan are examples of a delayed response and a failure to learn from the experience of heavily affected countries.

Overall, the world has become more vulnerable to HIV and AIDS. On the basis of the societal factors that create vulnerability to spread of HIV, *AIDS in the World* has identified 57 countries as *high risk* for HIV spread—including countries that have thus far escaped the brunt of the pandemic, such as Indonesia, Egypt, Bangladesh, and Nigeria. An additional 39 countries are considered to be at *substantial* risk of a major HIV epidemic, including 11 Latin American countries, 8 in the southeast Mediterranean, 7 in Asia (including China), 4 in the Caribbean, and 9 in other regions.

We *are* at a critical juncture in the confrontation with AIDS, but we are not helpless. By revitalizing leadership, by addressing prevention and the needs of the affected, by formulating clear, international strategies, by accelerating effective, safe, and affordable treatments and vaccines, it *is* possible to stall the future spread of the pandemic.

At a time when many countries are undergoing major geopolitical transitions and are facing severe economic recessions, HIV/AIDS is not simply fading away. The world will continue to experience a rapid increase in the number of people developing AIDS until there is a cure. In the meantime, a troubled world population can unite together to fairly and equitably make available prevention and treatment programs until that day comes.

THE LONG SHOT

What the world needs now, more than ever, is a good AIDS vaccine.
Why don't we have one?

Mark Caldwell

We're now well over a decade into the AIDS pandemic, and the dreadful clock hasn't stopped ticking. According to the World Health Organization, as many as 14 million adults and 1 million children have been infected by the AIDS virus, and a stunning total of up to 120 million is predicted for the year 2000. True, medicine has gotten better at treating the opportunistic infections of late-stage AIDS and has come up with a few stopgap drugs like AZT. And reports of vaunted new therapies regularly erupt in the press. But many of these remedies have proved disappointing at best and completely illusory at worst. Antibiotics have spoiled us with their power to knock bacteria to the canvas with a satisfying roundhouse punch. Drugs against viruses, unfortunately, have a hard time even landing their blows.

Vaccines should be another story. Vaccination has a long track record against viral diseases. From smallpox to polio to measles—Europe had a crude smallpox vaccine as long ago as the 1700s.

And, in principle, vaccination seems so beguilingly simple. By introducing the body to a harmless version of a virus (usually one that's been crippled or killed outright), you can whip the body's defense system into a state of active vigilantism. If the real virus later tries to invade, it will be smartly repulsed.

At least that was the way it had always appeared to work. Thus in 1983, when researchers confirmed that the cause of AIDS was a type of virus—the human immunodeficiency virus, or HIV—you could almost hear the sigh of relief. There seemed little reason to doubt that you could deploy the immune system's power against this new virus, no matter how peculiar it might be. (Our immune systems, after all, have been battle-trained by eons of evolution to fight off all kinds of nasty foreign agents.) A vaccine in ten years seemed a sensible forecast. Indeed, in early 1984 researchers told the *New York Times* that an AIDS vaccine might be ready for testing within two years. A decade later, of course, that kind of talk has begun to look like innocence, not to say naïveté. While about a dozen prototype vaccines have finally begun inching their way into human trials, they're purely experimental. Nobody's ready to claim they'll actually fend off AIDS.

So what went wrong? Where's our AIDS vaccine? Why are we still waiting?

It's not, after all, as if researchers have been sitting on their hands—never before has so much been learned about a virus so fast. Unfortunately, what they've learned is not nearly enough. Molecular biology can tell us a great deal about HIV's structure, its genes, and its rarefied life inside cells growing in lab dishes, but it tells us next to nothing about how the virus interacts with a warm human body, and in particular with the body's immune system. That's one of the major problems at the core of AIDS, of course—the virus attacks the very cells that are supposed to defend us from infectious invaders. Back in 1984, though, nobody could foresee just how insidious HIV was, how many feints it had to parry the thrusts that the immune system deployed against it. Nobody knew at first how genetically variable HIV was, constantly changing even after it infected a host. It was an incredibly elusive moving target, hard for any potential vaccine to hit. Nor was it understood how the virus could hide out, often for years at a time, invisible but nonetheless preparing the massive assault on the immune system that characterizes late-stage AIDS. It's a terrible disease for patients, and so far it hasn't proved a forgiving one for scientists.

John Moore, who studies the structure of HIV at the Aaron Diamond AIDS Research Center in New York, puts it this way: "The guys who were hoping for a vaccine in a couple of years were really working on the assumption that they would be able to take the obvious approach." In other words, they trusted dumb luck, the way they had with a lot of other, earlier vaccines. Unfortunately, with HIV it's not that simple. You can't just inject this virus into people and hope their immune systems will make the right antibodies against it. "What's emerging pretty clearly," says Moore, "is that the immune system is multifactorial and complicated." Antibodies are just one part of that complicated defense system, and in the case of HIV they may not be enough. When humans are infected with HIV, their immune systems make antibodies galore to the virus, but apparently those antibodies don't ultimately protect them. The question is: What other parts of the immune system will we have to stimulate to get protection against AIDS?

"We're really out there in the unknown," admits Murray Gardner, the director of the Center for AIDS Research at the University of California at Davis. "It's ten years since this thing started and in many ways we're still groping in the dark."

Perhaps worst of all, HIV is genetically unstable. In just a few years within a single individual, the virus can transmogrify itself so often that the human immune system can no longer keep up with it.

How did scientists involved in the vaccine race slip from the confidence of 1984 to the more chastened and tentative attitude prevalent today? It's a long story, but we can start by understanding just why virologists regard HIV as a far nastier customer than those they've traditionally dealt with. All viruses, including HIV, are primitive creatures: tiny bundles of genes wrapped in protein, quite unable to reproduce until they've infected their chosen host. Once inside the host's body, however, they show a remarkable range of different behaviors. Some viruses, like polio and smallpox, stumble into the immune system like dim-witted thugs, setting off alarms everywhere. But the AIDS virus is different. It's a retrovirus, one of the very few so far known to infect humans, and it steals into our cells like a master criminal. Once there, it hides in the cells' DNA, undetected by the immune system, covertly copying itself every time the cells divide. Worse, it eventually kills off our key sentinels against infection: the white blood cells, called T cells, that are crucial to an effective immune response. Worse yet, nobody knows exactly how the virus goes about its killing spree. Research published in the British journal *Nature* in March suggested it may hide for years in the lymph nodes (small but important immune system checkpoints found in the neck, armpits, and groin),

then emerge, either gradually or suddenly, to destroy T cells in the bloodstream.

Whatever the virus's modus operandi—and chances are it may have many tricks up its sleeve—by the late stages of the disease it's wiped out virtually all T cells. Lastly, and perhaps worst of all, HIV is genetically unstable. There are dozens of different known strains; in just a few years within a single individual, the virus can transmogrify itself so often that the human immune system can no longer keep up with it.

So unstable and dangerous is the virus that by the late 1980s most researchers felt you couldn't justify putting whole viruses—whether killed or disabled—into a vaccine. As Dani Bolognesi, a virologist at Duke University, puts it: "With a killed-virus vaccine, the worry is that you don't kill everything"—meaning that if even a single virus survives, it may sneak into a T cell, replicate, and begin the infection the vaccine is designed to prevent. "With an attenuated virus," Bolognesi continues, "the risk is different. Assume you really have made the virus nonpathogenic, unable to cause disease. Even so, we don't know the long-term consequences of having *any* retrovirus inside you for 20 years." Retroviruses can affect your genes, turning them on or off, and nobody's sure what tricks of this sort HIV might play, even if it didn't bring on AIDS. Over time, Gardner explains, "it might turn on oncogenes"—genes that cause cancer—"or God knows what."

That fear led to the first pothole on the road to a vaccine. To avoid such dangers, most researchers concluded, they'd have to turn to a brand-new vaccine technology. Rather than relying on whole virus, they pinned their hopes on using chunks of viral protein as harmless HIV stand-ins. These proteins—called antigens, because they *gen*erate *anti*body response in the host—could then be spliced into a harmless carrier organism like vaccinia, the non-disease-causing virus traditionally used in smallpox inoculations.

"Trying to make a recombinant vaccine work against this heterogeneous virus is asking a lot of a tiny clone, which is all a recombinant protein really is," says Gardner. None has shown lasting protection.

In fact, a successful vaccine against hepatitis B, using more or less this "recombinant" technology, had debuted in 1986. And by 1990 it looked as if the approach might really work for HIV too, thanks to a promising study by Marc Girard of the Pasteur Institute in Paris and Patricia Fultz of the University of

Alabama at Birmingham. Until that point, the most encouraging results had been achieved in macaques, using injections of whole virus to ward off a monkey version of AIDS. Fultz and Girard, working with chimpanzees, showed for the first time that you could raise a protective response to HIV using just pieces of protein from the outer envelope of the virus.

Their finding seemed to lift a huge cloud from the entire AIDS field. But the respite didn't last long. Within a year hope began to recede again, succumbing to the recurrent waves of pessimism that have characterized the AIDS battle. Experiments with recombinant vaccines just weren't going—and still aren't going—all that swimmingly. "We've been trying," Fultz says, "but the major problem has been that the chimps' response wanes very rapidly following immunization. The protection we *have* achieved requires multiple vaccinations." That's disappointing if you're trying to envision a useful human vaccine. "It would be impractical—particularly in developing countries—if you needed four initial vaccinations and then a booster every year," Fultz concedes.

"Trying to make a recombinant vaccine work against this heterogeneous virus is asking a lot of a little tiny clone, which is all a recombinant protein really is," adds Gardner. "I'm not saying recombinant work is invalid, but the fact is that there's something like six times as many studies in monkeys where recombinant envelope approaches haven't worked as there are studies where they have. And even where they have, it's usually when the experiments stack the deck in their favor by optimizing conditions. Recombinant vaccines have worked in the lab, but none of them has shown long-lasting, strong, or broad protection against mucosal challenge or cell-associated virus." In other words, they haven't demonstrated protection where it may count the most—against virus entering through mucous membranes, the major route for sexual transmission of AIDS, or virus transmitted in infected cells.

Even if the recombinant approach *does* eventually pan out, there are plenty of hurdles on the way. Which viral proteins will make the most potent vaccine? What strain (or strains) of virus should the proteins come from? There's a vast range of choices, and nobody really knows how many will have to be tried before somebody hits on the magically right combination. "For a successful vaccine we'll need to stimulate all the arms of the complicated immune system," says Moore. But in the meantime, he says, "biotech companies doing vaccine research have taken the what-you-need-is-what-we-can-give-you approach."

And just what are they giving? At the moment, most of the 11 recombinant vaccines in human trials use all or part of gp (for "glycoprotein") 160, a large, sugary protein found on the virus's outer surface. Without this protein, HIV can't lock onto—and therefore can't infect—T cells. Gp160 consists of two major portions—a protruding knob-like structure, called gp120 (which the virus uses to attach itself to host cells), and a smaller protein, gp41, which anchors the knob in the virus's outer wall. These envelope proteins act as particularly strong stimulants to the immune system, so they're natural candidates for a recombinant vaccine. Gp160, for instance, is the mainstay of the highly controversial vaccine from MicroGeneSys, a private biotech company.

MicroGeneSys first drew flak last year when it lobbied Congress to become the sole candidate in a massive $20 million trial to be conducted by the U.S. Army and paid for by the U.S. taxpayer. The move—widely criticized by scientists—didn't succeed; the Department of Health and Human Services stepped in and proposed instead that the National Institutes of Health run a study comparing the vaccine from MicroGeneSys with two gp120 vaccines, produced by Chiron and Genentech. Meanwhile, in February, in a stinging letter to *Nature,* Moore and two colleagues argued that the MicroGeneSys vaccine used a misshapen form of gp160. "Our opinion," these researchers concluded, "is that there could not be a worse choice from the current envelope glycoprotein vaccine candidates than MGS gp160 to stimulate at least one important arm of the human immune system"—that is, the production of antibodies to a particularly crucial part of the virus.

Another researcher, who would speak only off the record, points out yet another potential problem, this one common to virtually *all* the vaccine prototypes based on envelope proteins. "All these proteins," this researcher notes, "are derived from only three sets of lab isolates"—that is, harvested from only three individuals among the millions infected worldwide. Some of these viruses have been cultured and massaged in labs for as long as ten years. Could such hothouse products provoke an effective immune response against all the multiple types of HIV found in the real world? The question is particularly troubling when you consider that the viral gene that produces gp120 changes at the rate of about 1 percent a year in any given virus. Mightn't the real-world virus already be one step ahead of the vintage proteins slated for vaccines? Such concerns—and the worry that recombinant vaccines may not provoke a sufficient immune response to infected cells—have led at least one famed vaccinologist to reconsider what was unthinkable: Jonas Salk is conducting trials with a vaccine made from whole inactivated virus. Salk's approach is so far being tried only in HIV-positive patients, to see if it can give their ailing immune systems a boost. Still, his work could offer glimpses into how the virus interacts with living humans—insights that might also help researchers design better vaccines to protect the uninfected.

There are other troubling questions in the air. Beginning in late 1991 a series of research reports appeared that, according to an alarming headline from the pages of *Nature,* turned AIDS research "upside down." The most immediately eye-opening of these reports came from James Stott, a virologist at England's National Institute for Biological Standards and Control. He and his colleagues had been working on simian immunodeficiency virus, or SIV—the close analogue of HIV that infects monkeys, producing a rapid AIDS-like disease. As had previous investigators, they found they could protect macaques by vaccinating them with inactivated SIV; no surprise there. They also found they could achieve protection if they inoculated the monkeys with SIV-infected human T cells. Not amazing either: such cells most likely flaunt telltale signs of the virus lurking inside them and could thus prick the monkeys' immune systems into a defensive response.

The real stunner was Stott's third finding. As a control, he had also injected four macaques with *uninfected* human T cells. Amazingly, two of these monkeys produced a protective immune response not just against the foreign-looking injected cells (which you'd expect) but against SIV. What in thunder, Stott and his colleagues wondered, was going on? How could a normal, uninfected human T cell raise immunity against a monkey virus that the macaques had never seen before? It was almost as if you'd given a prisoner in a locked cell a cupcake and then found he'd suddenly acquired a bazooka.

Many investigators suspected the answer, but it was immunologist Larry O. Arthur of Program Resources (a contractor with the National Cancer Institute) who finally showed what was happening. Neither HIV nor SIV grows on its own. Both have to be bred in human cells growing in lab dishes. The virus reproduces and eventually buds out of these cells in large numbers—mimicking its behavior in the body of a host animal. Could these lab viruses, Arthur wondered, be grabbing proteins from their human incubator cells and then carrying them into the macaques? If so, it wouldn't be a surprise to find that the monkeys' antihuman immune response would also work against SIV: the virus was, thanks to its kleptomaniac habits, carrying stolen human proteins. Arthur actually found the proteins in question and proved that in fact the monkey virus does pick them up while incubating in human cells.

Stott's and Arthur's work jolted vaccinologists. Had all their experiments been bollixed up by proteins the virus filched from its human incubator cells? The new findings underlined again HIV's inherent deviousness—its ability to interact with living things in extraordinarily diverse and confusing ways.

The truth is that nobody really understands what's going on between these invading retroviruses and the host's immune system. Which of the many proteins in the virus set off which of the many trip wires in the immune system? Where do those proteins come from—the virus or the human cell it was bred in? And which

of the immune responses directed against the proteins fend off disease?

Even when researchers have raised some sort of defense against the AIDS virus, as they've done in chimpanzees, they don't really understand how it's worked. Your body has at least two major kinds of immune weapons, and they're quite distinct from each other. One system fastens antibodies to a foreign invader circulating in the blood, thus marking it for destruction. Another system relies on a network of killer cells to seek out the virus hiding inside infected cells. Until researchers know which of these systems is more important for neutralizing HIV infection, the quest for a vaccine will rely to a disquieting degree on trial and error.

Finally, as if all these doubts weren't enough, yet another lurking issue surfaced with a vengeance in 1991: autoimmunity. One of the fundamental mysteries of AIDS has been how HIV manages to destroy so many more T cells than it seems to infect—it's rather scarce in the bloodstream until the late stages of the disease. Moreover, you can produce large quantities of antibodies against the virus yet still succumb to the disease. The revelation this past March that HIV hides in the lymph nodes for years and multiplies there begins to explain some of these discrepancies—even in the early stages of infection, there's a surprisingly large covert reservoir of virus. But not everyone is convinced yet that these findings are sufficient to account for the massive T cell destruction and other cell damage caused by AIDS. Some researchers suspect that the virus may do part of its damage indirectly, by destabilizing the immune system, tricking it into an assault on itself, or causing T cells to commit suicide.

Might not a recombinant vaccine backfire? If it raises an immune response to gp120, couldn't it also trick the immune system into a devastating attack on itself? Hoffmann believes that it could.

There are several models for an autoimmune component in AIDS, but Geoffrey Hoffmann—a maverick theoretical immunologist at the University of British Columbia in Vancouver—offers one of the more intriguing. Hoffmann, a disarmingly straightforward Australian, frankly admits his ideas are difficult: "I have to do a lot of hand waving to explain it," he concedes. But the rudiments aren't too hard to grasp. They rest on a long-standing mystery of the immune system. Our T cells are designed to coordinate an attack against foreign invaders. But how do they know what's foreign?

PROBLEMATIC PROTEIN

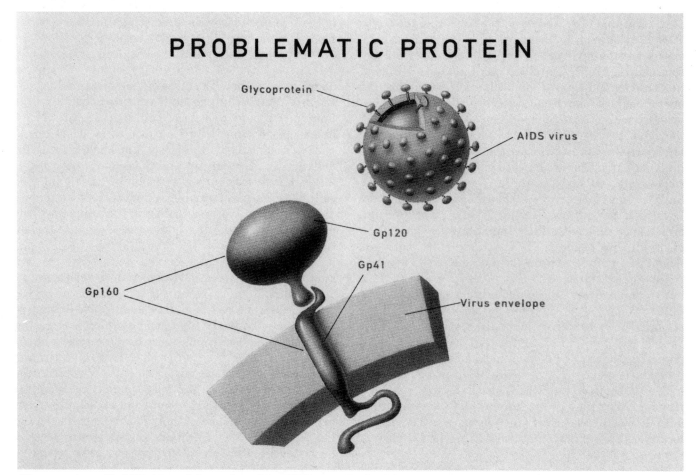

Glycoproteins called GP160 stud the surface of the AIDS virus. Each of these proteins has two parts: an outer knob called GP120 and a smaller anchor known as GP41. These envelope proteins form the basis of many vaccines to fend off AIDS—but some researchers worry that they could spell trouble.

Why don't they attack our own tissues as readily as they do marauding viruses?

Left to themselves, Hoffmann argues, they would. We all harbor some T cells that spring into action every time they meet a cell bearing a set of distinctive proteins that—just as a flag identifies a nation—brand us as ourselves. Many immunologists think our bodies destroy most such antiself cells before they mature. But Hoffmann thinks they're merely kept in check, diverted from committing mayhem by *other* cells, which carry proteins very similar to our own self-identifying badges. These counterbalancing cells preoccupy the potentially autoimmune cells and thereby stop them from launching an attack on us.

Fascinating—but what does it have to do with AIDS, autoimmunity, and vaccines? According to Hoffmann, the answer lies in an odd feature of a protein we've met before—gp120, the knob found on the envelope of the AIDS virus and in many of the recombinant vaccines now under development. Previous research has suggested that a key part of this protein strongly resembles the ID badge carried on the cells that restrain our autoimmune cells. Hoffmann argues that this similarity can, in the human body, lead to a Keystone

Kops–like series of mistakes that results in the collapse of the immune system. Think about it: to the body, a key part of the AIDS virus looks like—of all things—the "self" badge on a crucial subset of its own cells. The body, reasonably, launches an immune attack on HIV. But that means the immune system's attack on HIV also destroys some of its own cells. Worse, these cells are the very ones that restrain your potentially autoimmune cells from targeting the rest of your T cells. The immune system, its network of checks and balances disrupted, self-destructs.

This scenario has led Hoffmann to raise a frightening possibility. Might not a recombinant vaccine backfire? If it raises a strong immune response against gp120, couldn't it also trick the immune system into a devastating attack on itself, bringing on the very collapse the vaccine was designed to prevent? Hoffmann believes that it could. "At least," he says, "we need to be concerned about the possibility." This has led him to propose a counterintuitive strategy for AIDS vaccines. "Alternative vaccines are conceivable that do the opposite of what conventional vaccines do. That is, they'd make you tolerate something as well as fight against it."

A vaccine that makes you accept unprotestingly part of the germ that causes the disease? That would be a first, and many immunologists are frankly skeptical. "The experimental evidence is extremely poor for any of these autoimmune models," comments Moore. Hoffmann's best support so far comes from some intriguing experiments in mice that he reported in *Science* two years ago. He found that mice that hadn't been exposed to HIV could make antibodies against the virus if they were exposed to cells bearing proteins similar to their own "self" badges. That strongly suggested at least some kind of resemblance between HIV and mammalian "self" proteins—the sort of resemblance that could lead to the tragedy of mistaken identities Hoffmann thinks may happen in AIDS.

Yet despite their skepticism, few researchers will dismiss Hoffmann's ideas out of hand. AIDS, after all, is a difficult, many-faceted, still largely baffling disease. "Maybe those interested in autoimmunity are opening up the door to another piece of this huge picture," says Gardner. "And it's not unreasonable to suggest that vaccines could cause autoimmune phenomena—vaccines have been known to enhance infections before. Those ideas are perfectly reasonable as hypotheses. The problem is proving them."

By now you may think vaccine research has become hopelessly mired in a morass of doubts, conflicting theories, and complications. Yet the need for a vaccine seems more urgent than ever. The news that the virus hides in the lymph nodes during the early years of infection—invisible, growing, apparently unimpeded by the immune system—gave many researchers pause. What does such early, large-scale infection imply for drug treatments and vaccines? "It suggests you should probably do as much as you can as early as you can to prevent the seeding of the host," says Bolognesi, "because once the virus is in, it's hard to imagine any kind of treatment that would keep it from progressing. So it shows us once again that an AIDS vaccine will have to be extremely effective at blocking the virus from entry into the host."

At times it almost seems as if the only predictable theme in AIDS research is that AIDS is a subtler, more labyrinthine, and meaner disease than we'd thought. Does that imply we're not much further than we were in 1983, when we began? If you ask researchers for a vaccine timeline, you can't help noting a hint of déjà vu: "For a vaccine in widespread use, I'd say ten years," Fultz hazards, echoing what seemed like a safe bet a decade ago. Kathelyn Steimer, who led the research to develop Chiron's recombinant vaccine, one of the vaccines slated for the NIH trial, is a bit more optimistic. "I think it's not inconceivable to look at the year 2000 and see a first-generation vaccine—one that's, say, up to 50 percent effective. It wouldn't offer complete protection, but it would offer enough protection to have an impact on the epidemic," she says. "A lot can happen in seven years."

In fact, the mood among vaccine researchers, while chastened, isn't as pessimistic as the problems facing them might suggest. There have been *some* results that indicate it's worth gamely plodding on. Late in May, for example, researchers at the New Mexico Regional Primate Laboratory announced they had protected monkeys against infection in conditions that simulate sexual transmission—now the most common way of contracting the disease—by using the traditional approach of a whole but weakened virus. A certain professional stoicism has set in. "Maybe," says Moore, "the public gets skeptical because too many scientists shoot off and say, 'If you back me, I'll come up with the goods.' But if you're a scientist, you have to be optimistic. You have to do your experiments—without shouting out to the press every time you get a good result. You have to keep going. You can always think of a million reasons why something won't work. But if that stops you, you'll never get a result."

Gardner agrees. "Some people are pessimistic about ever getting a vaccine," he says, "but who knows what might work?" What worries him more in the meantime is the difficulty of reconciling the pressing needs of desperate patients, the competitiveness of companies, and the rigors of good research. "If it weren't for the urgency of the situation, right now we'd be demanding much more basic science," he says. In other words, more testing should really be done with animals before vaccines are tried in humans. "Even given the urgency, I think we should be careful—not skimp research at the basic level, not rush to spend all our money on premature clinical trials. If we're careful and go slowly, we won't wreak havoc and we'll prevent a great disaster." Nothing could be worse, from a vaccine researcher's point of view, than a dicey vaccine that gives people a false sense of security;

Success, in the end, is likely to come the slow, hard, punishing way. And—barring dumb luck—it won't come tomorrow or next month. Moore puts it very succinctly: "If we could have done this by the seat of our pants, we wouldn't be sitting here now."

Human Sexuality

Sexuality is one of the most basic aspects of self-awareness. How sex differences affect the behavior of human beings is a topic that scientists and lay persons have been considering for quite some time. That women and men do differ, behaviorally, cognitively, and biologically, cannot be disputed. Why they differ, and whether or not these differences matter, are questions that remain unanswered.

Men and women differ in the area of sexuality and mating. Evolutionary psychologists who have studied mating behaviors contend that men and women are as different psychologically as they are biologically. For example, women are attracted to men based on their status, ambition, and re-sources, whereas men are attracted to women based on their youthful appearance and attractiveness. Cross-cultural studies have validated the universality of these preferences, and evolutionary psychologists have theorized that they evolved in response to the differing biological demands faced by men and women in the process of having children. These psychologists say that even behaviors such as infidelity and jealously are still being shaped by the mating concerns of our ancient ancestors. "The Mating Game" examines various contemporary mating behaviors of both men and women and explains how these behaviors are an evolutionary throwback.

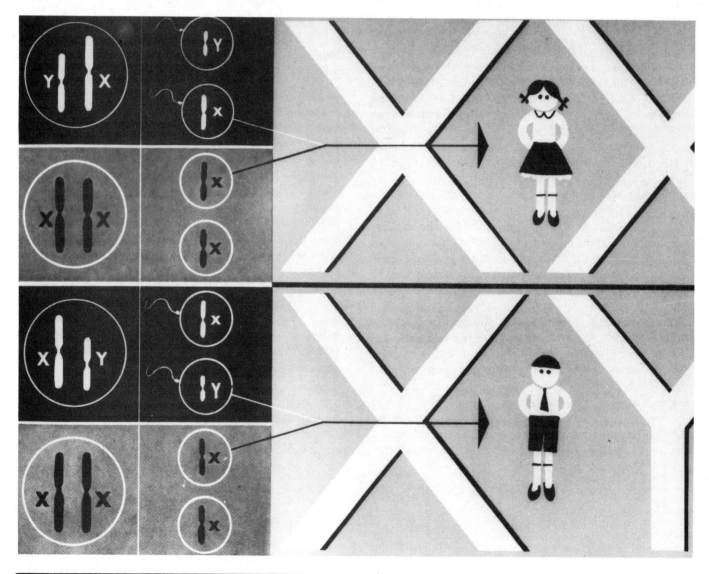

The menstrual cycle is one area of human sexuality that has been a significant source of conflict and confusion between the sexes, stemming from the profound behavioral and emotional changes that some women go through each cycle. For years men have nervously joked about these changes, while women have interpreted them as character flaws. Current evidence indicates that for many women the magnitude and severity of these changes are sufficient to constitute a clinical disorder, premenstrual syndrome (PMS). While there are over 150 different symptoms associated with it, the most common ones are mood swings, irritability, feelings of loneliness, and nervousness. Because of this diversity of symptoms, many women may mistakenly assume that they have PMS when in fact their medical problems may stem from other causes. This is an unfortunate situation because it may delay their seeking medical attention. Researchers are not sure what causes PMS, but estimate that between 16 and 80 percent of all menstruating women are affected by it. Paula Dranov's article "How Do You Know If It's PMS?" discusses the scope of the problem and analyses several of the most commonly prescribed treatments.

Three topics in human sexuality that have received considerable media attention are teenage pregnancy, abortion, and AIDS. As they all deal with reproduction, the standard approach to dealing with them has been to provide students with contraceptive-based sex education. How successful has this approach been? Statistics regarding the incidence of pregnancy, abortions, and AIDS among teenagers indicate its ineffectiveness. We must consider alternative strategies. Not only has this approach failed to reduce teenage pregnancies, abortions, and the spread of AIDS, but it may actually be contributing to the problem by fostering the expectation that it is normal for teenagers to experiment sexually. While it is true that many teenagers will experiment with sex regardless of whether they are knowledgeable about contraception, teens who receive contraceptive-based sex education are 53 percent more likely to become sexually active than are teens who do not. In fact, the majority of the teens choosing to become sexually active do not even use the contraceptives they have learned about. This poor showing has prompted a growing movement favoring abstinence-based sex education. "It's Not Just AIDS" by William Bergman discusses why contraceptive-based sex education is failing and suggests that the time is right to try teaching teens the value of virginity and abstinence.

The abortion issue involves an emotionally charged debate between pro-choice advocates, who defend individual freedom, and pro-life advocates, who defend the right to life—both of which are constitutional rights. Most pro-choice supporters feel that abortion should not be used as a form of birth control, but as a way to preserve a woman's rights if birth control fails and an accidental pregnancy results. The pro-life advocates argue that once the egg has been fertilized by the sperm, a life has been created, and any action on the woman's part to terminate the pregnancy is tantamount to murder. This debate has cooled off considerably since Bill Clinton was elected president, but it may heat up once again as this country prepares to legalize the abortion pill RU 486. Jill Smolowe's article "New, Improved and Ready for Battle" discusses how changes in the political climate with Clinton's election could make this pill available to all Americans within the next three years.

While the concept of "safe sex" is nothing new, the degree of open and public discussion regarding sexual behaviors is. With the emergence of AIDS as a disease of epidemic proportions, the surgeon general of the United States initiated an aggressive educational campaign based on the assumption that knowledge would change behavior. As has been the case with drug abuse, this approach, while logical, appears to have little impact on the targeted problem. Why has education failed? Most experts agree that for education to succeed in changing personal behaviors, (1) the recipients of the information must first perceive themselves as vulnerable and thus be motivated to explore replacement behaviors, and (2) the replacement behaviors must satisfy the needs that were the basis of problem behavior. To date, most AIDS education programs have failed to meet these criteria.

Given all the information that we now have on the dangers associated with AIDS, why is it that people do not perceive themselves at risk? It is not so much denial of risks as it is the notion that when it comes to choosing sex partners, we all think that we make good judgment decisions. Unfortunately, most judgment decisions regarding sexual behavior are based on subjective criteria that bear little or no relationship to the actual risks of contracting AIDS. Even when individuals do view themselves as vulnerable to AIDS, there are currently only two viable options for reducing the risk of contracting this disease through sexual behavior. The first is the use of a condom, and the second is sexual abstinence, neither of which are ideal solutions to the problem.

Looking Ahead: Challenge Questions

Do you feel that birth control has contributed to increased promiscuity and the rapid spread of sexually transmitted diseases? Why or why not?

What approach to sex education do you think would be most effective in reducing teenage pregnancies, abortions, and the spread of AIDS?

If you are sexually active, do you always practice safe sex? If not, why not?

Do you feel at risk of contracting AIDS? If not, why not? If you do, what are you doing to reduce your risk?

Do you think a female version of the condom would do much to slow the spread of AIDS?

THE
Mating
GAME

The sophisticated sexual strategies of modern men and women are shaped by a powerful Stone Age psychology.

It's a dance as old as the human race. At cocktail lounges and church socials, during office coffee breaks and dinner parties—and most blatantly, perhaps, in the personal ads in newspapers and magazines—men and women perform the elaborate ritual of advertisement and assessment that precedes an essential part of nearly every life: mating. More than 90 percent of the world's people marry at some point in their lives, and it is estimated that a similarly large number of people engage in affairs, liaisons, flings or one-night stands. The who, what, when and where of love, sex and romance are a cultural obsession that is reflected in everything from Shakespeare to soap operas and from Tristram and Isolde to 2 Live Crew, fueling archetypes like the coy ingénue, the rakish cad, the trophy bride, Mrs. Robinson, Casanova and lovers both star-crossed and blessed.

It all may seem very modern, but a new group of researchers argues that love, American style, is in fact part of a universal human behavior with roots stretching back to the dawn of humankind. These scientists contend that, in stark contrast to the old image of brute cavemen dragging their mates by the hair to their dens, our ancient ancestors—men and women alike—engaged in a sophisticated mating dance of sexual intrigue, shrewd strategizing and savvy negotiating that has left its stamp on human psychology. People may live in a thoroughly modern world, these researchers say, but within the human skull is a Stone Age mind that was shaped by the mating concerns of our ancient ancestors and continues to have a profound influence on behavior today. Indeed, this ancient psychological legacy

HOW WE CHOOSE

Women are more concerned about whether mates will invest time and resources in a relationship; men care more about a woman's physical attractiveness, which in ancient times reflected her fertility and health.

influences everything from sexual attraction to infidelity and jealousy—and, as remarkable new research reveals, even extends its reach all the way down to the microscopic level of egg and sperm.

These new researchers call themselves evolutionary psychologists. In a host of recent scientific papers and at a major conference last month at the London School of Economics, they are arguing that the key to understanding modern sexual behavior lies not solely in culture, as some anthropologists contend, nor purely in the genes, as some sociobiologists believe. Rather, they argue, understanding human nature is possible only if scientists begin to understand the evolution of the human mind. Just as humans have evolved

specialized biological organs to deal with the intricacies of sex, they say, the mind, too, has evolved customized mental mechanisms for coping with this most fundamental aspect of human existence.

Gender and mind. When it comes to sexuality and mating, evolutionary psychologists say, men and women often are as different psychologically as they are physically. Scientists have long known that people typically choose mates who closely resemble themselves in terms of weight, height, intelligence and even earlobe length. But a survey of more than 10,000 people in 37 cultures on six continents, conducted by University of Michigan psychologist David Buss, reveals that men consistently value physical attractiveness and youth in a mate more than women do; women, equally as consistently, are more concerned than men with a prospective mate's ambition, status and resources. If such preferences were merely arbitrary products of culture, says Buss, one might expect to find at least one society somewhere where men's and women's mating preferences were reversed; the fact that attitudes are uniform across cultures suggests they are a fundamental part of human psychology.

Evolutionary psychologists think many of these mating preferences evolved in response to the different biological challenges faced by men and women in producing children—the definition of success in evolutionary terms. In a seminal paper, evolutionary biologist Robert Trivers of the University of California at Santa Cruz points out that in most mammals, females invest far

From *U.S. News & World Report*, July 19, 1993, pp. 57-63. © 1993 by U.S. News & World Report. Reprinted by permission.

more time and energy in reproduction and child rearing than do males. Not only must females go through a long gestation and weaning of their offspring, but childbirth itself is relatively dangerous. Males, on the other hand, potentially can get away with a very small biological investment in a child.

Human infants require the greatest amount of care and nurturing of any animal on Earth, and so over the eons women have evolved a psychology that is particularly concerned with a father's ability to help out with this enormous task—with his clout, protection and access to resources. So powerful is this psychological legacy that nowadays women size up a man's finances even when, as a practical matter, they may not have to. A recent study of the mating preferences of a group of medical students, for instance, found that these women, though anticipating financial success, were nevertheless most interested in men whose earning capacity was equal to or greater than their own.

Healthy genes. For men, on the other hand, reproductive success is ultimately dependent on the fertility of their mates. Thus males have evolved a mind-set that homes in on signs of a woman's health and youth, signs that, in the absence of medical records and birth certificates long ago, were primarily visual. Modern man's sense of feminine beauty—clear skin, bright eyes and youthful appearance—is, in effect, the legacy of eons spent diagnosing the health and fertility of potential mates.

This concern with women's reproductive health also helps explain why men value curvaceous figures. An upcoming paper by Devendra Singh of the University of Texas at Austin reveals that people consistently judge a woman's figure not by whether she is slim or fat but by the ratio of waist to hips. The ideal proportion—the hips roughly a third larger than the waist—reflects a hormonal balance that results in women's preferentially storing fat on their hips as opposed to their waists, a condition that correlates with higher fertility and resistance to disease. Western society's modern-day obsession with being slim has not changed this equation. Singh found, for instance, that while the winning Miss America has become 30 percent thinner over the past several decades, her waist-to-hip ratio has remained close to this ancient ideal.

Women also appreciate a fair face and figure, of course. And what they look for in a male's physique can also be explained as an evolved mentality that links good looks with good genes. A number of studies have shown that both men and women rate as most attractive

---

WHOM WE MARRY

more than 90 percent of all people marry and, they typically choose mates who closely resemble themselves, from weight and height, to intelligence and values, to nose breadth and even earlobe length.

---

faces that are near the average; this is true in societies as diverse as those of Brazil, Russia and several hunting and gathering tribes. The average face tends to be more symmetrical, and, according to psychologist Steven Gangestad and biologist Randy Thornhill, both of the University of New Mexico, this symmetry may reflect a person's genetic resistance to disease.

People have two versions of each of their genes—one from each parent—within every cell. Sometimes the copies are slightly different, though typically each version works just as effectively. The advantage to having two slightly different copies of the same gene, the researchers argue, is that it is harder for a disease to knock out the function of both copies, and this biological redundancy is reflected in the symmetry in people's bodies, including their faces. Further evidence for a psychological mechanism that links attractiveness with health comes from Buss's worldwide study of mating preferences: In those parts of the world where the incidence of parasites and infectious diseases is highest, both men and women place a greater value on attractive mates.

Some feminists reject the notion that women should alter physical appearance to gain advantage in the mating game. But archaeological finds suggest that the "beauty myth" has been very much a part of the human mating psychology since the times of our ancient ancestors—and that it applies equally to men. Some of the very first signs of human artistry are carved body ornaments that date back more than 30,000 years, and findings of worn nubs of ochre suggest that ancient humans may have used the red and black chalklike

substance as makeup. These artifacts probably served as social signs that, like lipstick or a Rolex watch today, advertised a person's physical appearance and status. In one grave dating back some 20,000 years, a male skeleton was found bedecked with a tunic made from thousands of tiny ivory beads—the Stone Age equivalent of an Armani suit.

Far from being immutable, biological mandates, these evolved mating mechanisms in the mind are flexible, culturally influenced aspects of human psychology that are similar to people's tastes for certain kinds of food. The human sweet tooth is a legacy from a time when the only sweet things in the environment were nutritious ripe fruit and honey, says Buss, whose book "The Evolution of Desire" is due out next year. Today, this ancient taste for sweets is susceptible to modern-day temptation by candy bars and such, though people have the free will to refrain from indulging it. Likewise, the mind's mating mechanisms can be strongly swayed by cultural influences such as religious and moral beliefs.

Playing the field. Both men and women display different mating psychologies when they are just playing around as opposed to searching for a lifelong partner, and these mental mechanisms are also a legacy from ancient times. A new survey by Buss and his colleague David Schmitt found that when women are looking for "short term" mates, their preference for attractive men increases substantially. In a study released last month, Doug Kenrick and Gary Groth of Arizona State University found that while men, too, desire attractive mates when they're playing the field, they will actually settle for a lot less.

Men's diminished concern about beauty in short-term mates reflects the fact that throughout human evolution, men have often pursued a dual mating strategy. The most successful strategy for most men was to find a healthy, fertile, long-term mate. But it also didn't hurt to take advantage of any low-risk opportunity to sire as many kin as possible outside the relationship, just to hedge the evolutionary bet. The result is an evolved psychology that allows a man to be sexually excited by a wide variety of women even while committed to a partner. This predilection shows up in studies of men's and women's sexual fantasies today. A study by Don Symons of the University of California at Santa Barbara and Bruce Ellis of the University of Michigan found that while both men and women actively engage in sexual fantasy, men typically have more fantasies about anonymous partners.

Surveys in the United States show

that at least 30 percent of married women have extramarital affairs, suggesting that, like men, women also harbor a drive for short-term mating. But they have different evolutionary reasons for doing so. Throughout human existence, short-term flings have offered women an opportunity to exchange sex for resources. In Buss and Schmitt's study, women value an "extravagant lifestyle" three times more highly when they are searching for a brief affair than when they are seeking a long-term mate. Women who are secure in a relationship with a committed male might still seek out attractive men to secure healthier genes for their offspring. Outside affairs also allow women to shop for better partners.

Sperm warfare. A woman may engage the sexual interest of several men simultaneously in order to foster a microscopic battle known as sperm competition. Sperm can survive in a woman's reproductive tract for nearly a week, note biologists Robin Baker and Mark Bellis of the University of Manchester, and by mating with more than one man within a short period of time, a woman sets the stage for their sperm to com-

—— JEALOUS PSYCHE ——

Men are most disturbed by sexual infidelity in their mates, a result of uncertainty about paternity. Women are more disturbed by emotional infidelity, because they risk losing their mate's time and resources.

pete to sire a child—passing this winning trait on to her male offspring as well. In a confidential survey tracking the sexual behavior and menstrual cycles of more than 2,000 women who

said they had steady mates, Baker and Bellis found that while there was no pattern to when women had sex with their steady partners, having sex on the side peaked at the height of the women's monthly fertility cycles.

Since in ancient times a man paid a dear evolutionary price for being cuckolded, the male psychology produces a physiological counterstrategy for dealing with a woman's infidelity. Studying the sexual behavior of a group of couples, Baker and Bellis found that the more time a couple spend apart, the more sperm the man ejaculates upon their sexual reunion—as much as three times higher than average.

This increase in sperm count is unrelated to when the man last ejaculated through nocturnal emission or masturbation, and Baker and Bellis argue that it is a result of a man's evolved psychological mechanism that bolsters his chances in sperm competition in the event that his mate has been unfaithful during their separation. As was no doubt the case in the times of our ancient ancestors, these concerns are not unfounded: Studies of blood typings show that as many as 1 of every 10 babies born to couples in North America is not the offspring of the mother's husband.

Despite men's efforts at sexual subterfuge, women still have the last word on the fate of a man's sperm in her reproductive tract—thanks to the physiological effects of the female orgasm. In a new study, Baker and Bellis reveal that if a woman experiences an orgasm soon after her mate's, the amount of sperm retained in her reproductive tract is far higher than if she has an earlier orgasm or none at all. Apparently a woman's arousal, fueled by her feelings as well as her mate's solicitous attentions, results in an evolutionary payoff for both.

Cads and dads. Whether people pursue committed relationships or one-night stands depends on their perceptions of what kind of mates are in the surrounding sexual environment. Anthropologist Elizabeth Cashdan of the University of Utah surveyed hundreds of men and women on whether they thought the members of their "pool" of potential mates were in general trustworthy, honest and capable of commitment. She also asked them what kinds of tactics they used to attract mates. Cashdan found that the less committed people thought their potential mates would be, the more they themselves pursued short-term mating tactics. For example, if women considered their world to be full of "cads," they tended to dress more provocatively and to be more promiscuous; if they thought that the world was populated

—— BEAUTY QUEST ——

the most attractive men and women are in fact those whose faces are most average, a signal that they are near the genetic average of the population and are perhaps more resistant to disease.

by potential "dads"—that is, committed and nurturing men—they tended to emphasize their chastity and fidelity. Similarly, "cads" tended to emphasize their sexuality and "dads" said they relied more on advertising their resources and desire for long-term commitment.

These perceptions of what to expect from the opposite sex may be influenced by the kind of home life an individual knew as a child. Social scientists have long known that children from homes where the father is chronically absent or abusive tend to mature faster physically and to have sexual relations earlier in life. Psychologist Jay Belsky of Pennsylvania State University argues that this behavior is an evolved psychological mechanism, triggered by early childhood experiences, that enables a child to come of age earlier and leave the distressing situation. This psychological mechanism may also lead to a mating strategy that focuses on short-term affairs.

The green monster. Whether in modern or ancient times, infidelities can breed anger and hurt, and new research suggests subtle differences in male and female jealousy with roots in the ancient past. In one study, for example, Buss asked males and females to imagine that their mates were having sex with someone else or that their mates were engaged in a deep emotional commitment with another person. Monitoring his subjects' heart rates, frowning and stress responses, he found that the stereotypical double standard cuts both ways. Men reacted far more strongly than

Eroticism and gender

For insights into the subtle differences between men's and women's mating psychologies, one need look no further than the local bookstore. On one rack may be magazines featuring scantily clad women in poses of sexual invitation—a testimony to the ancient legacy of a male psychology that is acutely attuned to visual stimulus and easily aroused by the prospect of anonymous sex. Around the corner is likely to be a staple of women's erotic fantasy: romance novels.

Harlequin Enterprises Ltd., the leading publisher in the field, sells more than 200 million books annually and pro-duces about 70 titles a month. Dedicated romance fans may read several books a week. "Our books give women every-thing," says Harlequin's Kathleen Abels, "a loving relation-ship, commitment and having sex with someone they care about." Some romance novels contain scenes steamy enough to make a sailor blush, and studies show that women who read romances typically have more sexual fantasies and en-gage in sexual intercourse more frequently than nonread-ers do.

Sexual caricature. Since sexual fantasy frees people of the complications of love and mat-ing in the real world, argue psychologists Bruce Ellis and Don Symons, it is perhaps not surprising that in erotic mate-rials for both men and women, sexual partners are typically caricatures of the consumer's own evolved mating psycholo-gy. In male-oriented erotica, for instance, women are de-picted as being lust driven, ever willing and unencum-bered by the need for emo-tional attachment. In romance novels, the male lead in the book is typically tender, emo-tional and consumed by pas-sion for the heroine, thus en-suring his lifelong fidelity and dependence. In other words, say Ellis and Symons, the ro-mance novel is "an erotic, uto-pian, female counterfantasy" to male erotica.

Of course, most men also en-joy stories of passion and ro-mance, and women can be as easily aroused as men by sexu-ally explicit films. Indeed, sev-eral new entertainment ven-tures, including the magazine *Future Sex* and a video compa-ny, Femme Productions, are creating erotic materials using realistic models in more sensual settings in an attempt to appeal to both sexes. Still, the new re-search into evolutionary psy-chology suggests that men and women derive subtly different pleasures from sexual fantasy—something that even writing un-der a ghost name can't hide. According to Abels, a Harle-quin romance is occasionally penned by a man using a female pseudonym, but "our avid read-ers can always tell."

---

women to the idea that their mates were having sex with other men. But women reacted far more strongly to the thought that their mates were developing strong emotional attachments to someone else.

As with our evolved mating prefer-ences, these triggers for jealousy ulti-mately stem from men's and women's biology, says Buss. A woman, of course, has no doubt that she is the mother of her children. For a man, however, paternity is never more than conjecture, and so men have evolved psychologies with a height-ened concern about a mate's sexual infi-delity. Since women make the greater biological investment in offspring, their psychologies are more concerned about a mate's reneging on his commitment, and, therefore, they are more attentive to signs that their mates might be attaching them-selves emotionally to other women.

Sexual monopoly. The male preoccu-pation with monopolizing a woman's sexual reproduction has led to the op-pression and abuse of women world-wide, including, at its extremes, confine-ment, domestic violence and ritual mutilation such as clitoridectomy. Yet the new research into the mating game also reveals that throughout human evolution, women have not passively ac-quiesced to men's sexual wishes. Rath-

DUELING SPERM

If a couple has been apart for some time, the man's sperm count goes up during sex at their reunion—an ancient, evolved strategy against a female's possible infidelities while away.

er, they have long employed a host of behavioral and biological tactics to fol-low their own sexual agenda—behaviors that have a huge impact on men's be-havior as well. As Buss points out, if all women suddenly began preferring to have sex with men who walked on their hands, in a very short time half the hu-man race would be upside down.

With its emphasis on how both men and women are active players in the mating game, evolutionary psychology holds out the promise of helping negoti-ate a truce of sorts in the battle of the sexes—not by declaring a winner but by pointing out that the essence of the mating game is compromise, not vic-tory. The exhortations of radical femi-nists, dyed-in-the-wool chauvinists and everyone in between are all spices for a sexual stew that has been on a slow boil for millions of years. It is no accident that consistently, the top two mating preferences in Buss's survey—expressed equally by males and females world-wide—were not great looks, fame, youth, wealth or status, but *kindness* and *intelligence*. In the rough-and-tum-ble of the human mating game, they are love's greatest allies.

WILLIAM F. ALLMAN

The Female Condom

Reality is all about women protecting themselves

BETH BAKER

I t was really weird," says Deborah Keaton, of Phoenix, Arizona, recalling her initial reaction to the new female condom, Reality. "It was like . . . BIG. I showed it to my friends, and they couldn't believe it."

"Hilarious!" says Felicia Bembower, of Virginia Beach, Virginia, who also participated in the trial study for the new device. "It made for a lot of laughs."

But Dr. Mary Ann Leeper, senior vice president at Wisconsin Pharmacal, isn't laughing. She's responsible for developing the female condom for the United States market, with women's safety in mind. Reality has two flexible rings, one on either end of a six-inch polyurethane sheath. The sheath is wider than the male condom, but not longer. To use the condom, a woman must squeeze the ring at the closed end of the sheath and insert it into her vagina (similar to fitting a diaphragm). The other ring, at the open mouth of the sheath, extends about an inch beyond the vaginal opening. During intercourse, the prelubricated sheath fills the vagina while the outer ring lies flat against the labia, thus shielding the partners from skin-to-skin contact. Reality requires no prescription and may be used only once. One size fits all.

According to Dr. Leeper, the condom can be used in any coital position (except standing up) and, ideally, won't be felt by either partner during intercourse. The key is the proper amount of lubricant. Eighty percent of the women in the study said they were unaware of the condom during intercourse and some even said it actually increased their pleasure. Overall, 71 percent of the women liked Reality.

Then there's the other 29 percent: "It made me feel like an alien," says Michelle Smith, of Chesapeake, Virginia. "I tried to put it in in advance and the plastic swished when I walked. It's like having a plastic Baggie stuck in you." Others complained that the condom occasionally can become twisted or slip, and that the lubricant makes it messy. Some men said that they were more aware of the sheath than they are of the male condom.

If the Food and Drug Administration (FDA) gives the new device the go-ahead as expected, Reality, to be sold over the counter, will be in general distribution this summer. Each condom costs $2.50 and will be available in packets of three, with a tube of extra lubricant and a detailed instructional leaflet.

The price—nearly three times that of the male condom—reflects the higher cost of polyurethane compared to the latex used in most male condoms. (Perhaps the high price is also a result of the $7 million spent by Pharmacal over the past four years for research and testing to meet FDA requirements.)

Despite this higher cost, Reality does have advantages over the male condom. Polyurethane is a stronger yet thinner material that is a better conductor of heat than latex. Because it is not dependent on a male erection, a woman can insert the device ahead of time. But the most significant factor in its favor is that in covering the labia and the base of the penis, the female condom has the potential to offer the greatest protection against sexually transmitted diseases (STDs), including HIV/AIDS and herpes. As a result, women's health advocates and AIDS organizations have joined forces to put

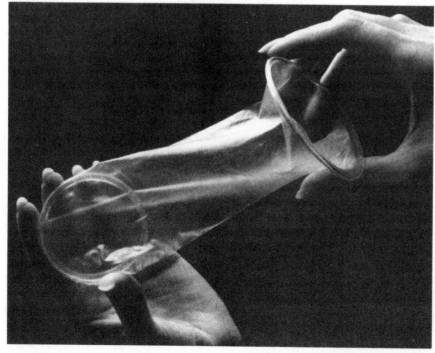

Reality on a fast track for FDA approval.

Last December, despite concerns about insufficient data verifying Reality's effectiveness against STDs, the FDA advisory panel recommended approval of the device, citing the "moral imperative" of HIV prevention. To ensure maximum protection against HIV, some health professionals suggest using a spermicide with the condom; Reality has a 15 percent failure rate. Although some may be tempted to use male and female condoms simultaneously, Dr. Leeper says it can't be done and not to try it.

Reality's biggest selling point is that it will be the first protection against disease—short of abstinence—that women can control themselves. The issue of control extends to its proper use. "With a male condom, I might not know if my partner has put it on properly," says a nurse who participated in the trial study in Virginia. "But with the female condom, I'd know right away if it were misplaced. I'd feel the ring inside me."

Assuming that the female condom is a reliable way to prevent pregnancy and the spread of disease, the big unknown remains public acceptance. Unfortunately, the product's targeted market was not included in the trials. Wisconsin Pharmacal wanted to test the product among women with multiple partners or among couples in which one partner is HIV-positive, but the FDA said no. "We were told, 'It's just not done,'" says Dr. Leeper. Instead, the FDA insisted that the trial study be conducted with monogamous, disease-free couples, whom the agency felt would be more likely to follow the test protocol.

As a result, a valuable opportunity to see how the new device would be accepted by the women most at risk was lost. The research was conducted among married couples, who presumably feel at ease with each other and can more readily deal with the woman emerging from the bathroom with her new appendage. But will young single women have enough self-confidence to use the condom? If her partner is convulsed with laughter, or if his ardor is cooled by her appearance, or if he just plain refuses, will she have the gumption to insist on using it? And will she be able to afford it?

Dr. Denese Shervington, a psychiatrist with Louisiana State University Medical Center, is optimistic. She conducted focus groups among low-income African American women in New Orleans and reports that the women knew the cost, and were still enthusiastic. Wisconsin Pharmacal, the distributor of Reality in the U.S., Mexico, and Canada, has agreed to sell the condom at a discount to public health providers in the U.S. A similar stance was taken by the primary international distributor as well.

Beth Baker is a writer living in Takoma Park, Maryland.

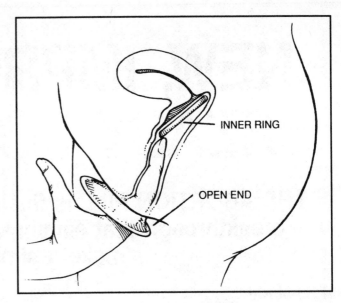

INNER RING

OPEN END

The Femidom In Europe

The female condom is marketed under the trade name Femidom in Europe. It is currently available in Austria, Holland, Switzerland, and the United Kingdom, but by the end of 1993, should be available in most of Western Europe. Femidom sells for about 30 to 45 cents less than Reality. Manufactured by the British firm Chartex International, Femidom is distributed through grocers, drugstores, pharmacies, and supermarkets.

Still new to women, Femidom has sparked an array of responses; initial reactions reflect a mixture of anxiety and naïveté. Women have described Femidom as "gross," "disgusting," "ridiculous," "huge," and "big enough for an elephant or rhinoceros"—responses not unlike their initial responses to other barrier methods.

On first use, women report that Femidom is slippery and sometimes hard to insert. Some find the lubricant too much and others say not enough. Some women complain that the outer ring rubs on the labia and clitoris, while others don't notice the ring at all. Then too there are reports that Femidom does not stay in place during intercourse.

Aesthetics are another consideration: many women do not like the way the device

Our Bodies, Ourselves

hangs out of the vagina and cite that as inhibiting foreplay. Some point out that it also can be noisy.

Reported advantages are that it virtually never breaks, women can insert it before lovemaking, and some men like this method better. Everyone agrees it takes some getting used to—at least three or four tries before couples feel comfortable and competent. Those who like Femidom best have had problems with other methods of birth control.

—The Boston Women's Health Book Collective

NEW, IMPROVED AND READY FOR BATTLE

THE ABORTION PILL is finally coming to the U.S., and a breakthrough that eliminates the follow-up shots will make it simpler to use

Jill Smolowe

Abortion is never easy. There is the anguish of the decision, the invasive nature of the procedure, and sometimes an ugly confrontation with right-to-life forces lying in wait outside the clinic door. But imagine if abortion could be a truly private matter. Say, something as easy as visiting a doctor, getting a few pills, returning home to swallow them, then checking back a few days later to make sure that all went as planned.

Science and politics are now conspiring to make that scenario—scary to some, a godsend to others—a reality, one that could allow abortion to be a truly private decision, albeit still not an easy one. Doc-

> ### "This new regimen is simpler and potentially allows greater privacy than any other abortion method."
> —Dr. Etienne-Emile Baulieu, Inventor of RU 486

tors have reported on a pivotal breakthrough in the use of the controversial French abortion drug known as RU 486: a woman who takes the drug will no longer have to go to a clinic for a follow-up injection to induce contractions. Instead, the entire procedure will involve simply taking two sets of pills. Concurrently, President Clinton has firmly signaled a willingness to reconsider the policies of the Reagan and Bush Administrations, which barred RU 486 from the U.S.

The resulting social upheaval could transform one of the nation's most divi-

sive political debates by making abortion far more difficult to regulate. And eventually it could mean abortions will become simpler, safer and more accessible not only throughout the U.S. but also around the world.

Dr. Etienne-Emile Baulieu, the inventor of RU 486, and his French colleagues describe the successful tests of the no-injection method in the *New England Journal of Medicine*. "This new regimen," they conclude, "is simpler and potentially allows greater privacy than any other abortion method." In a tough accompanying editorial, the *Journal* brands efforts to block use of the drug in the U.S. a "disgrace."

Those political barriers, however, are quickly crumbling. Two days after his Inauguration, President Clinton ordered his Administration to "promote the testing, licensing and manufacturing" of RU 486. Until then, the French manufacturer of the drug, Roussel Uclaf, and its German parent company, Hoechst AG, had steadfastly shied away from becoming involved in the American market for fear of infuriating antiabortion activists. But in April, at the instigation of the U.S. Food and Drug Administration, Roussel announced a compromise: it agreed to license RU 486 to the U.S. Population Council, a nonprofit organization based in New York City, which in turn would run clinical tests.

As a result, the abortion pill could become available through a testing program later this year. The Oregon and New Hampshire legislatures have already volunteered their states as test sites, and the FDA is enthusiastic. Says commissioner David Kessler: "If there is a safe and effective medical alternative to a surgical procedure, then we believe it should be available in this country." Although test-

ing a new drug generally takes seven to 10 years, RU 486 has been so widely used in France that U.S. approval could come in as little as two to three years. In the meantime, the testing will enable at least 2,000 women to use the pill.

These developments could change the nature of abortion and even of birth control by eventually permitting the widespread distribution of pills. Though the

> ### "When they invent new ways to kill children, we will invent new ways to save them."
> —The Rev. Keith Tucci, Operation Rescue National

Supreme Court's *Roe v. Wade* decision of 1973 made abortion legal in the U.S., the ruling was rendered moot in some places by the dearth of doctors willing to perform the procedure and by the fervor of demonstrators who frightened women away from clinics. Now the battleground may shift to the FDA, drug manufacturers and state legislatures.

"We will not allow anti-choice zealots to deny RU 486 to American women," vows Pamela Maraldo, president of the Planned Parenthood Federation of America. The pro-life forces are no less determined. "When they invent new ways to kill children, we will invent new ways to save them," warns the Rev. Keith Tucci of Operation Rescue National. A coalition of antiabortion forces has scheduled a demonstration in front of the French embassy in Washington on June 18, just three days before Roussel Uclaf holds its annual meeting in Paris.

THE ABORTION DRUG HAS BEEN A source of controversy ever since its invention was announced in 1982 by Baulieu, a French physician who worked as a researcher at Roussel Uclaf. The concept was rather simple: RU 486, an antiprogestin, could break a fertilized egg's bond to the uterine wall and thus induce a miscarriage. An injection two days later of prostaglandin, a hormone-like substance, would force uterine contractions and speed the ejection of the embryo. It took six more years and tests on more than 17,000 women before the French government announced that RU 486 would be made available for public use.

The news spawned furious reaction in the press, an outpouring of outraged letters from Roman Catholic doctors, and a church-sponsored protest through the streets of Paris. A month later, a shaken Roussel Uclaf yanked the drug from the market, saying the company did not want to engage in a "moral debate."

Doctors around the world certainly did. Thousands of physicians had convened that month at a medical congress in Rio de Janeiro, and most of them signed a petition demanding that the French government reverse Roussel's decision. Within 48 hours, Health Minister Claude Evin declared that once government approval had been granted, "RU 486 became the moral property of women," and he ordered Roussel to resume distribution. In 1989 RU 486 was made available to all licensed abortion clinics and hospitals in France. The results proved encouraging, save for a freak incident in 1991 when a woman who was an avid smoker suffered a heart attack while trying to use RU 486 to abort her 13th pregnancy. After that mishap, the government banned use of the pill by heavy smokers and women age 35 and older, who have a greater than usual risk of complications.

Using RU 486 was less painful, carried less risk of infection and gave women greater control over the process than a surgical procedure. Over the next 3½ years, 100,000 Frenchwomen used it successfully. Of those who made the decision early enough, about 85% chose RU 486 over surgery. (The pill is currently used in France only within seven weeks of the first day of a woman's last menstrual period; there is now talk of extending usage to a 10-week interval.) Almost all judged the method satisfactory.

Such promising results persuaded both Sweden and Britain to license RU 486; India is testing the drug. China is manufacturing clones that as yet are not widely available. Other countries, most notably Canada, are waiting for the U.S. to take the lead. "The U.S. is the leader in advanced research, the main source of development funds and the heart of worldwide

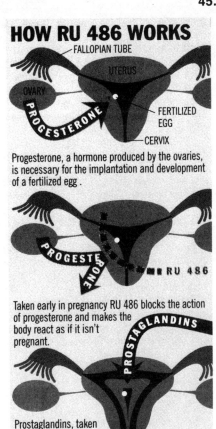

HOW RU 486 WORKS

FALLOPIAN TUBE
UTERUS
OVARY
PROGESTERONE
FERTILIZED EGG
CERVIX

Progesterone, a hormone produced by the ovaries, is necessary for the implantation and development of a fertilized egg.

PROGESTERONE
RU 486

Taken early in pregnancy RU 486 blocks the action of progesterone and makes the body react as if it isn't pregnant.

PROSTAGLANDINS

Prostaglandins, taken 2 days later, cause the uterus to contract and the cervix to soften and dilate. As a result, the embryo is expelled in 97% of the cases.

networks that can allow RU 486 to help women everywhere," explains Baulieu.

In 1991 the French began testing the new method of using RU 486 that does not require going to a clinic for a follow-up shot. An oral prostaglandin, commercially marketed as Cytotec by the American manufacturer G.D. Searle, enabled women to abort simply by swallowing a combination of pills. The efficiency rate rose from 95.5% to 96.9%, and the speed of the procedure improved. In 61% of the cases, the uterine contents were expelled within four hours after taking Cytotec, in contrast to 47% in the case of prostaglandin injections. Although there were instances of nausea and diarrhea, which are also common side effects with injections, those who took the pills reported considerably less pain. "Women tolerate it much better," says Dr. Elisabeth Aubeny of the Broussais Hospital in Paris, a testing ground for RU 486 in 1984. For French taxpayers, who foot 80% of the bill for each abortion through their national healthcare system, there is also an advantage: a dose of Cytotec costs only 72¢, vs. $22 for the prostaglandin shot.

Once again, controversy erupted. When Baulieu first began experimenting

with RU 486 in combination with an oral prostaglandin, Roussel balked. As a result, Baulieu had to persuade French public health officials to defray insurance costs. After preliminary trials, the government compelled Roussel to participate, arguing that the proposed testing of an oral prostaglandin was important for women. Although Searle raised no objections, its executives remain uncomfortable about being linked to the abortion business. "Searle has never willingly made [Cytotec] available for use in abortion," a company official wrote in a letter to the *Wall Street Journal* in February. "It is not Searle's intention or desire to become embroiled in the abortion issue." Searle's reservations echo that of Hoechst president Wolfgang Hilger, who has been open about his ethical objections to RU 486.

The uses of RU 486 could extend well beyond dealing with some of the 37 million abortions carried out around the globe each year. European studies have shown that it is an effective morning-after pill, inducing less nausea or vomiting than other drugs used for the same purpose. There are also indications that RU 486 can combat endometriosis, a leading cause of female infertility, and fibroid tumors, a condition that often necessitates hysterectomy. Thus the same drug that can help some women end unwanted pregnancies may enable others to bear children. Assorted studies have found that RU 486 may also combat breast cancer and Cushing's syndrome, a life-threatening metabolic disorder.

Despite the many potential uses for RU 486 and its effectiveness as an abortion method, efforts to legalize it in the U.S. have met with repeated failure. Last year a pro-choice group called Abortion Rights Mobilization decided to force a court challenge of the import ban imposed on RU 486 by the Bush Administration in 1989. The organization helped Leona Benten, a pregnant 29-year-old California social worker, fly to England, obtain a dose of RU 486, then try to bring it into the U.S. through New York City's Kennedy Airport. Customs officials seized the pills. The ensuing legal battle went up to the Supreme Court, which refused to order the government to return the pills. Benten subsequently had a surgical abortion.

The Clinton Administration has not yet revoked the ban, but its significance is minor. Because distribution of the pills is tightly controlled in Europe and they cannot easily be purchased and imported, the real issue is how quickly the Administration will encourage the manufacture and marketing of the drug in the U.S.

When the pill does become available in America, abortion will not be as easy as going to the doctor and taking some of the tablets home—at least not right away. In

France, for instance, a woman is required to pay four visits over a three-week period to one of the country's 800 licensed clinics or hospitals. The first step is a gynecological exam. Doctors make sure the pregnancy is in its early stages, and a social worker or psychologist discusses with her the decision to abort. Then the woman is sent home for a weeklong "reflection" period.

When she returns, she is required to sign a government form requesting the abortion. She must also sign a Roussel form that confirms her understanding that a malformed fetus might result if she does not see the abortion through to completion. (As yet no defects have been found in the small number of babies born to women known to have taken RU 486.) At that point, the woman is given three aspirin-like RU 486 tablets, each containing 200 mg of the drug. After swallowing the pills, she again goes home.

Except in the rare instance where the RU 486 is enough to induce a quick abortion, the woman must take two 200-mg Cytotec pills within the next 48 hours. Because the timing is critical and doctors want to monitor the effects of this contraction-inducing drug, women are required to return to the clinic. They are encouraged to remain for four hours, even if the expulsion happens earlier. Eight to 10 days later, they must pay a final visit for an exam to make sure no part of the egg remains.

Even with all these steps, the procedure seems blessedly simple to most women. "Taking a pill seems far less murderous and violent to the child than using a vacuum cleaner," says a 31-year-old woman who has had both types of abortion. "You feel so helpless when they put you to sleep and you know they're going to be using their tubes and knives on you." Some women, however, become traumatized by the thought of performing an abortion with their own hand. After her experience with RU 486, Joelle Mevel, 34, vows that if there is a next time, she will choose surgery. "I spent the whole time worrying that I would see the child in the basin, that I would be able to discern something human in the blood," she says. "I would rather have gone to sleep and awakened later knowing it was all over."

American abortion-rights advocates talk of boiling France's time-consuming RU 486 procedure down to just two visits to the doctor. It would be possible, though controversial, for the government to let RU 486 be administered in any doctor's office or possibly even by trained nurse practitioners. If that happened, many women could avoid running a gauntlet of protesters outside an abortion clinic. Still, it won't take all the anguish out of the procedure. "It's insulting to women to say that abortion now will be as easy as taking aspirins," says Baulieu. "It is always difficult, psychologically and physically, sometimes tragic."

—Reported by J. Madeleine Nash/Chicago, Frederick Painton/Paris, Janice C. Simpson/New York and Tala Skari/Paris

IT'S NOT JUST
AIDS

UNINFORMED AND MISINFORMED, TEENS FACE AN EPIDEMIC OF SEXUALLY TRANSMITTED DISEASES.

William L. Bergman, M.D.

William L. Bergman, M.D., is the medical director of Hahnemann Health Associates in New York and president of the World Medical Health Foundation.

While the sexually transmitted disease (STD) epidemic is a terrifying reality, in many ways it is a silent epidemic. In the privacy of their offices, doctors are seeing large numbers of STD patients. This new epidemic is a result of the increase in promiscuity that began with the sexual revolution of the 1960s.

One in five Americans between the ages of fifteen and fifty-five is infected with a sexually transmitted disease; 63 percent of the newly infected are under twenty-five.

As pointed out by Dr. Joe McIlhaney, Jr., president for Sexual Health, teenagers tend to think that STDs have always been around in the same numbers they are today. Looking at their parents' generation, who they know from accounts of the sixties have had multiple sexual partners, they may think that these older folk do not look like they were hurt by having sex as single people.

What the younger generation does not realize is that the older generation was not as likely to be infected with STDs as people are today. Centers for Disease Control (CDC) statistics reveal that one in five Americans between the ages of fifteen and fifty-five are infected with an STD, with 63 percent of the newly infected people under twenty-five years of age. The enormous increase in STD infection and of serious STDs makes it dangerous for anyone, especially young people, to have sex outside of marriage.

TRACKING THE INCREASE

Before 1960, syphilis and gonorrhea were the only important STDs, and the existing strains were easily treated. Today, however, Americans face over twenty significant STDs—some fatal, a few relatively harmless, but all contributing to the problem. It is estimated that twelve million people in the United States become infected each year.

The spread of STDs is alarming. In 1976, chlamydia was first reported; now it is the most common STD in the United States. In 1981, HIV was identified; today, between 1 and 1.5 million Americans are estimated to be infected and, in 1992, there were 140,000 deaths. Infection in the teenage population is increasing dramatically. In 1984, herpes became common, and today over thirty million Americans are infected with that virus. In 1985, we began to see an increasing incidence of human papilloma virus (HPV), which causes genital warts and cancers in both sexes.

In 1990, there was a 400 percent increase in the rate of tubal ectopic pregnancy. Not all tubal pregnancies are caused by STDs, but the huge increase is importantly the result of the rising rate of pelvic inflammatory disease (PID), which comes from chlamydia and gonorrhea. Scarred fallopian tubes caused by PID block the passage of fertilized eggs to the uterus; the growing embryo causes the tube to rupture. The April 1989 *Female Patient* reported that teens have the highest death rate from tubal ectopic pregnancy, which also can increase the incidence of infertility and subsequent tubal pregnancies. PID is painful and is the most common cause of hospitalization for women between the ages of fifteen and fifty-five, next to pregnancy.

YOUNG AT GREATER RISK

One reason teens are vulnerable is that people are likely to have more sexual partners the earlier they start having sex, according to a January 1991 study by the CDC.

OB/GYN reported in August 1990 that the lining of the cervix of a teenage girl produces extra mucus that nourishes STDs. As women reach their twenties or have babies, that lining is replaced by a tougher one. Also, during the first two years of menstrual periods, 50 percent occur without ovulation, making the cervical mucus more liquid and a better medium for disease-producing microorganisms.

A recent survey of high school students reveals that knowledge about AIDS or HIV infection and its prevention is not associated with any change in risk behavior.

Contraception (vol. 41, 1990) reports that women are more likely to have chlamydia or gonorrhea-induced PID if they begin having sex early. *Texas Medicine* (1987) reports that teens with PID are more difficult to treat than older patients. Teens have a 14 percent chance of not responding well to antibiotics and requiring major surgery involving the removal of the uterus, tubes, and ovaries. While most women survive tubal ectopic pregnancy, 70 percent who have never had a baby before their ectopic pregnancy will be infertile.

Medical Aspects of Human Sexuality (July 1990) states that "adolescent females appear to be at higher risk for HPV infection than most adult populations. Rates of HPV infection among teenage girls have been reported as high as 40 percent compared with 2 percent to 15 percent among adult women." *Pediatrics* reported in 1988 that teenagers are more likely to have precancerous and cancerous growths resulting from HPV than are adults with the same infection.

To what extent are STDs treatable? Chlamydia and gonorrhea can be cured by antibiotics, but after the microorganisms are killed, scars remain that can cause infertility, ectopic pregnancy, and pelvic pain. In 1990, penicillin-resistant strains of gonorrhea were identified in all fifty states; they can be cured, but only by fairly expensive drugs. Often, patients' inability to comply in taking prescribed medicine results in failure to successfully treat those disease for which there is a cure.

In 1990, syphilis, which is easy to diagnose and 100 percent sensitive to penicillin, reached a forty-year high. Babies are once again being born with syphilis. HIV, which causes AIDS, is, unlike syphilis, a very complex virus that mutates rapidly. The spread of syphilis indicates that any HIV cure may be only temporary if people continue their present sexual behavior.

SEXUAL 'LIBERATION'

What predisposing causes underlie our present patterns of sexual activity?

In the sixties, through an increase in social rebellion, alcohol, drugs, and free sex were increasingly condoned. "Sexual liberation" was justified as a kind of new morality: the idea that people were no longer bound or restricted by the traditional ethical standards of the past. Among the fast-breaking technological advances were new contraceptives that severed the link between sexual intercourse and procreation. In this environment, the sexual revolution was born. The idea that teenage sexual activity was inevitable was increasingly accepted. The popular culture, especially the entertainment industry, encouraged it.

The outcome was a kind of self-fulfilling prophecy in which the results reflected the expectations. With the widespread acceptance of the inevitability of premarital sexual activity, contraceptive-based sex education was embraced by many as a necessity.

A Harris poll found that after comprehensive sex ed emphasizing condoms, teens were 53 percent more likely to have intercourse than those whose sex ed did not discuss contraceptives.

As a result, in the early 1970s federal dollars began flowing into contraceptive approaches. Clinics were opened under Title X to provide birth control to teenagers as well as others. The problem was defined as teen pregnancy and STD, rather than as adolescent premarital sexual activity itself.

CONDOM EDUCATION FAILS

America now has a track record of approximately twenty years of contraceptive-based sex education, where the emphasis has been on knowledge about sexuality, contraceptive methods, and STDs (including HIV). However, during the period in which this knowledge has been disseminated, sexual activity has increased dramatically, and, with it, pregnancy rates and STDs.

A 1989 health risk survey of secondary school students states, "Responses show that nearly all students knew the two main modes of HIV transmission—intravenous drug use and sexual intercourse." *Pediatrics* (May 1992) states, "Knowledge about AIDS or HIV infection and its prevention was not associated with any change in risk behavior, nor were the number of sources of information about the epidemic, acquaintance with those who were infected, estimates of personal risk, or exposure to HIV test counseling."

A 1986 Harris poll reported that only 14 percent of sexually active teens not using contraceptives said they were not using protection due to a lack of knowledge or access. Clearly, knowledge alone has not been very useful in terms of actually making a difference in teenage sexual behavior. Similarly, a study of fourteen nationwide contraceptive-based sex education programs found that none had any impact in decreasing teen sexual involvement, as reported in *Sexuality Education and Evaluation of Programs and Their Effects* (Network Publications, Santa Cruz).

In Virginia, school districts that taught "comprehensive contraceptive-based sex education" experienced a 17.3 average percent increase in teen pregnancies, whereas school districts not offering such programs had a 15.8 average percent decrease, according to 1988 Virginia Department of Health statistics.

The April 1988 *American Journal of Public Health* reported that a study of condom education and distribution in San Francisco schools showed that a yearlong effort resulted in only 8 percent of males and 2 percent of females using condoms every time they had sex.

The overall pregnancy rate at a Dallas high school dispensing condoms was 1.47 times greater than the pregnancy rate at a similar school that did not (11.2 percent versus 7.6 percent), as reported in *Family Planning Perspectives* of January–February 1991.

In Adams High School in Commerce City, Colorado, which has had a condom distribution program since 1989, the pregnancy rate has risen 66 percent, to become 31 percent above the national average.

A Harris poll commissioned by Planned Parenthood in 1986 found that, after exposure to comprehensive sex education emphasizing condoms, teenagers were 53 percent more likely to have initiated intercourse than those whose sex education did not discuss contraceptives.

In spite of these appalling statistics, some still claim that we need to push the condom message even more and start introducing the message at earlier and earlier ages. This is advocated even though we have spent already about $2 billion on this type of education, which seems to have contributed to an increase in teen pregnancies and STDs.

PUSHING PLEASURE

Underlying assumptions of contraceptive-based sex education are that human nature is primarily sexual, that it is unnatural to sacrifice sexual desire, and that teens have a right to choose to be sexually active as long as they do it "properly."

In addition to advocating condoms, a goal of so-called protected sex education is to teach "outercourse," those sexual practices that are considered at low risk for HIV. Deborah Hafner, executive director of the Sex Informa-

tion and Education Council of the United States (SIECUS), says, "We should teach teens about oral sex and mutual masturbation in order to help them delay the onset of sexual intercourse and its resulting consequences." But HIV can be transmitted during oral sex if infected semen, vaginal secretions, or blood enters the bloodstream of the partner through cuts or sores in the mouth. In a society in which public acceptance of unmarried teenagers having intercourse and confidence in condoms is high, it should be pointed out that "outercourse" also may stimulate the desire for intercourse rather than delay it.

Peggy Brick of Planned Parenthood emphasizes the importance of helping adolescents understand "pleasure, sexual satisfaction and gratification and orgasm," whether carried out in the context of marriage or not.

Based on this mind-set, the Pennsylvania Department of Education includes in its publication "I Deserve Love," from the *Pennsylvania Health Curriculum Guide*, the following passage:

> "My lovers now approve of each other. My mother and father approve of my sex life. My minister approves of my sex life. God approves of my sex life. Christ intended for me to have abundance. I have the right to have multiple sex partners. I do not need to hold back and save my orgasms for someone special. I want to experience them now. . . . Oral stimulation can be very effective and I am delighted about it. I have no resistance to trying oral and anal sex. I have the right to enjoy my own genitals."

The New York City Department of Health has a Teenagers' Bill of Rights, funded by the CDC and the City of New York, which states, "I have the right to think for myself, I have the right to decide whether to have sex and who to have it with."

When parents express reservations about this kind of so-called safer sex education, they are accused of wanting to censor information, possibly due to their own sexual repression.

CONDOM FAILURE RATES

Latex condoms can help prevent the transmission of HIV. However, a significant problem with the contraceptive model of sex education is that while condoms are promoted as protecting against HIV, other STDs, and pregnancy, the facts concerning the high rate of condom failure due to product defects and difficulty of use are often never mentioned. This is justified on the assumption that young people are inevitably going to be sexually active and that some protection is better than none.

This point of view is widely held within the public health community. The April 1993 *American Journal of Public Health* states,

> We should be able to agree that premature initiation of sexual activity carries health risks. Therefore, we must exercise leadership in encouraging young people to postpone sexual activity. Adolescents are bombarded with

massages encouraging them to "do it." We need to strive for a climate supportive of young people who are not having sex and so help to create a new health-oriented social norm for adolescents and teenagers against sexuality. As we proceed toward this objective, we must be mindful that many will continue to engage in sexual activity. It is essential that these youngsters receive the message that they must practice safer sex and use condoms. The message that those who initiate or continue sexual activity must reduce their risk through correct and consistent condom use needs to be delivered as strongly and persuasively as the message "don't do it."

This approach is complicated by the fact that the risks in so-called protected sex are greater than is often admitted. Apart from moral considerations, why should teenagers be taught to abstain from sex until marriage? Because, quite simply, no other approach will sufficiently protect them. We need to look at the medical facts regarding condoms, since they are currently the centerpiece of educational policy with regard to HIV and other STDs.

Unless the sexually transmitted disease is localized directly beneath the condom, there is nothing separating the healthy teenager from the disease.

According to Dr. William R. Archer III, a former deputy assistant secretary for population affairs at the Department of Health and Human Services (HHS), "One out of three sexually active teenagers will acquire an STD before graduating from high school, and in most cases a condom would have done little to stop it. Condoms have an 18 percent failure rate for pregnancy for teenagers. Low-income adolescents, for reasons not fully understood, have a [much higher rate]. Studies suggest that condoms offer even less protection against STDs. A study which looked at a group of monogamous couples in which one partner was HIV positive found a 17 percent transmission rate of the virus at eighteen months, despite consistent use of a condom. Furthermore, many STDs can be passed by direct contact, even though the couple is using a condom. Unless the disease is localized directly beneath the condom, there is still nothing coming between the healthy teenager and direct contact with disease." Many STD sores are in areas of the genitals not covered by a condom.

A study at Rutgers University found that the rate of chlamydia transmission was exactly the same for couples using condoms as for those not using them.

Because of the mortal consequences of condom failure when one partner is HIV positive, it is crucial to understand how well condoms protect against the HIV virus. Consider that in pregnancy only the woman can become pregnant, but with HIV either partner can become infected. A woman is fertile approximately sixty days per year; HIV can be transmitted every day of the year.

Family Planning Perspectives (January–February 1992) expresses serious concerns regarding condoms. It reports "a sobering level of exposure to the risk of pregnancy and infection with HIV and other sexually transmitted diseases, even for those who most consistently use condoms."

A recent policy statement from the CDC entitled *Prevention of Heterosexual HIV Transmission: The Condom Strategy Reaffirmed* states that the partners of HIV-infected persons may consider the risk of transmission during sexual intercourse unacceptably high even if a condom *is* used:

> On the individual level, it means that the likelihood of acquiring HIV infection because of condom failure is largely dependent on the likelihood that the individual sexual partner is HIV-infected. Therefore, in the special circumstance in which one partner is known to be infected and the other is not, even the estimated 1 percent to 2 percent risk of condom failure [resulting from manufacture or product defect] may be unacceptably high. For this reason, persons in this category may be best advised to consider other expressions of intimacy and other methods of sexual gratification in lieu of intercourse even with condoms.

The April 1988 *Journal of the American Medical Association* reported, "Encouraging the use of condoms may in some circumstances even be harmful if it gives a false sense of security in a high-risk situation. . . . Instead of encouraging such couples where one partner is zero-positive to use condoms, the best advice may be that they should stop having vaginal intercourse."

In other words, authorities are saying that the level of risk is unacceptable if you know your partner is HIV-infected, yet somehow acceptable if you do not. If doctors will not recommend that an infected person or a person with an infected partner use a condom, how can this possibly be the basis of sound medical policy for America's youth?

MANY TEEN VIRGINS

According to studies done by the CDC and HHS, nearly half of all teens are virgins, and many others return to sexual inactivity. It is especially the sexually inactive teens who need to be supported in having made the optimum health choice.

If the schools teach so-called protected sex and the parents do not object, teenagers think they must be able to have sex safely because the adults in their lives are explaining how to do it or expecting them to do it. On the other hand, those students who, for whatever reason, are not sexually active may begin to feel abnormal if it appears that everyone expects them to be sexually active.

If contraceptive-based sex education is not effective, and even highly risky in an age of AIDS, what do we then do? What can be the basis for an effective approach?

A historical perspective may provide some clues. Over the period from 1970 to 1990, the rate of premarital sexual activity increased, except for a brief time in the early 1980s. What changes occurred then?

During that period, federal money going into contraceptive-based programs decreased, and federal funding for programs designed to teach adolescents to abstain from premarital sexual activity, the so-called Title XX funding, was instituted. During the mid and late 1980s, however, these policies were weakened or reversed. Why?

AIDS and the HIV crisis of the mid-1980s caused an increase in efforts to teach "safe" and then "safer" sex. Condoms were advocated as the solution, and, once again, funding for contraceptive sex education increased.

What, then, is the answer? An approach to sex education based on promoting abstinence from premarital sexual activity (that is, from the behavior that causes teen pregnancy and spreads HIV and other STDs) must be instituted. This approach can encourage attitudes that lead to marriage and the formation of stable families. We can teach single people that sex is a wonderful thing but that, like fire, it has a capacity for both constructive and destructive results. Almost all risk of STDs, including HIV, and all risk of out-of-wedlock pregnancy can be avoided by saving intercourse for marriage.

Abstinence education has achieved promising results. Americans need to acknowledge which approach has failed: contraceptive education or abstinence education.

But, some would argue, is teaching premarital abstinence realistic? Isn't it naive to propose delaying intercourse until one is older? About 50 percent of unmarried girls and 40 percent of unmarried boys aged fifteen through nineteen have not yet had intercourse. These people are practicing abstinence. Also, 83 percent of Japanese teenage girls are virgins, and 73 percent of America's highest achieving high school students never have had sexual intercourse. Saving sex for marriage was normal for most people until about thirty years ago and can become normal again.

Teens who have been sexually active can choose to stop. Secondary abstinence is based on the idea that

people can start over. Teenagers can protect their health. It is never too late to start saying no to premarital sex.

ABSTINENCE POSSIBLE

What, then, of the track record of premarital abstinence programs? After the San Marcos, Texas, unified school district used the Teen AID abstinence program, reported pregnancies dropped from 147 to 20, an 88 percent reduction. Similar programs—Sex Respect, Best Friends, Free Teens—have shown very promising results.

Students who receive the Sex Respect curriculum show significant changes in attitude over the course of their participation. There are consistent increases in the extent to which students (grades seven through nine) feel that sex among unmarried teens is wrong and that teens who have had sex outside of marriage would benefit by deciding to stop and wait for marriage.

Americans need to look at which approach has failed. Federal funding for contraceptive education per year is approximately $150 million, as opposed to about $2 million for abstinence education, a seventy-five to one ratio. It is time for a new approach.

Even if a perfect mechanical technique were invented that would eliminate the risk of pregnancy, HIV, and other STDs, research indicates still more reasons to support teen abstinence. Having sex as a teenager is linked to the use of drugs, alcohol, and tobacco. The February 1991 issue of *Pediatrics* states: "It is essential for health providers to explore the issue of sexual activity and the other risk factors that are strongly linked to it in adolescence. Engaging in one activity significantly increases the risk for the others, which carry additional biological and psychosocial risk."

Should a teenager's decision to be sexually active be affirmed and supported by the meaningful adults in that young person's life because "it's their decision"? Would we affirm teenagers' decisions to use drugs or drop out of school simply because they decided?

Teaching abstinence fits with what we have learned about drug, alcohol, and tobacco education. When we showed teens drug paraphernalia and let them smell marijuana, student drug use went up. When we started teaching that they should not use drugs, alcohol, and tobacco, use of those substances went down. We gave the teenagers the benefit of adult knowledge, and they listened. The same approach will work for sex education.

HOW DO YOU KNOW IF IT'S

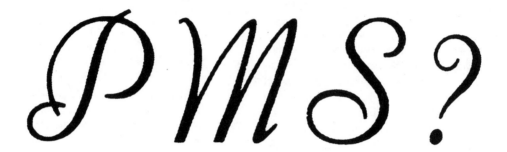

TRACKING SYMPTOMS HELPS YOU FIND THE RIGHT TREATMENT

PAULA DRANOV

Paula Dranov *is a New York City–based freelance writer who covers health and medicine.*

Lynne Adams* always had a difficult time just before her menstrual periods—terrible cramps, backaches, skin problems and, worse, a monthly change in personality she simply couldn't control.

"Ordinarily, I'm the rock of Gibraltar," says Adams, 41. "But I always felt tremendous anxiety before my period and would take it out on everyone. Once, I was driving a friend to the

*Not her real name

supermarket. Her voice got on my nerves, so I stopped the car and told her to get out. I drove away and left her there!

"I would have arguments with my family and apologize when I came to my senses. I broke off relationships with men. Nobody could deal with me, and I couldn't deal with myself."

Eventually, Adams heard about a treatment program for women with premenstrual syndrome (PMS) at Columbia Presbyterian Medical Center in New York. After a thorough physical and mental evaluation, her new psychiatrist prescribed an antidepressant, and her gynecologist started her on Anaprox, a drug for cramps.

"Everyone noticed the difference,"

Adams reports. "No more hand wringing, nail biting, snapping everyone's head off. I have a control over my life now I never thought I would have."

But while doctors today can more easily treat the symptoms, researchers still don't know what causes the problems women such as Adams experience. No one even knows for sure how many women are affected by the syndrome. Estimates range from 16% to 80% of all women, depending on who is doing the research and the criteria used to define PMS. What's more, 5% to 10% of these women have *very* severe symptoms, which some doctors are now called PMD, premenstrual disorder.

But classifying strong cycle shifts as

an illness at all is "anti-woman," says Esther Rome, coauthor of *The New Our Bodies, Ourselves.* Labeling PMS as an illness is political, she says, a way to deny normalcy to cycle changes. "We need to recognize there are cycle changes, which can be very uncomfortable and debilitating," she says. "Recognizing this as a fact of life for some women and not a defect in their characters is helpful and freeing."

In practical terms, however, if a woman suspects she has PMS she should track physical and emotional changes over the course of at least two cycles to verify that they occur only when she is premenstrual. The chart on p. 58 can help. While 150 signs have been documented, the 19 listed are the most common. The chart should serve as a springboard for discussions with a doctor.

Even women who don't have PMS may get mild versions of some symptoms when they begin menstruating or a few days before. But women with PMS may be plagued by discomfort or psychological distress for up to two weeks (from mid-cycle, when ovulation occurs, to the onset of menses).

The difference between mild premenstrual changes and PMS is one of degree. Severe symptoms that last days or even weeks, month after month, are more likely to be diagnosed as PMS than more tolerable versions of the same complaints.

"A woman's particular pattern tends to be consistent across cycles, but there is tremendous variability among women," notes Dr. Jean Endicott, a psychologist at a PMS evaluation unit affiliated with the New York State Psychiatric Institute. "If a woman is crying and terribly upset a week after her period ends—which should be the 'best' part of her cycle—chances are she's suffering from another chronic condition." Among the possibilities: depression, anxiety or an undiagnosed physical illness (including thyroid dysfunction, anemia, seizure disorders, chronic infections and endometriosis).

What About Hormones?

So far, the search for the cause of PMS itself has yielded only a few clues. Fluctuating levels of the ovarian hormones estrogen and progesterone

seem to play a key role: When production ceases after removal of the ovaries, symptoms disappear. The same thing happens if the hormone supply is suppressed with experimental hormone "agonists." These induce a "chemical menopause"—suitable only for people with the severest symptoms. For some women in the studies, symptoms inexplicably stayed at bay even when drugs were stopped and normal hormone production resumed, according to anecdotal reports.

Despite this evident hormonal connection, PMS sufferers have not been proven to have abnormally high or low levels of either estrogen or progesterone (or both). The same goes for all the other hormones that influence the menstrual cycle, says Dr. David Rubinow, NIMH clinical director. However, his PMS research team has turned up an intriguing new connection between PMS and thyroid hormones. About 35% of PMS patients produce either too much or too little thyroid-stimulating hormone in special tests. That finding has led Rubinow to begin looking at thyroid supplements.

Interestingly, about 25% of depressed patients given the same tests show the same abnormal thyroid reactions, he says. Rubinow is now investigating links between PMS and depression. Other studies have shown that PMS is more common among women who have suffered from major depression for more than a month. And because some women with PMS alternate between premenstrual depression and postmenstrual euphoria, some investigators feel PMS is related to manic depressive disorder.

What Helps

Whatever the underlying cause, PMS treatment depends on symptoms. No single drug works for everyone, and some that relieve one type of distress don't help others. "Many treatments are being offered for which there is no good scientific evidence and which are not without side effects," warns Endicott.

Magnesium supplements, for instance, have been touted because some PMS sufferers have low magnesium levels (though still within the normal range). There's little if any

evidence magnesium supplements relieve PMS symptoms, says Lilian Cheung, a nutrition specialist at Harvard's Center for Health Communications. Besides, magnesium can be toxic in high doses and may impair calcium absorption.

And though vitamin B6 supplements may help reduce some symptoms, they're not worth the risks, says Dr. Paula Schnurr, research assistant professor of psychiatry at Dartmouth Medical School. Even doses as low as 200 mg to 300 mg a day can cause nerve damage in some individuals, adds Cheung.

As for progesterone treatments, enthusiastic British claims for this hormone haven't panned out. Other tests suggest progesterone is no more effective than a placebo.

Then there's evening primrose oil. Proponents contend it boosts production of gamma-linoleic acid, which in turn restores prostaglandin balance. However, there's no evidence that women with PMS are prostaglandin-*deficient.* And it's never been clinically proven the substance relieves PMS symptoms.

Here's a rundown of what *may* help for physical and emotional problems:

■**Relaxation:** Women with severe PMS symptoms who practice relaxation-response techniques show a 60% reduction in overall symptoms, according to a new study by Dr. Irene Goodale and colleagues at Harvard University and New England Deaconess Hospital. Specifically, the women repeated a word, phrase, sound or prayer for 10 to 20 minutes twice a day, while passively disregarding everyday thoughts as they came to mind in order to elicit the relaxation response. (Progressive muscular relaxation is another technique that elicits the relaxation response, say investigators.) Dr. Herbert Benson, author of *The Relaxation Response* (Avon, $3.95), says that the techniques cause physiological and psychological changes, including decreased metabolism, rate of breathing, heart rate and blood pressure, and foster feelings of tranquility.

■**Exercise:** Although some athletes have PMS, exercise can help. It may stimulate the release of pain-relieving brain hormones called endorphins and can also help combat mild depression.

■**Ibuprofen:** Over-the-counter drugs containing ibuprofen combat cramp-causing prostaglandins. If they don't work, a stronger prescription version may. (Aspirin is a weak prostaglandin inhibitor and may help mild cramps.)

■**Diuretics:** They're sometimes prescribed for bloating and discomfort caused by premenstrual fluid retention. But do they really help? In five studies of diuretics' effectiveness against bloating and weight gain, only two showed any beneficial effect, according to a recent review. But these drugs don't affect depression and other mood disorders, notes Dr. Wilma Harrison, an associate professor of psychiatry at the Columbia University College of Physicians and Surgeons. What's more, according to a Mayo Clinic bulletin, diuretics seem to help only women who retain very large amounts of fluid.

■**Oral contraceptives:** Results are mixed. The Pill helps some women but worsens others' symptoms, Endicott and colleagues report.

■**Antibiotics:** One underlying cause of PMS may be low-grade infection of the pelvic organs, which can develop after sex, miscarriage, abortion or childbirth, according to a study by Dr. Attila Toth of New York's Cornell Medical Center. In such instances, treatment with the antibiotic doxycycline helps, he says.

■**Vitamin E:** There's no hard evidence vitamin E works, but a British study found that women who took 400 IU of vitamin E reported a 27% to 42% reduction in their symptoms' severity, particularly depression and anxiety, over a three-month period (see "The Oil of Relief," *AH*, April '88, p. 104).

No other drugs studied reliably affect PMS mood and behavior changes. While an antidepressant worked for Lynne Adams, there have been no controlled studies of antidepressants for PMS treatment. However, individual doctors may prescribe antidepressant or anti-anxiety drugs. In severe cases, when lethargy is incapacitating, stimulants may be prescribed.

Dietary changes may also help:

■**Avoid salt.** This can reduce the fluid retention that contributes to bloating and breast tenderness.

■**Cut down on caffeine.** Although it's no longer thought to aggravate harmless breast cysts that can cause pain premenstrually, many women are more comfortable when they do without the caffeine "jitters."

■**Watch out for sweets.** Many women have cravings when they're premenstrual, especially for simple carbohydrates and chocolate. If you overreact to sugar, avoid it, says Cheung. It may pick you up, but later it will bring you down, leaving you feeling worse than ever.

■**Avoid alcohol.** A drink may relax you, but too much alcohol and a hangover only add to menstrual miseries.

At whatever level PMS symptoms occur, most women learn to cope. Feminist author Esther Rome observes that despite severe premenstrual problems, many women continue to work and do a competent job. Whether or not it's best, she adds, women have learned as part of growing up to keep home and work place running—no matter how they feel.

But it's important for women not to dismiss the things that bother them premenstrually as "just my PMS." They may be symptoms of things that are troubling, though better tolerated, at other times, too, says Rome. "It's helpful to reflect on these problems when you're not premenstrual and try to find solutions."

ADAPTED FROM *THE AMERICAN MEDICAL ASSOCIATION ENCYCLOPEDIA OF MEDICINE.* NEW YORK, NY: RANDOM HOUSE, INC. 1989   AMY KEITH

THE MENSTRUAL CYCLE

Women with PMS tend to experience bodily discomfort or emotional distress for up to two weeks, from midcycle, when ovulation occurs and an egg is released, to the onset of menses, when the endometrium is shed. Fluctuating hormone levels do seem to play a key role in PMS, say researchers, but sufferers still have not been shown to have abnormally high levels of the ovarian hormones estrogen and progesterone.

A Nightly Checklist for PMS

If you think you have PMS and want to track your symptoms, you'll need a calendar (preferably one that shows dates in large boxes) and a separate note pad or diary for jotting down notes about particular days.

To begin, attach the instructions below to the bottom of the calendar. Every night before you go to bed, mark the letters that correspond to the symptoms or feelings you experienced during the day. Then, in parentheses, rate the severity of each problem as either: 1, minimal; 2, mild; 3, moderate; 4, severe; or 5, extreme. Note days on which you are menstruating with an X in the upper left corner of the box.

On a separate sheet of paper, keep a daily record of anything that happens that could affect you physically or psychologically, such as a cold or stressful situation. Be sure to mark the upper right corner of the appropriate calendar box with an asterisk to remind yourself to refer to this record.

After a couple of months, a premenstrual pattern should begin to emerge if you have PMS. In that case, take the calendar to your gynecologist. It will help the doctor decide how to treat physical complaints and may prompt a referral to a PMS expert to help with emotional or psychological problems. If, however, symptoms have no particular premenstrual pattern, another condition may be to blame. Even so, the calendar can help you and your physician diagnose the problem and decide on treatment.

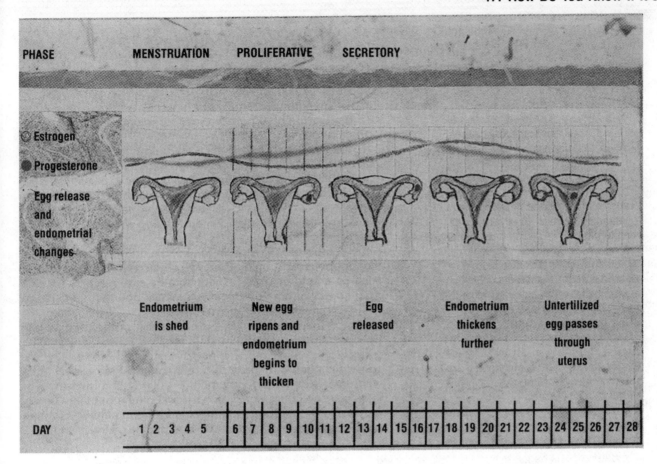

PHASE	MENSTRUATION	PROLIFERATIVE	SECRETORY		
Estrogen Progesterone Egg release and endometrial changes	Endometrium is shed	New egg ripens and endometrium begins to thicken	Egg released	Endometrium thickens further	Untertilized egg passes through uterus
DAY	1 2 3 4 5	6 7 8 9 10 11 12	13 14 15 16 17 18	19 20 21 22	23 24 25 26 27 28

Adapted from the daily ratings form developed by Dr. Jean Endicott and John Nee, Ph.D., of the New York State Psychiatric Institute; Jacob Cohen, Ph.D., of New York University; and Uriel
Halbreich, M.D., of the State University of New York at Buffalo.

Items Most Highly Associated:

A. Experienced mood swings.
B. Was irritable or angry.
C. Felt sad or lonely.
D. Felt anxious or nervous.
E. Wanted to avoid social activities.
F. Experienced abdominal heaviness or pain.
G. Had breast pain.
H. Was less interested in sexual
   activity.
I. Was more sexually active.
J. Had back or muscle pain.
K. Felt bloated.
L. Slept more or stayed in bed.
M. Felt impaired.
N. Had less energy.
O. Drank more coffee, tea or cold drinks.
P. Had increased appetite or cravings.
Q. Used alcohol or other drugs.
R. Couldn't sit still.
S. Had headaches.

Consumer Health

For many people, the term *consumer health* conjures up images of selecting health care services and paying medical bills. While these two aspects of health care are consumer health issues, the term consumer health encompasses all consumer products and services that influence people's health and welfare. The implications stemming from this broad definition suggest that almost everything we see or do may be construed to be a consumer health issue. Such is the case with media coverage of medical investigations. Over the last three years, millions of Americans have added food products that contain oat bran to their diets. Many of these people have now eliminated or are considering the elimination of oat bran products from their diets. They read reports claiming that oat bran could reduce blood cholesterol levels, and so they went out and bought products containing oat bran. When reports began to surface questioning the value of oat bran as a cholesterol reducer, many of these people stopped using it. This scenario is typical of the way American consumers respond to media reports on issues of health. If, at some future date, reports began to surface that reaffirmed the value of oat bran as a cholesterol reducer, how would these same individuals respond? Clearly, media reports such as this add to the confusion and fuel controversy, but they also sell newspapers, and that is, after all, a newspaper's bottom line.

There are a number of U.S. government agencies that serve to protect Americans from consumer health fraud, including the Food and Drug Administration, the Federal Trade Commission, the U.S. Postal Service, the Office of Consumer Education, the Office of Consumer Affairs, the Public Health Service, the National Institutes of Health, the Health Services Administration, and the Consumer Protection Agency. While these agencies play an active role in protecting the consumers' health, they are not able to keep pace with the number of products and services being marketed and sold. Remember, if the advertised claim sounds too good to be true, it probably is.

Of all the consumer health issues, the one that is the greatest source of confusion and controversy is nutrition. Numerous reports have been issued linking the typical American diet to both cancer and cardiovascular disease. On the basis of these reports, consumers have been encouraged to eat more fiber and reduce their intake of dietary fats, particularly saturated fats and cholesterol. The response of the food industry to these reports and recommendations has been mixed. On the positive side, they have introduced new products and modified their packaging so as to demonstrate their awareness of current dietary recommendations. On the negative side, many of the new products are only marginally better than their predecessors, even though the labeling suggests otherwise. Some food manufacturers have even resorted to changing the suggested serving size as listed on the label so that their products appear more nutritionally sound. " 'Nutrition Facts': To Help Consumers Eat Smart" by Paula Kurtzweil discusses how new labeling regulations will change the labeling format that appears on packaged goods and explains how this new format will serve as an educational tool that will help consumers evaluate food products in terms of their own diets.

On November 6, 1991 the Food and Drug Administration in conjunction with the U.S. Department of Agriculture announced proposed changes to existing food labeling laws that for 20 years had confused and deceived the American public. This announcement was unique in that the USDA, which regulates labeling on products such as raw and processed meats and poultry, hot dogs, luncheon meats, and convenience foods that contain meat, will for the first time adhere to the labeling guidelines set forth by the FDA. The guidelines, which took effect in May 1993, include (1) *Health Claims*—limited to only four areas and including messages about calcium and osteoporosis, fat and cardiovascular disease, fat and cancer, and salt and hypertension; (2) *Descriptors*—phrases used to describe a product's nutritional level are limited to a list of 22 words selected and clearly defined by the FDA. Under the new guidelines, words such as *lite* or *light*, regardless of spelling, can only mean reduced calorie and cannot refer to color, flavor, or texture. Any descriptive term not defined when the regulation went into effect will be deemed illegal; (3) *Serving Size*—the serving size is standardized for 131 foods and includes measurements in metric units; and (4) *Nutrients*—all product labels must disclose the total calories, calories from fat, protein, and carbohydrate, as well as information regarding the total amount of fat, saturated fat, cholesterol, dietary fiber, sodium, calcium, and vitamins A and C. The labels must also indicate how a particular product meets the Daily Values (DV), which replace the old RDA's. These rules apply to all processed foods, but labeling of fresh meat and poultry is voluntary. The article " 'Daily Values' Encourage Healthy Diet" explains how DV's are arrived at and how they can serve consumers in selecting foods to balance their diets.

A common consumer health issue that we all face from time to time is how to decide whether a particular ache or pain warrants a visit to a physician. Faced with the high cost of medical care, more and more people are trying home remedies in an attempt to avoid the expense of an unnecessary visit to the doctor. While home remedies may be an effective treatment for some ailments, they may also mask important symptoms signaling a medical emergency and could delay proper treatment. Should the use of home remedies be discouraged? Not necessarily. For the most part, home remedies are relatively safe as long as they are not used for more than a couple of days, and their use is restricted to treating minor disorders. "Patient, Treat Thyself"

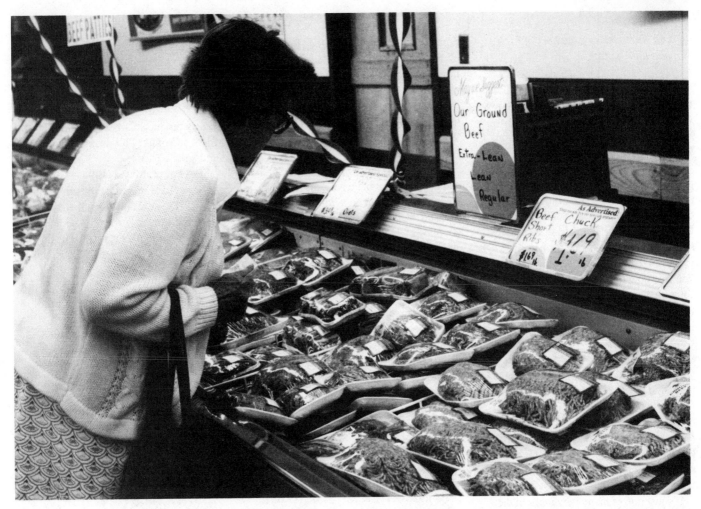

by Teresa Carr discusses several home remedies that may be used safely to treat minor ailments. She also discusses 10 home remedies that should never be used.

Suppose you needed major heart surgery or wanted a definitive answer on sleep disorders. Where would you go? When it comes to selecting medical care, few sources of information are readily available to consumers. Hospitals are like physicians in that some of them are specialized while others are generalists. The type of illness you have may warrant going to a hospital that functions as a specialist, but how do you know which ones are best? "Top Medical Centers" by David Levine provides a listing of the top medical centers for 16 different categories of illness.

Other consumer health issues covered by this unit include the testing of water quality, buying, storing, and using condoms to prevent the spread of AIDS, and helpful tips and information about selecting sunscreens and sunglasses. This unit is by no means exhaustive of all the possible topics that could be classified as consumer health issues, but it does demonstrate the diversity of such topics.

Looking Ahead: Challenge Questions

Should people be encouraged to try home remedies to treat minor ailments? If so, what precautions would you recommend?

What steps could be taken to eliminate deceptive advertising among food manufacturers? What should be done to those found guilty of deceptive advertising?

How would you decide which hospital to go to if you needed some form of specialized care?

Is the government doing enough to protect the consumer? If not, what recommendations would you make for changes?

'NUTRITION FACTS'

To Help Consumers Eat Smart

Paula Kurtzweil

Paula Kurtzweil is a member of FDA's public affairs staff.

Susan Thom, of Parma, Ohio, knows how important it is for people to know the number of calories from fat they eat each day.

As a registered dietitian, she counsels patients on the need to limit fat consumption to 30 percent or less of total daily calories. As a person with diabetes, and thus at increased risk for heart disease, she strives to do the same for herself.

But, in the past, obtaining that information from the food label has required some mathematical skill—namely, multiplying the total grams (g) of fat in a serving by 9, since 1 g of fat contains 9 calories.

"It does take time," Thom said. "But if you want to feed yourself well, you have to look at the label."

Help is on the way. For Thom and millions of other Americans who seek to restrict their fat intake to recommended levels, a new dietary component is being added to the food label—"calories from fat."

It's just one of many new items of diet-related information manufacturers are required to offer on their food products by 1994. There also will be information on saturated fat, cholesterol, dietary fiber, and other nutrients that relate to today's health concerns, such as heart disease, cancer, and other diseases linked, at least in part, to diet.

There will be more complete nutrient content information because almost all the required nutrients will have to be listed as a percent of the Daily Value. There will be more uniform serving sizes, too, which will make nutritional comparisons between foods easier. And, because nutri-

tion labeling is now mandatory for almost all processed foods, there will be a lot more products with this important information.

"The new information is going to be very helpful for consumers," said Virginia Wilkening, a registered dietitian in FDA's Office of Food Labeling.

"Some of the nutrients—saturated fat and cholesterol—have been allowed on the label before but on a voluntary basis," she said. "Dietary fiber and sugars were not allowed in the nutrition label. With the new label, consumers will soon have information about these and other nutrients, which can help them choose their foods more wisely."

The new requirements for nutrition labeling are spelled out in regulations issued in January 1993 by FDA and the U.S. Department of Agriculture's Food Safety and Inspection Service (FSIS). FDA's regulations meet the provisions of the Nutrition

Labeling and Education Act of 1990 (NLEA), which, among other things, requires FDA to make nutrition labeling mandatory for almost all processed foods. FSIS' regulations, which cover meat and poultry products, largely parallel FDA's. (Meat and poultry products were not covered by NLEA.)

FDA has set May 8, 1994, as the date by which food manufacturers must comply with the new nutrition labeling regulations. FSIS requires meat and poultry processors to relabel their products by July 6, 1994. However, some newly labeled products may begin appearing in grocery stores much sooner than the deadlines.

Dietary Components

What can consumers expect? First, they will see a new name for the nutrition panel. It used to go by "Nutrition Information Per Serving." Now, it will be called "Nutrition Facts." That title will

Old Label

NUTRITION INFORMATION	PER SERVING	PERCENTAGE OF U.S. RECOMMENDED DAILY ALLOWANCES (U.S. RDA)	
SERVING SIZE.................	5 OZ.	PROTEIN.............................	10
SERVINGS PER CONTAINER.........................	4	VITAMIN A.............................	*
		VITAMIN C.............................	*
CALORIES.........................	250	THIAMINE.............................	8
PROTEIN..............................	9g	RIBOFLAVIN........................	15
CARBOHYDRATE...............	19g	NIACIN................................	2
FAT......................................	11g	CALCIUM............................	20
SODIUM........................	530mg	IRON....................................	4

*CONTAINS LESS THAN 2% OF THE U.S. RDA OF THIS NUTRIENT

Starting this year, the 'old' nutrition label format above will be replaced by the one on the right. Both labels are for a frozen macaroni and cheese product.

   From *FDA Consumer,* May 1993, pp. 22-27. Reprinted by permission.

Key Aspects of the New Nutrition Label

A number of consumer studies conducted by FDA, as well as outside groups, enabled FDA and the Food Safety and Inspection Service of the U.S. Department of Agriculture to agree on a new nutrition label. The new label is seen as offering the best opportunity to help consumers make informed food choices and to understand how a particular food fits into the total daily diet.

New heading signals a new label. →

More consistent serving sizes, in both household and metric measures, replace those that used to be set by manufacturers.

Nutrients required on nutrition panel are those most important to the health of today's consumers, most of whom need to worry about → getting too much of certain items (fat, for example), rather than too few vitamins or minerals, as in the past.

Conversion guide helps consumers learn caloric value of the energy-producing nutrients.

New mandatory component helps consumers meet dietary guidelines recommending no more than 30 percent of calories from fat.

%Daily Value shows how a food fits into the overall daily diet.

Reference values help consumers learn good diet basics. They can be adjusted, depending on a person's calorie needs.

Nutrition Facts

Serving Size 1 cup (228g)
Serving Per Container 2

Amount Per Serving

Calories 260   Calories from Fat 120

	% Daily Value*
Total Fat 13g	**20**%
Saturated Fat 5g	**25**%
Cholesterol 30mg	**10**%
Sodium 660mg	**28**%
Total Carbohydrate 31g	**10**%
Dietary Fiber 0g	**0**%
Sugars 5g	
Protein 5g	

Vitamin A 4%	•	Vitamin C 2%
Calcium 15%	•	Iron 4%

* Percent Daily Values are based on a 2,000 calorie diet. Your daily values may be higher or lower depending on your calorie needs:

	Calories:	2,000	2,500
Total Fat	Less than	65g	80g
Sat Fat	Less than	20g	25g
Cholesterol	Less than	300mg	300mg
Sodium	Less than	2,400mg	2,400mg
Total Carbohydrate		300g	375g
Dietary Fiber		25g	30g

Calories per gram:
Fat 9 • Carbohydrate 4 • Protein 4

Types of Labels

A tabular format label (top) is allowed on packages, such as this can of tuna, that have less than 40 square inches for nutrition labeling. A simplified nutrition label (bottom), in which information about some nutrients otherwise required in nutrition labeling is omitted, will appear on labels of foods, such as this can of cola, that do not contain significant amounts of certain nutrients.

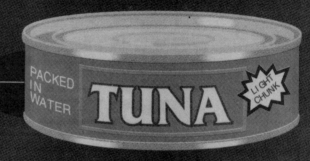

Nutrition Facts

Serv. Size 1/3 cup (56g)
Servings about 3
Calories 80
   Fat Cal. 10
*Percent Daily Values (DV) are based on a 2,000 calorie diet.

Amount/serving	%DV*	Amount/serving	%DV*
Total Fat 1g	**2%**	**Total Carb.** 0g	**0%**
Sat.Fat 0g	**0%**	Fiber 0g	**0%**
Cholest. 10mg	**3%**	Sugars 0g	
Sodium 200mg	**8%**	**Protein** 17g	

Vitamin A 0% • Vitamin C 0% • Calcium 0% • Iron 6%

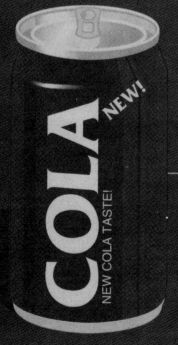

Nutrition Facts

Serving Size 1 can (360 mL)

Amount Per Serving	
Calories 140	
	% Daily Value*
Total Fat 0g	**0%**
Sodium 20mg	**1%**
Total Carbohydrate 36g	**12%**
Sugars 36 g	
Protein 0g	**0%**

* Percent Daily Values are based on a 2,000 calorie diet.

signal to consumers that the product is newly labeled according to FDA and FSIS' new regulations.

The new panel will be built around a new set of dietary components. (See graphic, page 209.) The mandatory (underlined) and voluntary dietary components and order in which they must appear are:

- total calories
- calories from fat
- calories from saturated fat
- total fat
- saturated fat
- stearic acid (on meat and poultry products only)
- polyunsaturated fat
- monounsaturated fat
- cholesterol
- sodium
- potassium
- total carbohydrate
- dietary fiber
- soluble fiber
- insoluble fiber
- sugars
- sugar alcohol (for example, the sugar substitutes xylitol, mannitol and sorbitol)
- other carbohydrate (the difference between total carbohydrate and the sum of dietary fiber, sugars, and sugar alcohol, if declared)
- protein
- vitamin A
- percent of vitamin A present as beta-carotene
- vitamin C
- calcium
- iron
- other essential vitamins and minerals.

If a food is fortified or enriched with any of the optional components, or if a claim is made about any of them, the pertinent nutrition information then becomes mandatory.

These mandatory and voluntary components are the only ones allowed on the nutrition panel. The listing of single amino acids, maltodextrin, calories from polyunsaturated fat, and calories from carbohydrate, for example, may not appear on the label.

The reason, according to Wilkening, is to help consumers focus on nutrients of public health significance. "Too much additional information could clutter the label or mislead or confuse the consumer," she said.

Nutrients required on the label, she pointed out, reflect current public health concerns and coincide with current public health recommendations. She noted that the order in which the food components and nutrients are required to appear reflects their public health significance and the order in which they were specified in NLEA.

On the new food label, the listing of thiamin, riboflavin and niacin will not be mandatory. Under the old nutrition labeling program, these vitamins were required to be listed. But because deficiencies of these are no longer a public health problem in this country, listing them is now optional.

New Format

Consumers also will see a new format, one that calls for many of the macronutrients (such as fat, cholesterol, sodium, carbohydrate, and protein) to be declared as a percent of the Daily Value—a new label reference value. The amount, in grams or milligrams per serving, of these nutrients still must be listed to their immediate right. But, for the first time, a column headed "%Daily Value" will appear.

According to Wilkening, the percent declaration of the Daily Value offers an advantage over amount declaration: The percent Daily Values put the nutrients on an equal footing in the context of a total daily diet.

For example, she said, a food is low in sodium if it has less than 140 mg of sodium. "But people look at that number, 140, and think it's a tremendous amount, when it actually is less than 6 percent of the Daily Value."

On the other hand, she said, a food with 5 g of saturated fat could be construed as being low in that nutrient just because 5 is a small number. Actually, that food would provide one-fourth the total Daily Value of 20 g of saturated fat for a 2,000-calorie diet.

"People are affected by the size of numbers," she said. "That's why percentages are helpful. They put all of the nutrients on a level playing field."

The percent Daily Value listing will carry a footnote stating that the percentages are based on a 2,000-calorie diet and that a person's individual dietary goal is based on his or her calorie needs. Some nutrition labels—at least those on larger packages—will list daily values for selected nutrients for a 2,000- and a 2,500-calorie diet and the number of calories per gram of fat, carbohydrate and protein. The calorie conversion information is required as a general guide about the caloric contributions of fat, carbohydrate and protein.

The content of micronutrients—that is, vitamins and minerals—will continue to be expressed as a percent, although the term "Daily Value" will replace "U.S. Recommended Daily Allowance."

Modifications

Some foods will carry a variation of this format. For example, the label of foods for children under 2 (except infant formula, which is exempt from nutrition labeling under NLEA) will not carry information about calories from fat, calories from saturated fat, saturated fat, polyunsaturated fat, monounsaturated fat, and cholesterol.

The reason, according to Wilkening, is to prevent parents from inadvertently assuming that infants and toddlers should restrict their fat intake, when in fact, they should not. Fat is important during this life stage, she said, to ensure adequate growth and development.

The labels of food for children under 4 cannot include percentages of Daily Values for macronutrients, except protein, nor any footnote information, including the lists of Daily Values for selected nutrients. The reason: Other than protein, FDA has not established Daily Values for macronutrients for this age group. The percent Daily Values for vitamins and minerals is allowed, however. The content of the other nutrients must be expressed as an amount by weight in a separate column to the right of the macronutrients.

Other foods may qualify for a simplified label format. (See bottom label, page 210.) This format is allowed when the food contains insignificant amounts of seven or more of the mandatory dietary components, including total calories. "Insignificant" means that a declaration of "zero" could be made in nutrition labeling or, for total carbohydrate, dietary fiber, and protein, a declaration of "less than 1 g."

For foods for children under 2, the simplified format may be used if the product contains insignificant amounts of six or more of the following: calories, total fat, sodium, total carbohydrate, dietary fiber, sugars, protein, vitamins A and C, calcium, and iron.

When the simplified format is used, information on total calories, total fat, total carbohydrate, protein, and sodium—even if they are present in insignificant amounts—must be listed. Calories from fat and other nutrients must be listed if they are present in more than insignificant amounts. Nutrients added to the food must be listed, too.

Serving Sizes

Whatever the format, the serving size remains the basis for reporting each nutrient's amount. However, unlike in the past, serving sizes now will be more uniform and closer to the amounts that many people actually eat. They also must be expressed in both common household and metric measures. (See accompanying table.)

Before, the serving size was up to the discretion of the food manufacturer. As a result, said Youngmee Park, Ph.D., a nutritionist in FDA's Office of Special Nutritionals, serving sizes often varied widely, making it difficult for consumers to compare nutritional qualities of similar products or to determine the nutrient content of the amount of food they normally ate.

The uniformity also is important, she said, for giving consistency to health claims and words describing nutrient content, such as "high fiber" and "reduced fat."

FDA and FSIS define serving size as the amount of food customarily eaten at one time. It is based on FDA- and USDA-established lists of "Reference Amounts Customarily Consumed Per Eating Occasion."

These reference amounts, which are part of the new regulations, are broken down into 139 FDA-regulated food product categories, including 11 groups of foods for children under 4, and 23 USDA meat and poultry product categories. They list the amounts of food customarily consumed per eating occasion for each food category, based primarily on national food consumption surveys. FDA's list also gives the suggested label statement for serving size declaration.

For example, the category "breads (excluding sweet quick type), rolls" has a reference amount of 50 g, and the appropriate label statement for sliced bread is "__ piece(s) __ (g)" or, for unsliced bread, "2 oz (56 g/__ inch slice)."

The serving size of products that come in discrete units, such as cookies, candy bars, and sliced products, is the number of whole units that most closely approximates the reference amount. For example, cookies have a reference amount of 30 g. The household measure closest to that amount is the number of cookies that comes closest to weighing 30 g. Thus, the

Metric Conversion Chart

Units as they will appear for serving sizes on label

Household Measure	Metric Measure
1 tsp	5 mL
1 tbsp	15 mL
1 cup	240 mL
1 fl oz	30 mL
1 oz	28 g

tsp = teaspoon

tbsp = tablespoon

fl oz = fluid ounce

oz = ounce

mL = milliliter

g = gram

serving size on the label of a cookie package in which each cookie weighs 13 g would read "2 cookies (26 g)."

If one unit weighs more than 50 percent but less than 200 percent of the reference amount, the serving size is one unit. For example, the reference amount for bread is 50 g; therefore, the label of a loaf of bread in which each slice weighs more than 25 g would state that a serving size is one slice.

For food products packaged and sold individually, if an individual package is less than 200 percent of the applicable reference amount, the item qualifies as one serving. Thus, a 360-milliliter (mL) (12 fluid-ounce) can of soda is one serving because the reference amount for carbonated beverages is 240 mL (8 fluid ounces).

However, if the product has a reference amount of 100 g or 100 mL or more and the package contains more than 150 percent but less than 200 percent of the reference amount, manufacturers have the option of deciding whether the product is one or two servings.

For example, the serving size reference amount for soup is 245 g. So a 15-ounce (420 g) can can be listed as either one or two servings.

Presentation

There also are rules governing how the nutrition information is displayed. Under existing FDA regulations, nutrition information must appear on the information panel to the immediate right of the principal panel. Thus, on boxed foods, for example, in which the principal panel is on the front of the box, the nutrition information appears on the right side of the box. Packages whose area to the immediate right is too small or not suited for such labeling may provide information on the next panel to the right.

FSIS allows nutrition information to be listed on the principal or information panels.

The new food labeling rules call for one additional variation: For packages that are 40 square inches or less, the nutrition information may be placed on any label panel.

The rules also address size and prominence of the typeface. For example, the heading "Nutrition Facts" must be set in the largest type on the nutrition panel and be highlighted in some manner, such as boldface, all capital letters, or another graphic to distinguish it from the other information. Such highlighting also is required for headings such as "Amount per serving" and "%Daily Value" and for the names of dietary components that are not subcomponents—that is, calories, total fat, cholesterol, sodium, total carbohydrate, and protein.

Exceptions and Exemptions

In some instances, special provisions

exist for providing nutrition information. For example:

• Nutrition information about game meat, such as deer, bison, rabbit, quail, wild turkey, and ostrich, may be provided on counter cards, signs, or other point-of-purchase materials. Because little nutrient data exists for these foods, FDA believes that allowing this option will enable game meat producers to give first priority to collecting appropriate data and make it easier for them to update the information as it becomes available.

• FDA-regulated food packages with less than 12 square inches available for nutrition labeling do not have to carry nutrition information. However, they must provide an address or telephone number for consumers to obtain the required nutrition information.

• Packages with less than 40 square inches for nutrition labeling may present nutrition information in a tabular format (see top label, page 210), abbreviate the names of dietary components, and omit the footnotes with the list of daily values and caloric conversion information but include a footnote stating that the percent Daily Values are based on a 2,000-calorie diet or place nutrition information on other panels.

Some foods are exempt from nutrition labeling. These include:

• food produced by small businesses. (As mandated by NLEA, FDA defines a small business as one with food sales of less than $50,000 a year or total sales of less than $500,000. FSIS defines a small business as one employing 500 or fewer employees and producing no more than a certain amount of product per year.)

• food served for immediate consumption, such as that served in restaurants and hospital cafeterias, on airplanes, and by food service vendors (such as mall cookie counters, sidewalk vendors, and vending machines)

• ready-to-eat foods that are not for immediate consumption, as long as the food is primarily prepared on site—for example, many bakery, deli, and candy store items

• food shipped in bulk, as long as it is not for sale in that form to consumers

• medical foods

• plain coffee and tea, flavor extracts, food colors, some spices, and other foods that contain no significant amounts of any nutrients

• donated foods

• products intended for export

• individually wrapped FSIS-regulated products weighing less than half an ounce and making no nutrient content claims.

Although these foods are exempt, they are free to carry nutrition information, when appropriate—as long as it complies with the new regulations.

But, there will be plenty of other foods carrying the new nutrition information. Dietitian Susan Thom sees that as a plus.

"We'll all know exactly what we're putting in our mouths," she said. "So there'll be little room for excuses."

'DAILY VALUES'

Encourage Healthy Diet

Paula Kurtzweil

Paula Kurtzweil is a member of FDA's public affairs staff.

I f you haven't added "DV" to your vocabulary yet, you probably will before long.

It stands for Daily Value, a new dietary reference value to help consumers use food label information to plan a healthy overall diet.

DVs actually comprise two sets of reference values for nutrients: Daily Reference Values, or DRVs, and Reference Daily Intakes, or RDIs. But these two sets are "behind the scenes" in food labeling; only the Daily Value term will appear on the label to make label reading less confusing.

In fact, said Christine Lewis, Ph.D., a registered dietitian and director of the division of technical evaluation in FDA's Office of Food Labeling, the Daily Value term is the only one of the terms that will be used in the government's food labeling education campaign. "The DV term is the one we expect consumers and professionals to use," she said.

FDA-regulated products must begin using the Daily Value as the basis for declaring nutrient content by May 8, 1994. U.S.

Department of Agriculture-regulated products—meat and poultry—have until July 6, 1994.

The move to Daily Values is due in large part to the Nutrition Labeling and Education Act of 1990. Among other things, the law requires nutrition label information to be conveyed in a way that enables the public to observe and comprehend the information readily and to understand its relative significance in the context of a total daily diet.

According to Lewis, the DV does that in two ways: First, it serves as a basis for declaring on the label the percent of the Daily Value for each nutrient that a serving of the food provides.

For example, the Daily Value for fat, based on a 2,000-calorie diet, is 65 grams (g). A food that has 13 g of fat per serving would state on the label that the "percent Daily Value" for fat is 20 percent.

Second, it provides a basis for thresholds that define descriptive words for nutrient content, called descriptors, such as "high fiber" and "low fat." For example, the descriptor "high fiber" can be used if a serving of food provides 20 percent or

more of the Daily Value for fiber—that is, 5 g or more.

What it is *not* intended to do is tell people what amounts of nutrients they should eat every day.

"They're not recommended intakes," Lewis said. "They're really just reference points to help people get some kind of perspective on what their overall daily dietary needs should be."

New References

Although they won't show up on the label, DRVs and RDIs have an important regulatory role. They serve as the basis for calculating percent Daily Values.

DRVs are for nutrients for which no set of standards previously existed, such as fat and cholesterol. RDIs, on the other hand, replace the term "U.S. RDAs" (Recommended Daily Allowances), which were introduced in 1973 as a reference value for vitamins, minerals and protein in voluntary nutrition labeling. Despite the name change, the actual values (except the value for protein) will remain the same—at least for the time being. FDA will consider revising these values in the near future.

From *FDA Consumer,* May 1993, pp. 28-32. Reprinted by permission.

Daily Reference Values (DRVs) *

Food Component	DRV
fat	65 grams (g)
saturated fatty acids	20 g
cholesterol	300 milligrams (mg)
total carbohydrate	300 g
fiber	25 g
sodium	2,400 mg
potassium	3,500 mg
protein**	50 g

*Based on 2,000 calories a day for adults and children over 4 only

**DRV for protein does not apply to certain populations; Reference Daily Intake (RDI) for protein has been established for these groups: children 1 to 4 years: 16 g; infants under 1 year: 14 g; pregnant women: 60 g; nursing mothers: 65 g.

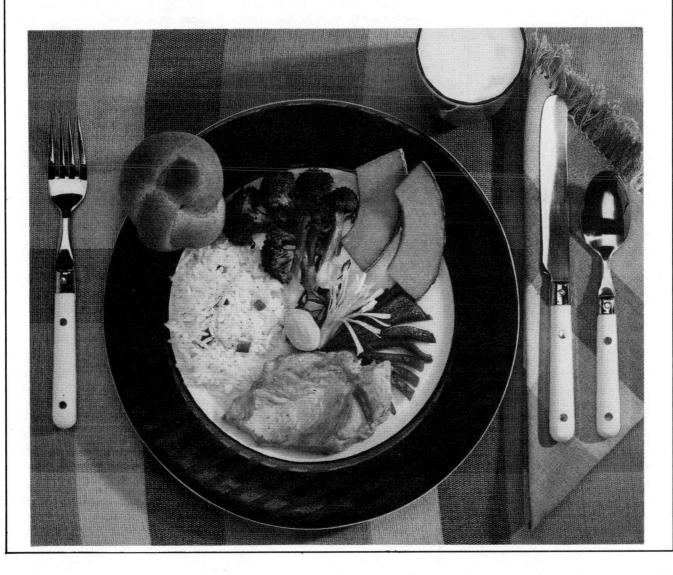

*Reference Daily Intakes (RDIs)**

Nutrient	Amount
vitamin A	5,000 International Units (IU)
vitamin C	60 milligrams (mg)
thiamin	1.5 mg
riboflavin	1.7 mg
niacin	20 mg
calcium	1.0 gram (g)
iron	18 mg
vitamin D	400 IU
vitamin E	30 IU
vitamin B_6	2.0 mg
folic acid	0.4 mg
vitamin B_{12}	6 micrograms (mcg)
phosphorus	1.0 g
iodine	150 mcg
magnesium	400 mg
zinc	15 mg
copper	2 mg
biotin	0.3 mg
pantothenic acid	10 mg

*Based on National Academy of Sciences' 1968 Recommended Dietary Allowances.

U.S. RDAs should not be confused with RDAs. The latter are short for Recommended *Dietary* Allowances, which are set by the National Academy of Sciences. FDA used the RDAs as the basis for setting U.S. RDAs (now called RDIs).

The confusion caused by the similarity of those terms was one of the reasons for the switch to RDI.

"The comments we received about the proposed name change generally agreed that there was a need to change the terminology," Lewis said. "People reported that it caused problems both in consumer education and with professional communication."

DRVs

DRVs for the energy-producing nutrients (fat, carbohydrate, protein, and fiber) are based on the number of calories consumed per day. For labeling purposes, 2,000 calories has been established as the reference for calculating percent Daily Values. This level was chosen, in part, because many health experts say it approximates the maintenance calorie requirements of the group most often targeted for weight reduction: postmenopausal women.

Also, unlike the 2,350-calorie reference that FDA used in its proposal, 2,000 calories is a rounded number, which makes it easier for consumers to calculate their individual nutrient needs.

The label will include—at least on larger packages—a footnote on the nutrition panel in which daily values for selected nutrients for both a 2,000- and a 2,500-calorie diet are listed. Manufacturers have the option of listing daily values for other calorie levels, if label space allows and as long as the Daily Values for the other two levels are listed, too.

Whatever the calorie level, DRVs for the energy-producing nutrients are always calculated as follows:
- fat based on 30 percent of calories
- saturated fat based on 10 percent of calories
- carbohydrate based on 60 percent of calories
- protein based on 10 percent of calories. (The DRV for protein applies only to adults and children over 4. RDIs for protein for special groups have been established. See table on previous page.)
- fiber based on 11.5 g of fiber per 1,000 calories.

Thus, someone who consumes 3,000 calories a day—a teenage boy, for example—would have a recommended intake for fat of 100 g or less per day. [0.30 x 3,000 = 900; 900 (calories) ÷ 9 (calories per g of fat) = 100 g]

The DRVs for cholesterol, sodium and potassium, which do not contribute calories, remain the same whatever the calorie level. (See table on previous page.)

Because of the links between certain nutrients and certain diseases, DRVs for some nutrients represent the uppermost limit that is considered desirable. Eating too much fat or cholesterol, for example, has been linked to an increased risk of heart disease. Too much sodium can heighten the risk of high blood pressure in some people.

Therefore, the label will show DVs for fats and sodium as follows:

Alphabet Soup Made Appetizing

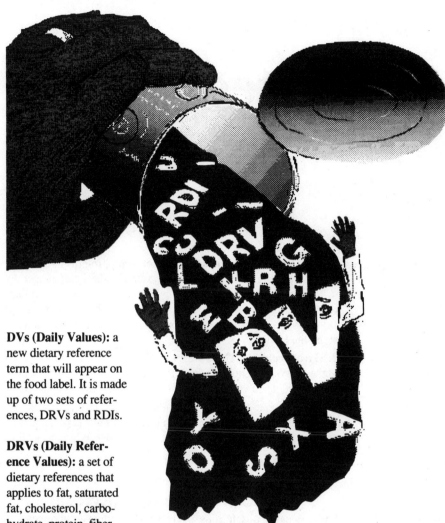

DVs (Daily Values): a new dietary reference term that will appear on the food label. It is made up of two sets of references, DRVs and RDIs.

DRVs (Daily Reference Values): a set of dietary references that applies to fat, saturated fat, cholesterol, carbohydrate, protein, fiber, sodium, and potassium.

RDIs (Reference Daily Intakes): a set of dietary references based on the Recommended Dietary Allowances for essential vitamins and minerals and, in selected groups, protein. The name "RDI" replaces the term "U.S. RDA."

RDAs (Recommended Dietary Allowances): a set of estimated nutrient allowances established by the National Academy of Sciences. It is updated periodically to reflect current scientific knowledge.

Although consumers will continue to see vitamins and minerals expressed as percentages on the label, these percentages now refer to the Daily Values.

- total fat: less than 65 g
- saturated fat: less than 20 g
- cholesterol: less than 300 mg (milligrams)
- sodium: less than 2,400 mg

RDIs Replace U.S. RDAs

Unlike DRVs, which are a new concept, many consumers may already have a good idea of what the RDIs are. That's because the RDIs (the former U.S. RDAs used by FDA) have been around for almost 20 years as the established estimated values for vitamins, minerals and protein.

The provisions of the Nutrition Labeling and Education Act and the Dietary Supplement Act of 1992 require FDA to retain these estimated values for at least another year.

Although consumers will continue to see vitamins and minerals expressed as percentages on the label, these percentages now refer to the Daily Values.

Getting to Know DVs

Like any new concept, DVs may take some getting used to but, through education and practice, FDA and USDA believe it soon will become second nature to many consumers.

"As more and more new labels make their way into the marketplace," Lewis said, "people will gradually become familiar with the DV term and be able to use the information effectively."

"I think consumers are going to find it very helpful," she said.

Full sun protection

There is no such thing as safe sunbathing. More and more people are getting the message that the sun causes skin cancer and premature aging of the skin. Plus, it's hard on your eyes.

Can you separate the myths from the facts below?

1. You can't get a sunburn on a cloudy day.

2. It's better to use a sunscreen with two active ingredients than just one.

3. If you freckle easily, you should not try to tan.

4. Sunglasses and a wide-brimmed hat may help prevent cataracts in later life.

5. Cheap drugstore sunglasses won't protect your eyes.

6. Self-tanning lotions, which darken your skin, prevent sunburn.

7. A high intake of vitamin C and beta carotene (as in carrots) will help prevent sunburn.

8. Very dark-skinned people don't need a sunscreen.

Answers

1. Myth. Clouds do filter a small percentage of the sun's ultraviolet (UV) radiation, but enough gets through to cause serious sunburns.

2. Fact. Two kinds of ultraviolet light damage the skin; it takes different ingredients to protect you from each of them.

3. Fact. A freckle is a patch of melanin, the pigment that absorbs UV rays and acts as the body's defense against the sun. If you freckle rather than tan, this is a sign that your skin lacks enough melanin to defend its whole surface against sunlight. The parts that don't freckle will burn.

4. Fact. Lifelong exposure to bright sunlight can promote cataracts. A hat with a brim not only protects your eyes, but also your face, neck, and lips.

5. Myth. When it comes to sunglasses, you can't always go by price. If you know what to look for, you can get adequate sunglasses for under $10.

6. Myth. Sunless tanning lotions contain a colorless dye (DHA) that turns a golden color when it reacts with proteins in the outer layer of the skin. The color fades in just a few days, but many fair-skinned people prefer self-tanning lotions to the risks of sunning. However, this is not a real tan and won't guard against burns and skin damage. A few of these lotions do contain a sunscreen and say so on the label.

7. Myth, probably. There are many good reasons to eat foods high in these two nutrients, but don't forsake your sunscreen. Research so far has not shown that diet has any effect in preventing sunburn.

8. Fact. African-Americans and other dark-skinned people have a high concentration of melanin, which absorbs UV rays. Thus they are less susceptible to sunburn, sun-induced wrinkling, as well as skin cancer.

Sunscreens: the full spectrum

Sunscreens are oils, lotions, or creams containing compounds that filter out UV rays. A sunscreen is a necessity, even if you're tan (unless you are naturally very dark-skinned). The good news is that sunscreens are better than they were even a few years ago. Most contain two or more active ingredients to protect against the two types of UV radiation (A and B) and most are water-resistant.

Screens with sun protection factors (SPFs) higher than 15 are now far less likely to cause skin irritation. PABA (para-aminobenzoic acid), once the most common ingredient, often caused itching or rashes. It has mostly been replaced with PABA derivatives, such as padimate-O, which are less likely to irritate. Other common and effective sunscreen ingredients are cinnamates (such as octyl methoxycinnamate) and salicylates.

Because sunburns in childhood are a risk factor for skin cancer much later in life, it's important to apply sunscreen with an SPF of at least 15 to fair-skinned children beginning at six months. (Keep small children out of the sun during peak hours.) Most sunscreens for children pose little risk of skin irritation.

What an SPF means

It tells you the relative length of time you can stay in the sun before you burn, compared to using no sunscreen. A product with an SPF of 8, for example, would allow you to remain in the sun without burning eight times longer than if you didn't apply it. Thus if you would burn in 10 minutes, a screen with SPF 8 would allow you 80 minutes before burning. Remember, these are only averages. The effectiveness of specific sunscreens varies from person to person—and also depends on how much you apply.

Studies have shown, however, that people tend to apply only about half the amount of sunscreen that the FDA uses to determine SPF. Thus SPF 15 would drop, in effect, to about SPF 8. So if you're fair-skinned or will be outside for hours, either use a high-protection sunscreen (SPF 20 or more) or apply your sunscreen at frequent intervals.

What the SPF doesn't tell you

The SPF, however, pertains only to ultraviolet B (UVB) rays—those mainly responsible for sunburn and skin cancer. Most of the active ingredients in chemical sunscreens effectively absorb UVB rays, but let through the longer-wavelength ultraviolet A (UVA) rays, which researchers once thought would help you tan without harming the skin. Now it appears that UVA radiation can damage the skin's connective tissue, leading to premature aging, and that it also plays a role in causing skin cancer. However, there is no rating system to indicate how well a sunscreen protects you from UVA. Thus two screens with the same SPF can offer very different UVA protection.

Protection against UVA

The chemical compound avobenzone offers the fullest protection against UVA rays. So far, the FDA has approved only two products that contain it. One is Photoplex, the other is Shade UVAGUARD. Both are broad-spectrum screens that also protect against UVB. Both have an SPF of 15. Of the common ingredients in other sunscreens, benzophenones (such as oxybenzone) offer some protection against UVA rays, but less than Photoplex and Shade UVAGUARD. Benzophenones are used together with anti-UVB chemicals, such as padimate-O.

New claims

At least one new sunscreen contains a synthetic form of melanin (the natural pigment that absorbs UV light and permits tanning). In theory, synthetic melanin should prevent sun damage, but there's no scientific evidence that it will retain its protective properties when smeared on your skin—in spite of manufacturers' claims.

You'll also see sunscreens that contain antioxidants—vitamins C and E, for example. (Sunlight produces highly reactive molecules called free radicals, which can damage the skin, and antioxidants "mop up" these free radicals.) The theory behind using these two antioxidants on the skin is that if—and that's a big if—they penetrate the outer layer of skin and settle in the dermis, they might prevent free-radical damage. Some preliminary research, still unpublished, is said to be promising. Other studies, mostly using animals, have had inconsistent results.

This doesn't mean that melanin or antioxidants may not be proved useful at some point. Meanwhile, the only sure thing is that most sunscreens that contain them are expensive. Other products will probably do the job just as effectively.

Sunblocks

The true sunblocks are the opaque creams or pastes containing zinc oxide or titanium dioxide. When properly applied, they prevent all light from reaching the skin; thus they carry no SPF rating. They are good for the nose, lips, or other sensitive areas, but they look like clown makeup and are messy to use. However, some chemical sunscreens now contain titanium dioxide or zinc oxide in highly pulverized form. These work just as well and are less messy and less opaque.

Even though screens with an SPF above 15 are sometimes referred to as sunblocks, they still allow some UV wavelengths to pass through to the skin.

How to select and use a sunscreen

■ **Choose a screen with SPF 15.** If you're fair-skinned or will be outdoors for long hours, use one with an even higher SPF. Look for the seal of approval from the Skin Cancer Foundation, which tests sunscreens with SPF 15 or higher for safety and effectiveness in blocking UVB.

■ **For greatest protection against both UVA and UVB rays,** use Photoplex or Shade UVAGUARD. Otherwise, look for a "broad-spectrum" sunscreen with two or more ultraviolet-absorbing ingredients. Many ingredient combinations work in concert to block a broad range of light waves.

■ **Apply the screen at least 30 to 45 minutes** before exposure to the sun; this allows it to penetrate the skin.

■ **Apply it frequently and generously.** If you swim or tend to sweat a lot, look for a waterproof or water-resistant screen.

■ **Take into account the time of day and your location.** UV rays are strongest between 10 A.M. and 3 P.M., so adjust your sunscreen strength and reapplication schedule accordingly. The sun is more intense the closer you are to the Equator and the higher the altitude. If you're fair-skinned, you may need to wear protective clothing, a hat, and a sunblock on your nose and lips.

■ **Don't assume that because your skin isn't red, it isn't getting burned.** A sunburn becomes most evident 6 to 24 hours after sunning.

■ **If you're taking medication,** ask your doctor or pharmacist about possible reactions to sunlight and interactions with sunscreens.

Sunglasses: safety and quality

Everybody needs sunglasses, and not just in the summer. Exposure to UV rays over the years can damage the lens, retina, and cornea. No one knows how many of the one million cataract cases reported each year in the U.S. are sun-related and thus preventable, but it can't hurt to take the precaution of wearing sunglasses year round when you're in the sun. *Any sunglasses are better than no sunglasses.* It's not true that sunglasses cause your eyes to dilate and thus admit more UV rays. Here's how to buy sunglasses:

■ **Choose sunglasses that block as much UV rays as possible and at least 75% of visible light.** The tint blocks some visible light, but not UV rays. Clear glass or plastic will absorb a certain amount of UV rays. But special chemicals need to be added to the lens when the glasses are made to do the best blocking job. (You can have your clear lenses treated so they also will block virtually 100% of UV rays.) Labeling for UV and visible light blockage is voluntary, and there are no government standards. If possible, buy glasses that meet the standards of the American National Standard Institute (ANSI). Look for the following ANSI labels: *General Purpose*—medium to dark tinted lenses for use in any outdoor activity. *Special Purpose*—for very bright environments, such as skiing, tropical beaches, and mountain climbing. *Cosmetic*—lightly tinted lenses for use in shopping and other around-town uses. Glasses without a label may be fine, but it's hard to be sure.

Some lenses may not block an adequate amount of visible light. Check this by trying on the glasses and looking in a mirror; if they're dark enough, you won't be able to see your eyes. Avoid glasses that are too dark, as they could cut your vision too much and contribute to falls or other mishaps. Ask the clerk if you may step outside for a moment to test the glasses in bright light.

■ **Select sunglasses that block at least part of the blue light.** These rays are lower in frequency than UV. There's controversy about the danger of blue light. Some scientists think that lifetime exposure may damage the retina and contribute to blindness; others think these fears are exaggerated. Still, any pair of sunglasses that blocks 75% of visible light will also block a significant amount of blue light. Brown or amber-tinted lenses screen blue light best, though they do produce some color distortion. Blue light is of most concern to the groups listed in the box below.

■ **Get glasses that don't distort colors excessively.** You should be able to distinguish the colors of traffic lights, for example. Gray lenses are the least distorting for most people; amber and brown are good, too. Blue and purple tend to distort too much.

■ **Check that the sunglasses don't distort shapes and lines.** Hold the glasses at arm's length and look at a straight line in the distance. Slowly move the lenses across that line; if it sways or bends, then the lenses are imperfect. Look through the outer edges as well as the center of the lenses.

■ **Make sure the sunglasses are large enough** to keep out light from above, below, and the sides of the frame. Wraparound styles are often quite protective. If you're going to use the glasses for driving, make sure the frames don't block your peripheral vision. Small round glasses are fashionable again, but they don't provide as much protection.

■ **Choose comfortable sunglasses that suit your activities.** Lens and frame type are largely a matter of personal choice. *Plastic* lenses are best for most people. *Glass* doesn't scratch as easily, but can be heavy. *Mirrored* lenses scratch easily. *Gradient* lenses (darker at the top than at the bottom) are useful for driving, since they let you see the dashboard more clearly.

Special needs

See an eye-care professional for sunglasses if:

■ you've had cataract surgery, which removes the eye's UV-absorbent lens.

■ you take medication that increases sensitivity to UV.

■ your sport or job keeps you outdoors much of the time, particularly in locations where sunlight is reflected off water, sand, or snow, or if you live at a high altitude.

the purist's guide to tap water

Worried about what's coming out of your faucet? We make it all perfectly clear.

John Poppy

John Poppy is a contributing editor.

Jack DeMarco thinks the tap water in Cincinnati is as safe as water can be made these days. He drinks it. His family drinks it. Of course, there might be a bit of a scandal if they didn't, since DeMarco is the guy responsible for keeping it clean—no small job in a city that draws most of its raw material from the Ohio River.

"An industrial river" is how DeMarco, superintendent of water quality and treatment for the Cincinnati Water Works, characterizes it. Flowing southwest from Pittsburgh through 460 miles of population, industry, and agriculture before reaching Cincinnati's intake pipe, the waterway contains traces of as many as 200 different chemicals on any given day. Among them are benzene, toluene, and others listed by the U.S. Environmental Protection Agency as causing nerve damage, cancer, and other grave illnesses. Also floating in the current: effluents from 120 city sewers and 150 factories.

So he wouldn't dip his coffee cup into the Ohio and drink from it? "No," he says, recoiling in mock horror. But only because of the bacteria—a hazard in any raw river water—not the chemicals. Since last October, the city has handily met that challenge with the world's largest, most elaborate water-scrubbing carbon filters.

Not that chemicals aren't an increasingly common worry around the country. When DeMarco's son and daughter-in-law moved to a Southern city he doesn't want to name, that city's own reports on the lead and toxic chemicals coming out of its taps prompted him to suggest that his grandchildren drink only bottled water until the city cleaned up its act. And just this April investigators from the U.S. General Accounting Office cast doubt on the effectiveness of the state inspections that are supposed to assure the 232 million Americans who slake their thirst at the municipal trough that their water is safe. People served by small systems with fewer than 3,300 customers—28 million people in all—are particularly at risk. But nearly everyone has reason to worry. Twenty-three states inspect less frequently now than they did five years ago, and some consumers are drinking from systems that haven't been inspected in ten years. Among the more egregious goofs the investigators cited, regardless of system size, were cross-connections that let sewage and industrial pollutants leak into pipes carrying drinking water.

No wonder sales of bottled water have more than doubled in the past ten years. No wonder the nation's water suppliers are scrambling to find ways to deliver a cleaner, safer product.

One particularly vexing problem confronts all comers: what to do about the potentially hazardous chemical byproducts that form when chlorine, the major germ-killer in nearly all treated water, comes in contact with dissolved particles of decaying leaves, dead animals, and other natural debris that fall into reservoirs and rivers. One of those byproducts, chloroform, is suspected of increasing the risk of cancer of the bladder and rectum.

The solution certainly isn't to throw out the chlorine with the drinking water. There's no telling how many people it has saved since 1908, when it was introduced in New Jersey, from swallowing armies of bacteria, viruses, and molds that would have killed them or at least made them feel wretched. What's needed, nearly everyone agrees, is a way to filter out more of the organic debris before chlorine hits it.

Since last October, Cincinnati's answer has been to run its water through the usual settling ponds and sand filters and then through 12 deep pools of black, sandy carbon. Actually crushed coal riddled with chemical-adsorbing pores, the carbon does a great job of trapping organic chemicals—the toxic troublemakers that lurk in much of the nation's drinking water. Because it also removes most of the organic matter that slips through in other systems, Cincinnati uses less chlorine than it did before—about one-fourth as much. That means less chloroform and other chlorination byproducts.

Scores of other cities around the country, DeMarco says, have long used carbon filters to remove pesticides and sweeten up water that smells of chlorine and other unpopular flavors. As it happens, those filters also remove other chemicals—for the first few months. But DeMarco's counterparts replace their carbon only once every three years or so, long after it's become so coated with gunk it can't trap most contaminants.

Cincinnati refreshes its filters every four to six months. Their sheer size (each could swallow a two-story house) and their mission (wiping out most of the chemicals in the city's water) are what make the Cincinnati Water Works unusual. But what makes it unique is two giant 1,500-degree furnaces that "reactivate" old carbon, burning off the gunk the filters collect and destroying the poisonous vapors.

Cincinnati built its carbon filters and furnaces for $60 million; running them adds about six cents a day to an average family's water bill. Admittedly Cincinnati's monument to water purity isn't the answer to every problem. It would be an expensive choice for systems less focused on chemical pollutants—many of those in the West, for example, with access to more pristine watersheds. Nor would it have been much use this past April against a tiny parasite called *Cryptosporidium parvum*, which sickened as many as 370,000 people in and around Milwaukee, sent nearly 2,000 to doctors with severe diarrhea, caused one death, and contributed to five others after millions of its "eggs," or cysts, slipped through the city's sand filters. But for the 120 million or so Americans in Cincinnati's boat— those who live on industrial rivers such as the Ohio, Missouri, Mississippi, and their feeder streams, and in factory and farm areas where chemicals seep into underground water supplies—it's clearly worth a long look. Cincinnatians, DeMarco figures, get a lot of peace of mind for $22 a year.

That's fine for them, but what about the rest of us? What if the water tastes odd? How worrisome, really, are the reports of leaking gas tanks, neighborhood cancer clusters, and cities in the throes of diarrhea? Plenty worrisome, obviously, if you're sitting down-faucet from a pocket of high pollution. In general, though, the picture is not as dark as it often appears.

WHAT'S THE WORST THAT CAN HAPPEN IF I DRINK AVERAGE AMERICAN TAP WATER ALL MY LIFE?

Probably nothing you should lose sleep over. The three threats that worry water experts most are these: microbes (viruses, bacteria, and intestinal parasites such as cryptosporidium and giardia); chemicals (inorganic, such as lead and nitrate, and organic, such as benzene and several dozen others on the EPA health advisory list); and disinfection byproducts (what chlorine, for example, gives off when it mixes with the

---

| HOW TO | Avoid Troubled Waters at Home

IF YOU'RE WORRIED about what might be in your tap water, there are a lot of places to turn for help. Make your calls in this order:

YOUR LOCAL WATER SUPPLIER

If you pay a water bill, the phone number is on it. Most water companies will send someone to try to fix a problem or at least explain what's going on.

The law says your water company must test its finished product regularly and make the results available to you. (Ask also for a test of water from your own faucets to see if something is harming it between the treatment plant and you. Most water districts will test for free.) On the printout they send you, look for the detected levels of the big five—bacteria, lead, nitrate, radium, disinfection byproducts—and for any other substances that exceed Environmental Protection Agency standards, usually printed alongside the actual level in your water.

YOUR CITY, COUNTY, OR STATE WATER AGENCY

You can usually find these in the government section of the phone book under the health or environmental department. If you don't get satisfaction from your local supplier, these are the highest levels to which you can appeal for help with problems such as taste or smell that the EPA considers undesirable but not a threat to health.

AN INDEPENDENT LABORATORY

If your water comes from a private well, you should probably have it tested by an independent lab every year for bacteria, metals, and radon. Rather than order up scattershot tests, it's more efficient and less expensive to think about what specific substances you're after. If the well is within a couple of miles of a gas station, refinery, chemical plant, landfill, or military base, have it tested for organic chemicals. If you live near a farm or ranch, have it tested for nitrate and pesticides. Shop around. Lab charges can run from $35 for a lead test to around $100 for a broad-spectrum scan for chemicals and bacteria; for around $45 to $135 more, they'll check for pesticides. Don't bother with giardia and cryptosporidium; only a few labs in the country test for them, the tests require a suitcase-size piece of equipment (which the lab will lend you), they cost at least $200, and they're inaccurate. The best labs estimate they catch only one out of every five cysts in 100 gallons of water.

THE EPA SAFE DRINKING WATER HOTLINE

If you feel your problem isn't being solved, and it concerns a contaminant the EPA regulates, the hotline will relay your complaint to an EPA enforcement officer. The hotline, at 800/426-4791, is open weekdays, 9 A.M. to 5:30 P.M., EST. —*J. P.*

---

residue of decaying leaves and other organic debris).

Microbes are the most likely to make you suddenly sick, but your risk is low unless something in the water supply leaps out of control, as it did in Milwaukee this April. At the right concentration, chlorine kills the bacteria that used to cause epidemics of cholera and typhoid, and filters are supposed to take out bad actors that chlorine doesn't kill, including most parasite cysts.

Less serious dangers may be another story. In a 1988–89 study, Canadian researcher Pierre Payment found more cases of diarrhea, vomiting, and nausea among tap water drinkers in a middle-class suburb of Montreal than among people using home filters, even though the straight tap water met government standards (generally parallel to those in the United States). "We don't have a clue about the cause," he says. "It might have been a few viruses or parasites getting through the water treatment system. Or it might be bacteria regrowing in the water pipes in the houses." Payment will soon repeat the study in another Canadian city.

Nobody counts how many intestinal miseries people blame every year on flu or indigestion, but the number actually caused by tap water may be "non-trivial," in Payment's words. "People think, It's only diarrhea," he says. "But if you look at the economic impact in the U.S. of just what we found in our study—infectious gastrointestinal illness—it's about $30 billion a year, ranging from hospital care to loss of productivity."

Chemicals attract more attention than microbes because so many are linked to cancer and other diseases. Hexachlorocyclopentadiene sounds a lot scarier than a bug. Yet few of the chemicals on the EPA's most-dangerous list have been shown beyond a doubt to harm humans through drinking water. Those that have—chiefly nitrate, lead, and copper—don't cause cancer. They damage the blood, heart, and nervous system. Several others—among them benzene and vinyl chloride—do have a history of causing cancer, but almost entirely in people who inhale them or get splashed in factories or on farms. Most connections between human cancer and chemicals in drinking water are extrapolated from experiments on laboratory animals, and critics say that's a toxicological leap in the dark.

The dose of chemicals that gives a lab rat cancer, says Lois Swirsky Gold, a University of California cancer hazard expert, is often thousands of times higher than the lifetime dose for an American human. Gold and her associates ranked "possible carcinogenic hazards" by comparing doses of chemicals that caused cancer in rats and mice to the daily doses of those chemicals a human being can expect over a lifetime. Their results: Something called furfural in two slices of white bread rates twice the known hazard of the average dose of chloroform in water; caffeic acid in a handful of lettuce, 300 times more; ethyl alcohol in two glasses of wine, 4,700 times more than water.

Others remain wary. "We take the prudent position," says Jennifer Orme-Zavaleta, a top EPA risk assessor for drinking water. "These chemicals might cause a human health effect, and we don't want them to do that, so we try to control them." It's also the law: Allowable levels of possibly dangerous impurities must be set below a point at which no health effect can be seen.

Disinfection byproducts became suspect when several long-term health studies suggested increased cancer rates among drinkers of chlorinated surface water. But the International Agency for Research on Cancer says the data aren't good enough to prove a cancer connection. The risks of not chlorinating far outweigh any proven risks of doing it. Still, the EPA plans to cut the allowable limits of disinfection byproducts by about 20 percent by 1995.

~~~~~

OKAY, SO THE WATER IN MY HOUSE HAS THINGS IN IT. WHICH ONES SHOULD I BE MOST WARY OF?

The four troublemakers that turned up most frequently in violations of EPA standards last year were bacteria, lead, nitrate, and radium. Nitrate can only get into drinking water at the source—before it arrives at the treatment plant. Bacteria and lead get in after the water leaves the plant, while it travels through service pipes to your house, and, in the case of lead, through household plumbing. Radioactive minerals can come from natural or human-made radium or uranium concentrations in the ground.

Bacteria cause diarrhea, dysentery, hepatitis, typhoid fever, and cholera. Lead damages the brain and kidneys, especially in fetuses and children. In children, who absorb lead more efficiently than adults do, it causes learning disorders and behavior problems. In adults, it causes nerve damage and hypertension. Nitrate, in children under a year old, can cause "blue-baby" anemia, a potentially fatal blood disorder. And radium causes cancer, especially of the bone.

~~~~~

ISN'T BOTTLED WATER SAFER THAN TAP WATER?

Not necessarily. Bottled waters (except for soda water) are classed as food, so the Food and Drug Administration sets quality standards for them almost identical to EPA tap water standards. As it turns out, about 25 percent of the "bulk" water sold in jugs is essentially tap water, usually filtered to make it taste better; the FDA rules that went into effect in July require labeling it "municipal water" when that's so. "Mineral" water gets the same FDA scrutiny as bulk water, except that it's allowed to have more of some ingredients such as chloride, iron, manganese, sulfate, and zinc, because the EPA considers them aesthetic problems instead of health threats. In any case, the label has to carry a list of the minerals in the water. Fine, except that the FDA admits it lacks the resources for annual bottling-plant inspections—even though the International Bottled Water Association, which represents and polices most of the water bottlers in the United States, wants them. The Association does require members to be inspected by the private NSF International, a food equipment inspection company. To find out if a particular brand is a member, write to the IBWA at 113 North Henry St., Alexandria, VA 22314.

Pierre Payment, the Canadian researcher, found bacteria counts in bulk water even higher than in the tap water that made his study subjects sick. "You can flush the water from your pipes by letting it run a while," he says. "With bottled water, you can't."

~~~~~

HOW CAN I TELL IF THE WATER IN MY HOUSE NEEDS TESTING?

If your senses tell you something is off, call your water company. Sulfur's distinctive rotten-egg smell is more an aesthetic nuisance than a health hazard. But other odors or persistent stains on sinks or laundry can mean there's something in it that shouldn't be—perhaps excess copper, iron, or manganese. Cloudy water is a really bad sign. Turbidity, as it's called, interferes with disinfection. Also, it showed up in the cryptosporidium outbreak in Milwaukee; filters unable to remove visible particles weren't doing a very good job of removing parasite cysts either.

You might want to test for lead even if you think everything else is okay, because lead gets into tap water for reasons that can vary from house to house. It might be lead solder in your pipes or lead in a supply line leading to your house. A recent EPA survey found excess levels of lead in 819 different water systems serving 30 million people.

~~~~~

WHAT'S THE SIMPLEST THING I CAN DO TO REDUCE MY FAMILY'S EXPOSURE TO BACTERIA, LEAD, AND DISINFECTION BYPRODUCTS?

Let your water run for at least 30 seconds any time it's been sitting for several hours. Water sitting in pipes can pick up lead, and it collects some lead in faucets. Run it until it's as cold as it can get, a sign that you're drawing from the service pipe outside the house. You can use this "first draw" to water houseplants.

You can disinfect water by boiling it for ten minutes. That also evaporates chlorine and its suspect cousins; letting water stand in an open pitcher for a day or two accomplishes the same thing.

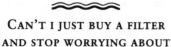

CAN'T I JUST BUY A FILTER AND STOP WORRYING ABOUT ALL OF THIS?

Sure, you can buy a filter. And no, you can't buy one that handles everything. If you're thinking of getting one, first find out what's in your water that you don't want—lead? chloroform? benzene?—then find the one that best removes those specific substances.

To make sure the filter you buy delivers on its promise, shop for a unit certified by the nonprofit NSF International. NSF charges manufacturers big bucks to run their devices through rigorous tests. Those it certifies carry an NSF label listing the contaminants a device actually removes. Not having the label doesn't mean a device won't work, but having it is an assurance that it will. For $10, NSF will mail you a list of the drinking water treatment units it currently certifies. (Its address is 3475 Plymouth Rd., Ann Arbor, MI 48105. Or call 313/769-8010.)

Your best bet is probably one of the many activated carbon filters on the market. Miniature versions of the big ones in Cincinnati, these can remove bad tastes, odors, and organic compounds including pesticides, chloroform, and solvents. They won't remove bacteria, nitrate, sodium, or fluoride, and most won't trap heavy metals (though NSF now certifies several for lead reduction).

A typical under-sink model with a cartridge about three inches in diameter and six to ten inches high will give you a generous flow of water on demand. You'll need to replace the cartridge after about 500 gallons, a year's drinking and cooking supply for a family of four.

Carbon can harbor bacteria, so flush the system for 30 seconds to a minute after it has sat unused for more than a few hours—the water is fine for plants.

Good units cost between $190 and $380. Replacement cartridges cost from $30 to $70. You can expect to spend about $70 a year for upkeep.

If you want almost complete removal of lead—along with arsenic, asbestos, parasite cysts, and nitrate—you might want to look into reverse osmosis filters. But be forewarned: they're slower, fussier to main-tain, more expensive than carbon, and more wasteful.

Remember, any home filter has to be cleaned or changed regularly to work right and keep it from becoming a health hazard in itself. Properly maintained, though, it's like having a little bit of the Cincinnati Water Works under your sink.

FOR MORE HELP

THE SAFE DRINKING WATER HOTLINE at 800/426-4791 will answer your questions. They'll also send you Environmental Protection Agency publications, including

Is Your Drinking Water Safe?, a booklet on what the government is doing to monitor the safety of drinking water and why.

Citizen Monitoring: Recommendations to Public Water System Users, a fact sheet describing potential contaminants and "action steps" for consumers.

Lead and Your Drinking Water, a question-and-answer pamphlet explaining lead contamination and what individuals can do about it.

patient, treat thyself

HOME REMEDIES

You don't always have to see a doctor to get the care you need

Teresa Carr

Teresa Carr is a freelance writer specializing in health, science and technology.

We all have our favorite home remedies, those traditional poultices and practices we call on to soothe life's minor ills. Some have their basis in scientific fact; others appear to work even though no one is exactly sure why. A few medical experts swear by the healing properties of gel from freshly cut leaves of the aloe plant, for example, though they aren't sure which are the active ingredients.

There are also heartfelt testimonials for remedies that the experts say shouldn't work—which is not the same as saying that they *don't* work. The placebo effect can be strong medicine. Pondering the medicinal merit of applying chewed tobacco to a bee sting, Dr. Varro Tyler, a professor of pharmacognosy at Purdue University in West Lafayette, Ind., chuckles and says, "It probably works more as a distraction than anything else." But for a teary child who's just wandered barefoot into the clover, a distraction may prove just the ticket.

A few household items are so widely known and used for their medicinal properties that they would probably qualify as old-fashioned cure-alls. Yogurt, especially with active acidophilus cultures, is one; it appears to be good for everything from preventing yeast infections to soothing a sunburn. Likewise you can use a wet tea bag to take the sting out of a fever blister, freshly brewed tea to soak smelly feet, or a tea compress to relieve eyestrain. Ever useful baking soda not only cleans your cabinets and deodorizes your refrigerator, but it's also touted for treating bleeding gums (when paired with hydrogen peroxide and salt), insect bites and athlete's foot. Tyler says that in his 30-odd years of exploring natural remedies, garlic and onions, used against everything from colds to cancer, have come up more often than anything else, though it's doubtful you'll find them recommended as remedies for bad breath.

All the remedies that follow should be taken with a generous application of common sense. In general, seek medical advice if your ailment doesn't improve within a day or two or is accompanied by inexplicable symptoms.

skin care

▶**ITCHY, DRY SKIN AND ECZEMA.** All dry skin remedies, from the fanciest to the most humble, work by keeping the skin moist, either by attracting water from the atmosphere or keeping it from evaporating, says Dr. Esta Kronberg, a staff physician at the Women's Hospital of Texas in Houston. Hot water dries the skin, so take tepid baths or showers. Avoid soap, which also dries the skin, or use it sparingly (substitute oatmeal or lipid-free soaps such as Cetaphil). Pat yourself dry, then apply a moisturizer while your skin is still damp. Humidity helps, so if you live in an arid climate, try using a humidifier.

To soothe the itchy, red breakouts of eczema, try cold milk compresses or a bath product containing finely ground oatmeal that forms a suspension in water (Aveeno is the most common brand). Or grind your own oatmeal, using a blender or food processor. For severe outbreaks of eczema, see a doctor.

▶**SUNBURN.** Apply compresses soaked in cool water, milk, witch hazel or tea. Or try cool water run through oatmeal (use a colander or cheesecloth). Yogurt and shaving lotion are also soothing. For extra relief, immerse yourself in a cool bath doctored with finely ground oatmeal or baking soda. Many people also swear by aloe. Tyler suggests getting the gel straight from the plant; commercial processing may render it less effective.

▶**POISON IVY AND OAK.** The culprit here is urushiol, found in the sap of these three-leaved plants. Urushiol is potent—so potent, in fact, that you can get a bad rash just by petting a dog who has run through the weeds. So the first thing you need to do is banish the offending sap from your skin, clothes, pet, furniture, car door or anything else you or it may have touched. Soap and water work best, but plain water will do.

Oral antihistamines such as Chlor-Trimeton and Benadryl will lessen the severity of minor breakouts. Calamine lotion, that old standby, cools, relieves some of the itch and helps dry up oozing blisters. Other drying agents to try include zinc oxide, witch hazel, baking soda, aluminum acetate solutions (Bluboro and Domeboro are two brands) and the ever versatile oatmeal.

Don't try to treat a severe rash yourself, especially if it comes on within a

A few household items are so widely used they qualify as cure-alls.

few hours of exposure and is accompanied by swelling. These symptoms signal a more serious allergic reaction; you need to get to a doctor for treatment.

▶**DIAPER RASH.** The enzymes that cause this bane of babyhood thrive in the moist, alkaline environment of soiled diapers. Your first task, then, is to keep Baby's bottom clean and dry by changing diapers often. An old-time remedy for stubborn rashes is to soak gauze or

cosmetic cotton squares in an aluminum acetate solution, place them on the rash, then diaper the baby as usual to hold the compresses in place. This dressing soothes the rash and at the same time makes the diaper area less alkaline. If you use cloth diapers, adding vinegar to the final rinse when you wash them will keep the acidity of the diapers more in line with Baby's skin.

tummy treatments

▶**DIARRHEA.** An occasional bout of diarrhea is your body's way of cleaning out bacteria or viruses infecting your bowel. For mild cases, your best bet may be just to let the bug run its course.

Most important, you need fluids. Diarrhea depletes your supply of sodium and potassium, so a sports drink such as Gatorade, which contains these two elements, is a good choice. You can also drink bouillon (for sodium) and fruit juice (for potassium). If you can't tolerate the juice, try adding some "light" salt to your broth, suggests Dr. John Rogers, vice chairman of family medicine at Baylor College of Medicine in Houston. Most brands of this supermarket item contain both sodium and potassium salts. Because diarrhea causes a temporary deficiency in the enzyme lactase, needed to digest the milk sugar lactose, Rogers also recommends avoiding milk and other dairy products—except yogurt—for at least a week. (The active cultures in yogurt may help because they start breaking down lactose. Some people believe yogurt also restores "good" bacteria to the bowel—a theory many experts find plausible, especially in diarrhea caused by antibiotics such as amoxicillin, which don't discriminate between good and bad bacteria.)

Stick to clear liquids—gelatin, juice and broth—for 12 to 24 hours to give the bowels a chance to rest. When you venture back to solid foods, remember the acronym BRAT—*bananas, rice, applesauce* and *toast.* Bananas contain potassium and they are binding, as is the pectin in applesauce; rice is easily digested; and toast (no butter) adds bulk to the stool.

If you must stem the tide, fiber sup-

plements such as Metamucil add bulk to the stool. The anitdiarrheal medication Imodium is also very effective.

Most bouts of diarrhea aren't serious. You should seek medical help, however, when:

• Diarrhea occurs in the very young, the elderly or those with already compromised immune systems.

• Symptoms don't improve in a couple of days.

• Diarrhea is accompanied by prolonged fever and severe abdominal cramps, rashes, jaundice or extreme weakness.

• Stools contain blood, pus or mucus.

• The person can't keep food and liquids down.

▶ **CONSTIPATION.** What you absolutely shouldn't do, say the experts, is rely heavily on chemical laxatives. Your intestines may grow dependent on them for normal function. What you need more than anything for constipation is water.

You also need to eat plenty of fiber in the form of whole grains, fruits, vegetables and beans. But be careful: If your intake of fiber is low to begin with, you need to increase it gradually, since too much too fast will result in gas, cramping, bloating and even diarrhea. The oldest constipation remedy in the book is prunes (or prune juice), which function as natural bowel stimulants. Just don't overdo it with more than a serving (four to six large prunes).

And remember to exercise. When you get moving, so do your bowels. Walking seems to be particularly effective.

If you must use a laxative on an occasional basis, pick a high-fiber bulking agent (such as FiberCon or Fiberall), or one based on the psyllium seed (Metamucil). You can also use a stool softener such as Colace or Dialose. These products, whose active ingredient is docusate sodium, attract water to the stool and increase bulk.

▶**HEMORRHOIDS.** These varicose veins around the rectum are often caused by straining during bowel movements. To a large extent, then, the remedies for constipation may help you avoid hemorrhoids too.

Americans spend $200 million a year on over-the-counter hemorrhoid preparations, most of which do little lasting good. The main ingredient in most of these preparations is a lubricant that eases friction and irritation. Petroleum jelly works just as well. Some preparations also include a topical anesthetic to ease the pain temporarily and an astringent to relieve secondary swelling around the hemorrhoids (despite advertising claims, the preparations don't "shrink" the hemorrhoid itself). Hot water relieves pain and increases the blood flow to the area, and this reduces swelling. Try sitting in a shallow, hot bath for 15 minutes. Don't use bubble bath or oils, as they can irritate sensitive tissue. Many people add Epsom salts, but the experts we talked to say it's the hot water, not the salts, that do the trick.

▶**HEARTBURN.** Normally a valve between the esophagus and the stomach prevents stomach acid from leaking into the esophagus. But when stomach acid is increased by chocolate, coffee or cigarettes (to name a few), the acid can surge up and irritate the delicate lining of the esophageal tube, causing the burning sensation for which this common

Be aware that what you drink is just as important as how much you drink.

misery is named. Popping an antacid (such as Tums or Rolaids) to neutralize the acid is an effective remedy. If you don't have any, try drinking a large glass of cold water, which washes the acid back down into the stomach and dilutes it there.

You want gravity working against stomach acid, so don't lie down or bend over for a couple of hours after you eat. If nighttime heartburn is a problem, try elevating the head of your bed a couple of inches by putting two-by-four planks at that end. (Don't just pile on the pillows, as you'll only strain your neck.)

One common, though unproven, digestive (and motion sickness) aid is ginger. But you won't get enough from a slice of gingerbread or a glass of ginger ale. Instead take ginger capsules or eat raw or crystallized ginger, available at most grocery stores. Two other well-known remedies, milk and mints, will only make you feel worse: Mints tend to relax the valve that keeps acids out of the

esophagus, and though milk soothes initially, its calcium induces the stomach to secret even more acid. Antacid mixtures containing calcium carbonate can also cause excess acid to be secreted, but the antacid portion neutralizes it.

headaches

At one time or another you've probably experienced the tightness and pressure spanning the forehead characteristic of a tension headache. The dull ache may even extend down the sides of your head and across your shoulders or neck. Less common but more debilitating are migraine headaches, in which severe, throbbing pain, usually on one side, is often accompanied by nausea and a heightened sensitivity to light and sound.

For both types of headache, relaxation techniques—massage, a warm bath, meditation, biofeedback or whatever else works for you—often eliminate the headache at its source by dissipating stress. Other nonchemical remedies include either ice or heat on the forehead or the back of the neck. You can also try acupressure: Apply firm pressure to the web between your forefinger and thumb or on either side of your spine at the base of your neck.

If you opt for a pain reliever, take it at the first hint of symptoms. Pain is much harder to control once it's allowed to become intense. A cup of coffee may help as well. Caffeine constricts blood vessels and is an ingredient in some over-the-counter analgesics and prescription migraine medications. Beware the caffeine backlash, however. Your body quickly grows dependent on daily caffeine. Skipping your morning coffee, or even cutting back, can lead to a headache from caffeine withdrawal.

▶**HEADACHE TRIGGERS.** After a bad day at the office, when the baby won't stop crying, or when your car is on the fritz again, the cause of your headache may be painfully obvious. If you can't discern where your headaches are coming from, however, consider these possible triggers:

• Food additives including monosodium glutamate (MSG), sulfites, nitrites and aspartame (NutraSweet).

• Foods that contain the amino acid tyramine, including chocolate, aged cheeses, cured meats, yeast products and nuts.

• Environmental factors such as noise, exposure to chemicals or pollution, or an abrupt change in the weather.

• Eyestrain or poor posture.

• A variety of common medications, including oral contraceptives and high–blood pressure drugs that contain reserpine and hydralazine. Even pain relievers, taken chronically, can cause so-called rebound headaches.

▶**THE HANGOVER HEADACHE.** Because alcohol is a powerful diuretic, most of the cause of a hangover headache is dehydration, so drink several glasses of water. Eating a light, nongreasy snack, such as toast, cereal or crackers, will help combat nausea. The infamous "hair of the dog" cure, drinking something alcoholic, apparently works for some people—at least temporarily. But most experts say it probably just delays the inevitable pain.

Be aware that what you drink can be just as important as how much. The worst offenders include brandies, whiskey and champagne. Red wine is notorious for causing headaches, possibly because it contains both tyramine and sulfites. To avoid, or at least diminish, morning-after misery, eat some honey on crackers or drink a glass of juice before going to bed. The fructose in these foods may help metabolize the alcohol.

first aid

▶**NOSEBLEEDS.** The best remedy for a minor nosebleed is to sit up straight, squeeze your nose closed, and hold it for five to 15 minutes. If the bleeding doesn't stop within 20 minutes, seek medical attention.

Slight bleeding is common in the winter when dry, warm air dries out delicate nasal passages; humidifying your surroundings can help. High levels of estrogen increase blood flow to mucous membranes in the nose, so pregnancy and oral contraceptives can also cause minor nosebleeds. Keep in mind that aspirin, which interferes with clotting, will make bleeding worse. Though anecdotal support for vitamin C as a remedy is strong, experts say it probably doesn't help except in rare cases of gen-

10 Home Remedies You Should Never Use

1 **DON'T APPLY BUTTER, GREASE OR OTHER FOODS TO A BURN.** These substances tend to hold in the heat and can even cause infections. Also don't use adhesive bandages or fluffy materials such as cotton balls. For minor burns, cool the heat with ice or cold water, then cover the wound with a gauze pad. Don't try to self-treat third-degree burns (which are charred and white), burns that are larger than a quarter on a child or a silver dollar on an adult, or *any* burns on infants younger than a year old.

2 **DON'T USE ALCOHOL BATHS TO REDUCE A FEVER.** A sponge bath with cool water works better, plus you don't inhale noxious fumes.

3 **DON'T GIVE ASPIRIN TO CHILDREN UNDER THE AGE OF 15 TO REDUCE FEVERS.** In kids with upper respiratory tract infection, chicken pox or the flu, aspirin can trigger Reye's syndrome, a rare but potentially deadly neurological illness. Acetaminophen is safe.

4 **DON'T TREAT ULCERS WITH MILK OR BAKING SODA.** Milk feels good going down, but the fats, protein and especially the calcium trigger the release of stomach acid. And using baking soda repetitively can lead to a sodium overload, which increases blood pressure and exacerbates heart disease. The often used combination of milk and baking soda is particularly hard on the kidneys, where calcium buildup can cause kidney stones or even kidney failure.

5 **DON'T TREAT HYPOTHERMIA (BODY TEMPERATURE BELOW 95°) BY DRINKING ALCOHOL.** You'd be better off putting warm cocoa in the St. Bernard's flask. Alcohol dilates blood vessels and thus speeds the release of body heat. You should also avoid piling on heavy layers of clothes or blankets and rubbing or massaging cold limbs. If rewarming is done too quickly, it dilates the blood vessels near the skin, further lowering blood pressure and sending even colder blood to vital organs. Get the chilled person into a warm bed, cover his head, give him a warm—not hot—drink if he's conscious and not coughing or vomiting, and get medical help. A good way to help prevent hypothermia is to wear a warm hat, since as much as 20% of body heat is lost through the head.

6 **DON'T WEAR A PATCH OVER A RED, ITCHY EYE.** If the irritation arises from a bacterial infection, the warmth and moisture behind the patch will only serve to incubate the bacteria and worsen the condition.

7 **DON'T ATTEMPT TO CUT OFF FOOT CORNS OR CALLUSES.** Although you may be tempted to hack away at the offending skin, such bathroom surgery can lead to serious infection. Also avoid medicated pads and over-the-counter corn removal treatments, which can cause ulcerations in the corn and may damage surrounding healthy tissue.

8 **DON'T TREAT SPRAINS OR STRAINS WITH HEAT.** Or at least wait 48 to 72 hours after the injury before you do. Heat will increase circulation to the injured area, and thus increase swelling. To treat sprains, remember the acronym RICE: *Rest* to take the pressure off; apply *ice* to relieve pain and reduce the swelling; wrap with a *compression* bandage to prevent further swelling and provide support; and *elevate* the sprain above the heart, again to reduce swelling.

9 **DON'T SLAP A CHOKING PERSON ON THE BACK.** If the person is able to cough, leave him alone. Hitting a coughing victim on the back may drive the obstruction further down the airway. If the person is not coughing or breathing, or is breathing only with great difficulty, you need to perform the Heimlich maneuver to dislodge the blockage. Stand behind the victim and, with your arms around him, clench one fist and place it, thumb-knuckle inward, at a spot above the navel and below the rib cage. Hold your fist with the other hand and pull both hands toward you with a quick upward thrust into the abdomen. (The procedure is slightly different for infants and children. All parents and anyone who cares for children should know the basics of infant and child first aid and cardiopulmonary resuscitation. Contact your local Red Cross for details.)

10 **DON'T BREAK BLISTERS CAUSED BY BURNS OR FRICTION.** A blister forms a natural bandage that allows a wound to heal and prevents infection. If the blister is in such an awkward spot that you have to break it, insert a sterile needle in one end and let the fluid ooze out. But be sure to leave the skin flap intact, or the area will be painful and vulnerable to infection.

uine deficiency. Finally, don't pick at the small scabs inside your nose.

▶**INSECT STINGS AND BITES.** First get the stinger out. If you were stung by a bee (wasps don't leave their stingers behind), take care not to squeeze the stinger or venom sac, as this just pumps more poison into the skin. Don't pull out the stinger with your fingers or tweezers; instead, gently scrape it out with a fingernail or the edge of a credit card or a sterilized knife.

Experts say the best remedy for easing the pain of a sting is a meat tenderizer containing the enzyme papain. Applied immediately, papain breaks down the protein-based venom. Other common remedies, which also work for mosquito or fly bites, include heat, ice, a drop of household ammonia, a paste of baking soda and water, and an aspirin rubbed on the moistened sting. An oral antihistamine will also help minimize pain and swelling. Caution: One of every 250 people is allergic to insect attacks, and a sting can send an allergic person into life-threatening anaphylactic shock. Seek medical help immediately if the victim develops chest tightness, hives, nausea, vomiting, wheezing, hoarseness, dizziness, a swollen tongue or face, fainting or shock.

If a tick bites you, don't try to pluck it out; you'll probably leave its mouth parts embedded in your skin, and they could cause infection. To remove a tick safely, ease it out *slowly* with tweezers, or heat a needle or nail in a flame and place it against the tick's backside to make it let go. The head of a match that's been lit and blown out will also work. Kerosene, gasoline and alcohol can irritate a tick into releasing its grip on you, but don't use these flammable liquids in conjunction with heat. You can also suffocate a tick with paraffin, petroleum jelly or fingernail polish, which should make it fall off in about 30 minutes.

the common cold

Mom was probably onto something when she gave you chicken soup and tea with honey and lemon. You need to drink plenty of liquids to replace lost fluids and loosen mucous secretions. Chicken soup seems to be particularly efficient at increasing the flow of nasal secretions and decreasing nasal congestion, perhaps because of its pungent aroma. Honey soothes your throat, and lemon adds a touch of vitamin C. A cup of tea may ease bronchial spasms. Caffeine, which is in the same family as the asthma drug theophylline, can lessen wheezing and coughing.

Vitamin C is many people's first choice for a cold, although evidence for its efficacy is mixed. It certainly won't hurt to increase your intake moderately for the duration of a cold by taking a supplement or drinking juice that is rich in the vitamin, such as orange, grapefruit or cranberry. Researchers in both the U.S. and Great Britain have shown that for some people, zinc shortens the duration of a cold. Sucking on flavored zinc lozenges relieves a sore throat. Just don't take megadoses: Zinc can be toxic if taken in large amounts for a long period of time.

Salt water is another time-honored cold remedy. Add one-quarter teaspoon of salt to eight ounces of warm water to make a soothing gargle for a sore throat. Use the same recipe with cool water to make saline nose drops, especially effective for nasal congestion in infants.

Lozenges of all types can soothe your sore throat and help relieve that cough-inducing tickle. Licorice, in the form of lozenges or tea, works as a natural expectorant to help you clear your lungs and throat of mucus. Some cough drops still contain this old-time remedy; just make sure you're getting real licorice and not anise flavoring. Another way to relieve congestion and moisten your throat is to take a hot shower; better still, boil a pot of water, make a tent over your head and the pot with a towel, and inhale the warm vapor.

corns and calluses

These are your body's responses to excessive pressure from ill-fitting shoes or a misalignment of the foot. Podiatrist Mark Sussman of Wheaton, Md., coauthor of *The Family Foot Care Book,* says most remedies aimed at dissolving corns and calluses, particularly medicated pads and creams, are just too aggressive. "These products can eat into good tissue and even cause allergic reactions," he warns. Instead, soften the thickened skin by adding two tablespoons of mild detergent to half a gallon of warm water and soak your feet for at least 10 minutes. Dry them thoroughly and rub in a couple of drops of vegetable oil to soften the area even more. Then gently file down the top layer of the corn or callus using a pumice stone or special callus file. Never use a sharp instrument, such as a knife or razor blade. Clean the area with soap and water using a gauze pad.

For corns on the top of a toe, take the pressure off by applying a doughnut-shaped (nonmedicated) corn pad. Stretch the pad so that it clears the corn by at least an eighth of an inch on all sides. Then apply petroleum jelly to the hole, cover it with a gauze square and wrap the toe with adhesive tape. For corns between toes, daub on petroleum jelly and place a plug of lamb's wool between the toes to keep them from rubbing.

odds and ends

▶**HICCUPS.** Everyone has a favorite hiccup treatment, although the one involving standing on your head while drinking a glass of water is probably mostly for the entertainment of other people. The odds-on favorite? Eating a teaspoon of granulated sugar, which may work by interfering with nerve impulses in the mouth that signal the diaphragm to contract and so trigger an attack. Also, carbon dioxide in the blood inhibits hiccups, so many remedies are simply creative ways to get victims to hold their breath. Some of the more popular include:
- Drinking water slowly.
- Bending forward at the waist and drinking water.
- Bending at the waist and drinking water from the opposite side of the glass (harder than it sounds).
- Yanking on your tongue.
- Sucking on ice cubes.
- Scaring the victim (makes him inhale suddenly).

9. CONSUMER HEALTH

• Breathing in and out of a paper bag (never use plastic).

▶ **INSOMNIA.** For the occasional sleepless night, a sleeping pill or a hot toddy probably won't hurt. But if poor sleep is a frequent problem, those remedies will only make matters worse.

What does it take to get to dreamland? One British study showed that a group of volunteers slept better when they drank warm malted milk before bedtime than after they took what they thought was a sleeping pill but was actually a placebo. Some researchers attribute all milk's beneficial effect to the amino acid L-tryptophan, also found in poultry, fish and eggs.

While sipping your milk, examine your life for factors that may be interfering with sleep. Alcohol, caffeine and nicotine are common culprits. Antihistamines, decongestants, antidepressants, beta-blockers (drugs for high blood pressure and heart ailments) and other medications can also stimulate the nervous system at the wrong time of day, and cause sleep problems. Lifestyle factors that adversely affect sleep include varying your sleep routines from day to day, not getting enough exposure to daylight, and eating a large meal too close to bedtime. You'll rest better if you exercise during the day to make yourself physically tired, then follow a regular, relaxing routine each night.

▶ **JET LAG.** Anyone who's traveled across time zones has experienced the disorientation, sleeplessness and fatigue collectively called jet lag. Night workers have similar problems, especially when they change shifts regularly or try to return to a daytime schedule on their days off.

One theory has it that a strict diet alternating large and small high-carbohydrate, high-protein meals will reduce jet lag. When researchers from the U.S. Army Institute of Environmental Medicine in Natick, Mass., and the New York Hospital/Cornell Medical Center in New York City subjected a group of Marines to simulated changes in time zones, however, they found that those on the diet were just as jet lagged as those who weren't, and the special dieters were even more sleep deprived to boot.

The best cure for jet lag, say sleep researchers, is to reset your internal body clock at your destination by getting outside to expose yourself to as much daylight or darkness as possible and trying to sleep during the local nighttime.

PREVENTING STDs

This article is part of a [continuing FDA Consumer] series with important health information for teenagers. Unlike previous articles, however, it contains sexually explicit material in an effort to reduce the incidence of STDs among teens. Parents and teachers may want to review the article before giving it to teenagers.

Judith Levine Willis

Judith Levine Willis is editor of FDA Consumer.

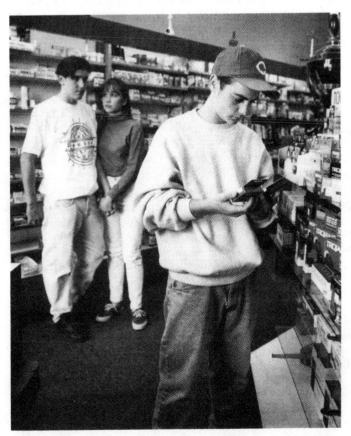

It's important to read the information printed on the package to make sure a condom's made of latex and labeled for disease prevention. The label may also give an expiration date and tell you if there is added spermicide or lubricant.

You don't have to be a genius to figure out that the only sure way to avoid getting sexually transmitted diseases (STDs) is to not have sex.

But in today's age of AIDS, it's smart to also know ways to lower the risk of getting STDs, including HIV, the virus that causes AIDS.

Infection with HIV, which stands for human immunodeficiency virus, is spreading among teenagers. From 1990 to 1992, the number of teens diagnosed with AIDS nearly doubled, according to the national Centers for Disease Control and Prevention. Today, people in their 20s account for 1 out of every 5 AIDS cases in the United States. Because HIV infection can take many years to develop into AIDS, many of these people were infected when they were teenagers.

You may have heard that birth control can also help prevent AIDS and other STDs. This is only partly true. The whole story is that *only one form of birth control—latex condoms* (thin rubber sheaths used to cover the penis)—is highly effective in reducing the transmission (spread) of HIV and many other STDs.

(When this *FDA Consumer* went to press, the Food and Drug Administration was preparing to approve Reality Female Condom, a form of birth control made of polyurethane. It may give limited protection against STDs, but it is not as effective as male latex condoms.)

So people who use other kinds of birth control, such as the pill, sponge, diaphragm, Norplant, Depo-Provera, cervical cap, or IUD, also need to use condoms to help prevent STDs.

Here's why: Latex condoms work against STDs by keeping blood, a man's semen, and a woman's vaginal fluids—all of which can carry bacteria and viruses—from passing from one person to another. For many years, scientists have known that male condoms (also called safes, rubbers, or prophylactics) can help prevent STDs transmitted by bacteria, such as syphilis and gonorrhea, because the bacteria can't get through the condom. More recently, researchers discovered that latex condoms can also reduce

From *FDA Consumer*, June 1993, pp. 33-35. Reprinted by permission.

231

the risk of getting STDs caused by viruses, such as HIV, herpes, and hepatitis B, even though viruses are much smaller than bacteria or sperm.

After this discovery, FDA, which regulates condoms as medical devices, worked with manufacturers to develop labeling for latex condoms. The labeling tells consumers that although latex condoms cannot entirely eliminate the risk of STDs, when used properly and consistently they are highly effective in preventing STDs. FDA also provided a sample set of instructions and requested that all condoms include adequate instructions.

Make Sure It's Latex

Male condoms sold in the United States are made either of latex (rubber) or natural membrane, commonly called "lambskin" (but actually made of sheep intestine). Scientists found that natural skin condoms are not as effective as latex condoms in reducing the risk of STDs because natural skin condoms have naturally occurring tiny holes or pores that viruses may be able to get through. Only latex condoms labeled for protection against STDs should be used for disease protection.

Some condoms have lubricants added and some have spermicide (a chemical that kills sperm) added. The package labeling tells whether either of these has been added to the condom.

Lubricants may help prevent condoms from breaking and may help prevent irritation. But lubricants do not give any added disease protection. If an unlubricated condom is used, a water-based lubricant

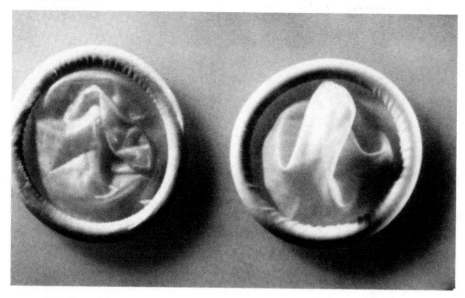

If a condom is sticking to itself, as is the one on the left, it's damaged and should not be used. The one on the right is undamaged and okay to use.

New Information on Labels

Information about whether a birth control product also helps protect against sexually transmitted diseases (STDs), including HIV infection, is being given added emphasis on the labeling of these products.

"In spite of educational efforts, many adolescents and young adults, in particular, are continuing to engage in high-risk sexual behavior," said FDA Commissioner David A. Kessler, M.D., in announcing the label strengthening last April. "A product that is highly effective in preventing pregnancy will not necessarily protect against sexually transmitted diseases."

Labels on birth control pills, implants such as Norplant, injectable contraceptives such as Depo Provera, intrauterine devices (IUDs), and natural skin condoms will state that the products are intended to prevent pregnancy and do not protect against STDs, including HIV infection (which leads to AIDS). Labeling of natural skin condoms will also state that consumers should use a latex condom to help reduce risk of many STDs, including HIV infection.

Labeling for latex condoms, the only product currently allowed to make a claim of effectiveness against STDs, will state that if used properly, latex condoms help reduce risk of HIV transmission and many other STDs. This statement, a modification from previous labeling, will now appear on individual condom wrappers, on the box, and in consumer information.

Besides highlighting statements concerning sexually transmitted diseases and AIDS on the consumer packaging, manufacturers will add a similar statement to patient and physician leaflets provided with the products.

Consumers can expect to see the new labels by next fall. Some products already include this information in their labeling voluntarily. FDA may take action against any products that don't carry the new information.

FDA is currently reviewing whether similar action is necessary for the labeling of spermicide, cervical caps, diaphragms, and the Today brand contraceptive sponge.

Looking at a Condom Label

Like other drugs and medical devices, FDA requires condom packages to contain certain labeling information. When buying condoms, look on the package label to make sure the condoms are:
- made of latex
- labeled for disease prevention
- not past their expiration date (EXP followed by the date).

(such as K-Y Jelly), available over-the-counter (without prescription) in drugstores, can be used but is not required for the proper use of the condom. Do *not* use petroleum-based jelly (such as Vaseline), baby oil, lotions, cooking oils, or cold creams because these products can weaken latex and cause the condom to tear easily.

Condoms with added spermicide give added birth control protection. An active chemical in spermicides, nonoxynol-9, kills sperm. Although it has not been scientifically proven, it's possible that spermicides may reduce the transmission of HIV and other STDs. But spermicides alone (as sold in creams and jellies over-the-counter in drugstores) and spermicides used with the diaphragm or cervical cap do not give adequate protection against AIDS and other STDs. For the best disease protection, a latex condom should be used from start to finish every time a person has sex.

FDA requires condoms with spermicide to be labeled with an expiration date. Some condoms have an expiration date even though they don't contain spermicide. Condoms should not be used after the expiration date, usually abbreviated EXP and followed by the date.

Condoms are available in almost all drugstores, many supermarkets, and other stores. They are also available from vending machines. When purchasing condoms from vending machines, as from any source, be sure they are latex, labeled for disease prevention, and are not past their expiration date. Don't buy a condom from a vending machine located where it may be exposed to extreme heat or cold or to direct sunlight.

Condoms should be stored in a cool, dry place out of direct sunlight. Closets and drawers usually make good storage places. Because of possible exposure to extreme heat and cold, glove compartments of cars are *not* a good place to store condoms. For the same reason, condoms shouldn't be kept in a pocket, wallet or purse for more than a few hours at a time.

How to Use a Condom
• Use a new condom for every act of vaginal, anal and oral (penis-mouth contact) sex. Do not unroll the condom before placing it on the penis.

STD Facts

• Sexually transmitted diseases affect more than 12 million Americans each year, many of whom are teenagers or young adults.
• Using drugs and alcohol increases your chances of getting STDs because these substances can interfere with your judgment and your ability to use a condom properly.
• Intravenous drug use puts a person at higher risk for HIV and hepatitis B because IV drug users usually share needles.
• The more partners you have, the higher your chance of being exposed to HIV or other STDs. This is because it is difficult to know whether a person is infected, or has had sex with people who are more likely to be infected due to intravenous drug use or other risk factors.
• Sometimes, early in infection, there may be no symptoms, or symptoms may be confused with other illnesses.
• You cannot tell by looking at someone whether he or she is infected with HIV or another STD.

STDs can cause:
• pelvic inflammatory disease (PID), which can damage a woman's fallopian tubes and result in pelvic pain and sterility
• tubal pregnancies (where the fetus grows in the fallopian tube instead of the womb), sometimes fatal to the mother and always fatal to the fetus
• cancer of the cervix in women
• sterility—the inability to have children—in both men and women
• damage to major organs, such as the heart, kidney and brain, if STDs go untreated
• death, especially with HIV infection.

See a doctor if you have any of these STD symptoms:
• discharge from vagina, penis or rectum
• pain or burning during urination or intercourse
• pain in the abdomen (women), testicles (men), or buttocks and legs (both)
• blisters, open sores, warts, rash, or swelling in the genital or anal areas or mouth
• persistent flu-like symptoms—including fever, headache, aching muscles, or swollen glands—which may precede STD symptoms.

• Put the condom on after the penis is erect and before *any* contact is made between the penis and any part of the partner's body.

• If the condom does not have a reservoir top, pinch the tip enough to leave a half-inch space for semen to collect. Always make sure to eliminate any air in the tip to help keep the condom from breaking.

• Holding the condom rim (and pinching a half inch space if necessary), place the condom on the top of the penis. Then, continuing to hold it by the rim, unroll it all the way to the base of the penis. If you are also using water-based lubricant, you can put more on the outside of the condom.

• If you feel the condom break, stop immediately, withdraw, and put on a new condom.

• After ejaculation and before the penis gets soft, grip the rim of the condom and carefully withdraw.

• To remove the condom, gently pull it off the penis, being careful that semen doesn't spill out.

• Wrap the condom in a tissue and throw it in the trash where others won't handle it. (Don't flush condoms down the toilet because they may cause sewer problems.) Afterwards, wash your hands with soap and water.

Latex condoms are the only form of contraception now available that human studies have shown to be highly effective in protecting against the transmission of HIV and other STDs. They give good disease protection for vaginal sex and should also reduce the risk of disease transmission in oral and anal sex. But latex condoms may not be 100 percent effective, and a lot depends on knowing the right way to buy, store and use them.

Top Medical Centers

A consumer's guide to hospitals offering state-of-the-art care

DAVID LEVINE

David Levine writes about medicine and health and is a contributing editor at Physician's Weekly.

Some physicians are generalists; others are highly specialized. Hospitals too come in many varieties, from small community clinics to major teaching centers to facilities focusing on a specific disorder, such as cancer. If you (or a family member) have to be hospitalized for a serious illness, have an ailment no one can diagnose, or need specialized outpatient treatment, it may pay to seek care from an institution known for its expertise and up-to-date technology.

From the thousands of diseases that afflict us, we created 16 major groupings, then compiled a list of hospitals or centers most likely to offer specialized care in these categories. Some names—Johns Hopkins, Massachusetts General, the Mayo Clinic, for example—cropped up re-

peatedly because the very best teaching hospitals tend to be strong in all areas. (The absence of a description for certain centers indicates broad expertise in the field.)

A variety of criteria were used in making our choices. We evaluated existing hospital rating lists and spoke to medical professional societies, health care agencies and patient advocacy groups. We tried to offer as much geographic spread as possible, which sometimes meant eliminating a facility in an already well-represented region.

Also, by "best," we didn't mean which facility has the nicest grounds or the tastiest food. The choices were based on medical factors such as the quality of staff and expertise in diagnosis and treatment. At

the end of this list, you'll find "Hot Spots," a brief round-up of hospitals offering help for special problems, such as Lyme disease.

There are approximately 6,700 hospitals and medical centers in the U.S. We apologize to the more than 6,600 hospitals we may have unintentionally offended by omission. Some hospitals, however, were excluded because their representatives never got back to us or we were unable to reach them by telephone. If on two occasions no one picked up after the 20th ring, we gave up.

Keep in mind that this guide has no listings for trauma centers, burn units or emergency rooms. The reason is simple: We cannot stress strongly enough that when you're having a heart attack or you've had an accident, the best hospital is the *nearest* hospital. Delay in getting help can be deadly.

There are also practical considerations. If, say, you are part of a health maintenance organization (HMO), you may have no choice about which hospital you go to. Also, remember that you can rarely check yourself into a hospital on your own. You usually need a doctor's referral, so call ahead to find out what's required. Finally, use this list as a guide, not a bible. A community hospital near your home and family may be just fine for your needs.

HOSPITALS BY SPECIALTY

(listed alphabetically)

AIDS

• **Beth Israel Medical Center,** New York City, 212-420-2000. Beth Israel's doctors were among the first to identify and treat clusters of infections caused by HIV. Beth Israel offers comprehensive services for adults and children with AIDS.

• **Jackson Memorial Hospital,** Miami, 305-585-1111. The main hospital for the South Florida AIDS Network, Jackson Memorial provides comprehensive inpatient and outpatient services.

• **Johns Hopkins Hospital,** Baltimore, 410-955-5000. Hopkins is one of several institutions approved to test AIDS vaccines and experimental AIDS drugs. The hospital is also a major research center.

• **Massachusetts General Hospital,** Boston, 617-726-2000. Affiliated with Harvard Medical School, Mass. General's staff includes top AIDS specialists and researchers.

• **St. Luke's-Roosevelt Medical Center,** New York City, 212-523-4000. The center is designated by the state as an AIDS treatment facility. Because of the scope of the AIDS problem in New York City, doctors here have gained considerable expertise at treating the disease and its complications.

• **St. Vincent's Hospital and Medical Center,** New York City, 212-790-7000. St. Vincent's, another state-designated AIDS facility, was the first Catholic hospital in the country to take a leadership role in treating the illness. It has since gained a national reputation for its quality of care.

• **San Francisco General Hospital,** 415-206-8000. Doctors at this hospital, all of whom are on the University of California at San Francisco (UCSF) Medical Center faculty, are among the top AIDS researchers in the country. San Francisco General is also known for its quality of care and compassionate staff.

• **UCSF Medical Center,** 415-476-1000. Merged in 1990 with Mount Zion Hospital and Medical Center, UCSF offers a wide range of services to AIDS patients and their families.

ALLERGY AND ASTHMA

• **Brigham and Women's Hospital,** Boston, 617-732-5500. Affiliated with Harvard Medical School, Brigham and Women's is known for all-around excellence in patient care, research and education in this field.

• **Johns Hopkins Hospital,** Baltimore, 410-955-5000. This hospital is chosen for its excellent treatment and research programs in allergy and asthma.

• **Mayo Clinic,** Rochester, Minn., 507-284-2511. Like Hopkins, Mayo is known for overall excellence in treatment and research.

• **National Jewish Center for Immunology and Respiratory Medicine,** Denver, 303-388-4461. National Jewish is a treatment and research center for respiratory and immune system disorders, and it's particularly renowned for diagnosing and treating tuberculosis. The "Lung Line" is staffed by registered nurses to help patients and families (call 800-222-LUNG).

• **Northwestern Memorial Hospital,** Chicago, 312-908-2000. A large teaching hospital, this center is known for general excellence in allergies and asthma.

• **UCLA Medical Center,** 310-825-9111. UCLA is one of the nation's top centers for the diagnosis and treatment of allergies.

• **University of Michigan Medical Center,** Ann Arbor, 313-936-4000. Researchers here are currently studying the adverse effects of certain airborne pollutants on asthmatics and nonasthmatics as well as conducting clinical research on drugs that not only treat the symptoms but also may cure asthma.

CANCER

• **Comprehensive Cancer Center,** University of Wisconsin, Madison, 608-263-8600. Wisconsin is known for prevention and treatment of breast and prostate cancers.

• **Dana-Farber Cancer Institute,** Boston, 617-732-3000. Originally established as the Children's Cancer Research Foundation, this Harvard Medical School–affiliated facility is known for its pioneering work in treating lymphoma and leukemia and for its bone marrow transplant program. It's also strong in gynecological and pediatric oncology, and cancers of the head, neck and lungs.

• **Duke Comprehensive Cancer Center,** Durham, N.C., 919-684-2748. Duke is world renowned for quality cancer care, especially for tumors of the brain, breast, colon and kidney.

• **Fox Chase Cancer Center,** Philadelphia, 215-728-6900. Fox Chase is known for its treatment programs for ovarian, esophageal and prostate cancer. The center also has prevention programs for breast, liver and ovarian cancer.

• **Fred Hutchinson Cancer Research Center,** Seattle, 206-667-5000. Devoted exclusively to bone marrow transplants for a variety of adult and pediatric cancers, this institution is the largest bone marrow transplant center in the world.

• **Johns Hopkins Oncology Center,** Baltimore, 410-955-8638. Hopkins is a top treatment and research facility with special recognition for its bone marrow transplant program.

• **Kaplan Comprehensive Cancer Center,** New York University Medical Center, New York City, 212-263-7300. Kaplan specializes in breast cancer, melanoma, pediatric cancers, childhood central nervous system malignancies, and lung and ovarian cancer.

• **Massachusetts General Hospital,** Boston, 617-726-2000. This facility is known for strength in all areas of cancer treatment and research.

• **Mayo Clinic Comprehensive Cancer Center,** Rochester, Minn., 507-284-4718. This is where Jordan's King Hussein had surgery for urinary tract cancer. The center is outstanding in cancer surgery and in research on new drug therapies. Mayo is developing a special clinic to centralize care for cancers that primarily affect women.

• **Memorial Sloan-Kettering Cancer Center,** New York City, 212-639-2000. Memorial is the country's oldest and largest privately operated cancer center. It's the leading cancer surgery center in the U.S. and has a large bone marrow transplant program. A new outpatient breast cancer and diagnostic imaging center opened last fall.

• **Norris Cotton Cancer Center,** Dartmouth-Hitchcock Medical Center, Lebanon, N.H., 603-650-5527. The Norris Center specializes in autologous (self-donated) bone marrow transplants and in treating cancers of the lung, ovary and prostate.

• **Stanford University Medical Center Oncology Clinic,** Stanford, Calif., 415-723-7621. A pioneer in treating Hodgkin's disease, Stanford also specializes in prostate cancer and lymphoma.

• **University of Chicago Cancer Research Center,** 312-702-9200 or 800-289-6333. The center specializes in cancers of the breast, colon, liver, kidney and pancreas, and in treating leukemia and lymphoma.

• **University of Texas M.D. Anderson Cancer Center,** Houston, 713-792-7000. Strong in treating all kinds of cancer, this facility is known for innovative reconstructive surgery for patients with disfiguring cancers. It also conducts many clinical trials of new cancer drugs and treatments.

CARDIOLOGY

• **Brigham and Women's Hospital,** Boston, 617-732-5500. Affiliated with Harvard Medical School, this hospital did the first heart transplant in New England. It also conducts the ongoing Nurses' Health Study, an analysis of risk factors for cardiovascular disease, cancer and other women's diseases.

• **Cedars-Sinai Medical Center,** UCLA, 310-855-5000. Cedars-Sinai is one of the leaders in developing heart attack treatments, such as delivering clotbuster drugs via catheters inserted into an artery in the groin and using lasers to unclog coronary arteries.

• **Cleveland Clinic,** 216-444-2200 (with a center in Fort Lauderdale, Fla., 800-359-5101 or 305-978-5000). Known as *the* heart center, the Cleveland Clinic was a pioneer in developing coronary arteriography, the heart-lung machine, heart valve repair and bypass surgery. Its rate of mitral valve repairs is one of the highest in the U.S., and 1,500 coronary balloon angioplasties are done there annually.

• **Columbia-Presbyterian Heart Institute,** New York City, 212-305-2500. In addition to routine open-heart surgery, the institute treats high-risk cases of valvular and coronary artery disease. It does surgery on patients turned down elsewhere and specializes in electrophysiology, congestive heart failure and pediatric cardiology and surgery.

• **Johns Hopkins Hospital,** Baltimore, 410-955-5000. Hopkins is a pioneer in both cardiovascular surgery and cardiopulmonary resuscitation.

• **Krannert Institute of Cardiology,** Indianapolis, 317-630-7261. Echocardiography, an ultrasound technique for diagnosing heart disease, was developed here. Krannert specializes in diagnosing and treating heart arrhythmias.

• **Lenox Hill Hospital,** New York City, 212-439-2345. This hospital is a leader in interventional cardiology and cardiovascular surgery. The first balloon angioplasty in the country was done here in 1978. (One was done simultaneously on the West Coast.) The hospital offers coronary artery bypass surgery, valve repair and replacement, and surgical management of arrhythmias.

• **Massachusetts General Hospital,** Boston, 617-726-2000. Mass. General has overall strength in cardiac diagnosis and treatment.

• **Mayo Clinic,** Rochester, Minn., 507-284-2511. Mayo is known for its echocardiography labs and is strong in all areas, including diagnosis and surgery.

• **Mount Sinai Medical Center,** New York City, 212-241-6500. Major research is under way here on the application of molecular biology to cardiology and on strategies for preventing and treating blood clots. The Children's Heart Center does transplants as well as other complex cardiac surgery on infants and children.

• **Parkland Memorial Hospital,** Dallas, 214-590-8000. Parkland has a center for arrhythmia management that provides evaluation, counseling and treatment services. The center specializes in using electrophysiological techniques that are more sophisticated than conventional noninvasive cardiac tests.

• **Texas Heart Institute,** St. Luke's Episcopal Hospital, Houston, 800-292-2221. This institute has done the most open-heart procedures in the U.S. It's currently developing portable heart-assist devices designed to prolong transplant patients' lives while they wait for donors.

• **UCLA Medical Center,** 310-825-9111. Known for heart transplants, UCLA is strong in all cardiological areas. It specializes in treating critically ill heart-failure patients.

• **University of Pittsburgh Heart Institute,** 412-647-6000. Pittsburgh specializes in heart and heart-lung transplants (as well as other organ transplants). The institute is a leader in developing temporary and permanent artificial organs, and it has used more temporary artificial hearts for patients awaiting a donor than any other institution.

• **University of Washington Medical Center,** Seattle, 206-548-3700. This institution was one of the first centers to use clotbuster drugs to help save the lives of heart attack patients.

ENDOCRINOLOGY

• **Cleveland Clinic,** 216-444-2200. Chosen for overall excellence in treatment and research, Cleveland specializes in diabetic neuropathy (nerve damage).

• **Jackson Memorial Hospital,** Miami, 305-585-1111. One of the best teaching hospitals in the Southeast, Jackson has earned a reputation for treating diabetes and other diseases of the endocrine system. Its excellent clinical staff attracts patients from all over the U.S., as well as from the Caribbean and Latin America.

• **Mayo Clinic,** Rochester, Minn., 507-284-2511.

• **Mount Sinai Medical Center,** New York City, 212-241-6500. Mount Sinai researchers have made important advances in diabetes and liver disease. A special program treats patients with thyroid disease or thyroid cancer.

• **Stanford University Medical Center,** Stanford, Calif., 415-723-4000. Doctors' special interests include pituitary and adrenal gland disorders, thyroid disease, gonadal abnormalities and hypertension of endocrine origin.

• **UCLA Medical Center,** 310-825-9111. UCLA treats patients for problems related to the entire spectrum of endocrine diseases.

• **University of Chicago Medical Center,** 312-702-1000 or 800-289-6333. This facility is world-famous as a center for diabetes research.

GASTROENTEROLOGY

• **Brigham and Women's Hospital,** Boston, 617-732-5500. This hospital did the first successful human kidney transplant in 1954 and was also the first to use a cadaver kidney successfully, which opened up a whole new era in transplantation.

• **Cleveland Clinic,** 216-444-2200. Cleveland does more than 15,000 procedures on digestive system diseases annually. Its endoscopy unit, which uses tube-like scopes to view body cavities, is one of the world's largest and most sophisticated. Cleveland is known for innovative treatments for inflammatory bowel disease, colorectal cancer and polyps, and motility disorders, such as gastric emptying problems.

• **Johns Hopkins Hospital,** Baltimore, 410-955-5000.

• **Massachusetts General Hospital,** Boston, 617-726-2000.

• **Mayo Clinic,** Rochester, Minn., 507-284-2511.

• **Mount Sinai Medical Center,** New York City, 212-241-6500. Mount Sinai pioneered the use of the transplant immunosuppressive drug cyclosporine in the treatment of inflammatory bowel disease in America.

• **Parkland General Hospital,** Dallas, 214-590-8000. Parkland provides state-of-the-art diagnostic, therapeutic and consultative management of patients with gastrointestinal disorders. It uses endoscopic retrograde cholangiopancreatography, a nonsurgical procedure, to treat gallbladder, liver and pancreas ailments. Its kidney transplant success rate is among the best in the nation.

•**University of Chicago Medical Center,** 312-702-1000 or 800-289-6333. This center is outstanding for treating inflammatory bowel disease among all age groups.

•**University of Pittsburgh Medical Center,** 412-648-9115. Pittsburgh's transplantation program is the largest and busiest in the world. The hospital is best known for liver, kidney and intestinal transplants and is a leader in trying to perfect immunosuppressant therapy.

NEUROLOGY

• **Cleveland Clinic,** 216-444-2200. Its Amyotrophic Lateral Sclerosis (ALS, or Lou Gehrig's disease) Center treats patients from all over the world. Researchers here are seeking a cause for the illness and better ways to treat it.

•**Columbia-Presbyterian Medical Center,** New York City, 212-305-2500. Columbia is strong in research and management of patients with ALS, and Alzheimer's and Parkinson's diseases.

•**Hospital for Joint Diseases,** New York City, 212-598-6000. This facility specializes in sports neurology, movement and seizure disorders, neuropsychology and neurophysiology.

•**Jackson Memorial Hospital,** Miami, 305-585-1111. Jackson's Ryder Trauma Center is the largest independent facility of its type in the world. The hospital is known for treating neurological and spinal cord injuries.

•**Johns Hopkins Hospital,** Baltimore, 410-955-5000.

•**Massachusetts General Hospital,** Boston, 617-726-2000. The hospital excels in neurosurgery.

•**Mayo Clinic,** Rochester, Minn., 507-284-2511.

•**New England Medical Center,** Boston, 617-956-5000. This center offers comprehensive evaluation and management of diseases of the nervous system. Special areas of expertise: strokes, seizures and memory and neuromuscular disorders.

•**Swedish Hospital Medical Center,** Seattle, 206-386-6000. This hospital has just opened a new comprehensive center for diagnosis, evaluation and treatment of patients with epilepsy and epilepsy-like disorders.

•**University of California at San Francisco (UCSF) Medical Center,** 415-476-1000. UCSF is known for neurosurgery. The Brain Tumor Research Center is the largest center of its kind in the world and has been especially successful in treating cancers of the central nervous system. The Pediatric Neurosurgery Program treats 10% of the nation's childhood brain tumors.

•**University of Pittsburgh Medical Center,** 412-647-3000. Doctors here treat brain tumors and vascular malformations, once considered inoperable, with the so-called gamma knife, which directs gamma radiation to a target point and spares patients open-skull procedures.

OBSTETRICS / GYNECOLOGY

•**Brigham and Women's Hospital,** Boston, 617-732-5500. This center is a designated regional center for high-risk pregnancies and neonatology and is involved in research in human reproduction and reproductive biology.

•**Johns Hopkins Hospital,** Baltimore, 410-955-5000.

•**Lenox Hill Hospital,** New York City, 212-439-2345. Lenox Hill has a national reputation for exceptional obstetrical and neonatal care. The Prenatal Testing Center is one of the largest and most comprehensive in the country.

•**Mount Sinai Medical Center,** New York City, 212-241-6500. The ob/gyn department here specializes in infertility, menopause and high-risk pregnancies. Mount Sinai also established the first egg donation program in the city.

•**Ohio State University Hospitals,** Columbus, 614-293-8937. Ohio State specializes in treating infertility and offers an in-vitro fertilization and embryo transfer program.

•**St. Barnabas Medical Center,** Livingston, N.J., 201-533-5280. Its high-risk pregnancy referral service offers genetic counseling, in-vitro fertilization and other services (such as birthing rooms). The hospital has one of the largest regional gynecologic oncology centers in the Northeast, as well as a division of reproductive endocrinology and infertility.

•**Swedish Hospital Medical Center,** Seattle, 206-386-6000. Couples faced with high-risk pregnancies come here for genetic counseling, testing services and obstetrical care. For couples having difficulty conceiving, the center offers fertility evaluation for both men and women, assisted reproductive procedures and a donor sperm bank.

•**University of Southern California Medical Center,** Los Angeles, 213-226-2345.

•**Yale–New Haven Hospital,** New Haven, Conn., 203-785-4242. Yale specializes in managing high-risk pregnancies.

OPHTHALMOLOGY

•**Bascom Palmer Eye Institute,** Miami, 305-326-6190. Internationally recognized as one of the most advanced centers in ophthalmology, the institute does more than 10,000 surgeries annually and is a leader in the treatment of retinal diseases, eye tumors and pediatric ophthalmology.

•**Massachusetts Eye and Ear Infirmary,** Boston, 617-523-7900. A Harvard Medical School teaching facility, this hospital has the world's largest assemblage of scientists and physicians doing research on all aspects of the visual system. The institution literally is writing the book on the field with its upcoming four-volume text, *Principles and Practices of Ophthalmology: The Harvard System.*

•**Mayo Clinic,** Rochester, Minn., 507-284-2511.

•**Wills Eye Hospital,** Philadelphia, 215-928-3041. Wills offers cataract and primary eye-care service, as well as special services for contact lenses, diseases of the cornea and retina, neuro-ophthalmology, glaucoma, oncology and pediatric ophthalmology. It also has sports vision and low vision centers.

•**Wilmer Eye Institute,** Johns Hopkins Hospital, Baltimore, 410-955-5650. This institute was one of the first to use lasers to treat macular degeneration, a common form of blindness. Its researchers established the role of vitamin A supplements in treating corneal diseases and linked cataracts to ultraviolet rays and alcohol consumption.

•**UCLA Medical Center,** 310-825-9111. UCLA's Jules Stein Eye Institute attracts patients from all over the country.

ORTHOPEDICS

•**Columbia-Presbyterian Medical Center,** New York City, 212-305-2500. Columbia is a leader in the Northeast for custom-made hip replacements. The first shoulder joint replacement was developed here.

•**Hospital for Joint Diseases,** New York City, 212-598-6000. This hospital specializes in joint replacement, reconstructive and spinal surgery, pediatric orthopedics and hand, foot and ankle surgery. It also has sports medicine and dance injury programs.

•**Hospital for Special Surgery,** New York City, 212-606-1000. This is an outstanding place for orthopedic surgery. It specializes in joint replacement and hand surgery, as well as sports injuries.

•**Lenox Hill Hospital,** New York City, 212-439-2345. The Nicholas Institute of Sports Medicine and Athletic Trauma here was the first hospital-based center dedicated to sports medicine in the U.S.

•**Mayo Clinic,** Rochester, Minn., 507-284-2511.

•**Ohio State University Hospitals,** Columbus, 614-293-8000. Ohio State's new sports medicine center offers help to professional and weekend athletes alike and boasts a staff with experience on the professional, collegiate and Olympic level.

●**St. Luke's-Roosevelt Medical Center,** New York City, 212-532-4000. St. Luke's Miller Institute for Performing Artists specializes in injuries common to actors, dancers, musicians and singers.

●**UCLA Medical Center,** 310-825-9111.

●**University of Washington Medical Center,** Seattle, 206-548-3300. The center's strengths include shoulder surgery, trauma care and treatment of bone tumors.

PEDIATRICS

●**Children's Hospital,** Boston, 617-735-6000. Affiliated with Harvard Medical School, Children's is the largest pediatric medical center in the U.S. Its doctors conduct major organ and bone marrow transplantation on children of all ages. Hypothermia techniques (and others) developed here allow cardiovascular surgeons to operate on newborns with life-threatening heart defects.

●**Children's Hospital Medical Center,** Cincinnati, 513-559-4200. The oral polio vaccine was developed here, as well as the bubble oxygenator, which made possible the first open heart surgery. Most recently, the first bone marrow transplant for sickle-cell disease was done here.

●**Children's Memorial Medical Center,** Chicago, 312-880-4000. This center is a leader in inpatient and outpatient treatment of cancer and related blood diseases, including bone marrow transplants. Affiliated with Northwestern University Medical School, it's one of the largest centers for spina bifida, pediatric cardiology, organ transplantation, orthopedics and genetic diseases. It's also a national pediatric arthritis center designated by the National Arthritis Foundation.

●**Johns Hopkins Children's Center,** Baltimore, 410-955-2000. Hopkins specializes in difficult-to-diagnose pediatric illnesses.

●**Mount Sinai Medical Center,** New York City, 212-241-6500. Mount Sinai excels in the care of high-risk infants, patients with juvenile diabetes and children with respiratory disease.

●**New England Medical Center,** Boston, 617-956-5000. The center was founded in 1796 as the Boston Dispensary and includes the Floating Hospital for Children, which began in 1894 as a hospital ship serving the city's indigent children. Now permanently on land, it's a specialized diagnostic and referral center, offering comprehensive inpatient and outpatient care.

● **New York University (NYU) Medical Center,** New York City, 212-263-7300. NYU's division of pediatric neurosurgery does more than 600 surgical procedures and 3,000 consultations annually. It treats more spinal cord tumors than any other factility in the world and is one the largest U.S. centers for pediatric brain tumor surgery.

●**University of California at San Francisco (UCSF) Medical Center,** 415-476-1000. UCSF has gained a worldwide reputation for highly specialized diagnosis and treatment of children and seriously ill newborns.

●**Yale–New Haven Hospital,** New Haven, Conn., 203-785-4242. In 1960 Yale established the first neonatal intensive care unit in the world. Its new Children's Hospital [opened in 1993].

PSYCHIATRY

●**Columbia-Presbyterian Medical Center,** New York City, 212-305-2500. Columbia is a pioneer in treating depression and anxiety disorders and runs large clinical trials to test new psychiatric drugs. Another asset: The New York State Psychiatric Institute is based here.

●**Fair Oaks Hospital,** Summit, N.J., 800-526-4494. This hospital is a leader in research on panic disorders and substance abuse. It offers both full-time inpatient care and partial hospitalization programs, allowing patients to work and be with their families.

●**Johns Hopkins Hospital,** Baltimore, 410-955-5000.

●**McLean Hospital,** Belmont, Mass. 617-855-2000. Affiliated with Massachusetts General Hospital and Harvard Medical School, McLean is one of the most renowned psychiatric hospitals in the country. It offers inpatient and outpatient services, a Women's Treatment Network and various specialized programs, including a brain imaging center, a sleep disorders center and an eating disorders program.

●**Menninger Clinic,** Topeka, Kan., 913-273-7500. Patients from around the world have come for help since the Menninger Clinic opened in 1925. The facility treats schizophrenia, eating disorders, marriage and family problems, sexual dysfunction, professionals in crisis and alcohol and drug abuse. Menninger offers a separate women's program for eating disorders, headache, anxiety/panic and depression. This program can be reached by calling 800-351-9058, x6140.

●**Ohio State University Hospitals,** Columbus, 614-293-8000. This hospital offers treatment programs for sleep, eating and anxiety disorders and schizophrenia. It also has a children's psychiatric unit and is a research center.

●**Payne Whitney Psychiatric Clinic,** New York Hospital–Cornell Medical Center, New York City, 212-746-3800. The world-famous clinic offers comprehensive psychiatric and neurological services.

●**Sheppard and Enoch Pratt Hospital,** Towson, Md., 410-938-5000. This hospital offers a wide range of treatment options, including inpatient, outpatient, day hospital (patients go home at night) and supervised housing services. Programs for children and adolescents cover eating, attention deficit, mood and personality disorders. There's also a school on the hospital grounds.

●**University of Pittsburgh Medical Center,** 412-624-2100. Its Western Psychiatric Institute and Clinic is a world leader in the diagnosis and treatment of mood disorders. Researchers here discovered sleep pattern changes in depressed patients, indicating for the first time the biological nature of the illness.

● **University of Washington Medical Center,** Seattle, 206-548-3300. The center specializes in panic, anxiety and depressive disorders, geriatric problems and psychopharmacological therapy.

●**Yale–New Haven Hospital,** New Haven, Conn., 203-785-4242. Affiliated with Yale Medical School, this hospital treats children and adults (inpatient and outpatient). Its doctors are part of the sexual abuse team that investigated the Woody Allen/Mia Farrow charges.

REHABILITATION

●**Hospital for Joint Diseases,** New York City, 212-598-6000. This hospital offers inpatient rehabilitation and outpatient physical and occupational therapy. It also has a pain center.

● **Institute for Rehabilitation and Research,** Houston, 713-799-5000. Affiliated with Baylor College of Medicine, the institute offers programs in amputee rehabilitation, brain and spinal cord injuries, musculoskeletal and pediatric problems and stroke recovery.

● **Jackson Memorial Hospital,** Miami, 305-585-1111. Its Ryder Trauma Center is the largest and most comprehensive trauma center in the world. The hospital specializes in rehabilitating patients with difficult orthopedic and spinal cord injuries.

●**Mayo Clinic,** Rochester, Minn., 507-284-2511.

●**National Rehabilitation Hospital,** Washington, 202-877-1000. This hospital has special amputation, stroke, spinal cord and brain injury recovery programs. It also recently opened three outpatient units: the Center for Back Injury Prevention and Rehabilitation, the Center for Repetitive Motion Disorders and the National Arts Medicine Center.

● **Ohio State University Hospitals,** Columbus, 614-293-8000. This center offers programs for patients disabled by head and spinal cord injuries, chronic pain or strokes, plus a specialized program for multiple sclerosis and muscular dystrophy patients. New features include a spine clinic, a chronic pain management program and a concussion clinic.

● **Rehabilitation Institute of Chicago,** 312-908-6000. The institute offers programs for amputees and for patients with arthritis or brain injuries, geriatric and stroke rehabilitation and help for the special injuries of performing artists. Its Center for Pain Studies treats spinal and musculoskeletal problems. The hospital also has a sports rehab program and services for children and adolescents.

● **Rusk Institute of Rehabilitation Medicine,** New York City, 212-263-6208. Named after Dr. Howard Rusk, the father of rehabilitation medicine, Rusk was the first facility of its kind when it opened in 1948. Today it's the world's largest university-based center (it's part of New York University Medical Center) for treating and training disabled adults and children.

● **University of Chicago Medical Center,** 312-702-9200 or 800-289-6333. Chicago has an electrical trauma center for people who have been struck by lightning or who have sustained a severe electrical injury.

RHEUMATOLOGY

● **Brigham and Women's Hospital,** Boston, 617-732-5500. This major center for joint replacement surgery developed the Brigham knee and the first and most successful elbow replacement. It also has allergy and lupus clinics and Lyme disease specialists.

● **Duke University Arthritis Center,** Durham, N.C., 919-684-5093. Duke offers special clinics for chronic pain, lupus and rheumatoid arthritis.

● **Johns Hopkins Hospital,** Baltimore, 410-955-5000. Hopkins is outstanding in the diagnosis and treatment of rheumatic diseases, especially Raynaud's disease, a circulatory disorder. It also has developed special treatment procedures for pregnant lupus patients.

● **Hospital for Joint Diseases,** New York City, 212-598-6000. This hospital has specialists in arthritis, rheumatic diseases, lupus and Lyme disease and offers a comprehensive arthritis management program.

● **Hospital for Special Surgery,** New York City, 212-606-1000. This center is regarded as one of the best orthopedic surgery hospitals in the country. Its unique computerized system makes it possible for doctors to offer patients custom-designed artificial joints.

● **Mayo Clinic,** Rochester, Minn., 507-284-2511. Mayo specializes in treating unusual rheumatic disorders, such as vasculitis and transient osteoporosis syndrome.

● **University of California at San Diego Medical Center,** 619-543-5982. This center is known for treating patients with early rheumatoid arthritis and other rheumatoid diseases, including gout and ankylosing spondylitis.

● **University of Colorado Health Sciences Center,** Denver, 303-399-1211. The division of rheumatology here is studying new drugs for scleroderma, lupus and rheumatoid arthritis.

● **University of Connecticut Health Center,** Multipurpose Arthritis Center, Farmington, 203-679-2160. This center has a program for fibromyalgia (a rheumatic disorder affecting the muscles and tendons) and specializes in treating lupus, scleroderma and Lyme and Raynaud's diseases.

● **University of Washington Medical Center,** Seattle, 206-548-3300. One of this center's specialties is testing new drugs for osteoarthritis and rheumatoid arthritis.

● **Washington University Barnes Hospital Rheumatology Clinic,** St. Louis, 314-362-5058. Barnes is known for its expertise in treating angioedema, a hereditary condition characterized by swelling in various parts of the body. It holds a weekly clinic for patients with lupus.

SUBSTANCE ABUSE

● **Betty Ford Center,** Rancho Mirage, Calif., 310-477-3997. Not just for the rich and famous, this center's patients are mainly ordinary people. It provides topnotch treatment, and as a private, nonprofit hospital, its fees are comparable to those of most of the hospitals listed here.

● **Beth Israel Medical Center,** New York City, 212-420-2000. Beth Israel's methadone maintenance program is the largest drug treatment program in the U.S. The hospital recently established the Chemical Dependency Institute, where researchers are designing innovative treatment programs for drug abuse and associated conditions, such as AIDS and tuberculosis.

● **Fair Oaks Hospital,** Summit, N.J., 800-526-4494. Fair Oaks gained national recognition when it began its toll-free cocaine hotline (800-COCAINE) in 1983. The hospital offers inpatient and outpatient programs for teenagers, adults and their families.

● **Father Martin's Ashley,** Havre de Grace, Md., 410-273-6600. This nonprofit center treats alcoholics and chemically dependent people. It features primary, aftercare and relapse prevention programs and has a 24-hour help line: 800-848-8177.

● **Hazelden Foundation,** Center City, Minn., 800-257-7800. Founded in 1949, Hazelden is an internationally recognized, nonprofit organization for treating chemical dependency and related addictive behaviors. It offers residential programs, aftercare services, an adolescent program and a family center for those with friends or relatives who are substance abusers.

● **Menninger Clinic,** Topeka, Kan., 913-273-7500. This famed psychiatric clinic has a special unit for patients with drug- and alcohol-related problems.

● **McLean Hospital,** Belmont, Mass., 617-855-2000. This hospital's alcohol and drug abuse program treats patients and their families. It offers inpatient treatment, a transitional house on the hospital grounds and outpatient programs.

● **Smithers Alcoholism Treatment and Training Center,** New York City, 212-523-6491. Smithers, which specializes in alcohol and drug detoxification, provides inpatient and outpatient rehab services.

● **Sheppard and Enoch Pratt Hospital,** Towson, Md., 410-938-5000. This hospital provides a range of addiction recovery services, including detox and dual diagnosis (for people with psychiatric and substance abuse problems). There's also a program for child and adolescent substance abusers.

UROLOGY

● **Cleveland Clinic,** 216-444-2200. Cleveland treats large numbers of patients with complex kidney disorders, many of whom undergo reconstructive surgery to prevent kidney failure.

● **Columbia-Presbyterian Medical Center,** New York City, 212-305-2500. The center has an excellent reputation in diagnosing and treating urinary tract disorders.

● **Duke University Hospital,** Durham, N.C., 919-684-8111. This hospital's particular areas of expertise are in urologic oncology, male sexual dysfunction, reconstructive urologic surgery and the management of a wide range of complex urological malignancies.

● **Johns Hopkins Hospital,** Baltimore, 410-955-5000. The Brady Urological Institute here includes the Male Sexual Dysfunction Clinic, for men who have become impotent. A procedure to remove cancerous prostate glands without impairing sexual function was developed here.

●**Massachusetts General Hospital,** Boston, 617-726-2000.

●**Mayo Clinic,** Rochester, Minn., 507-284-2511.

●**Memorial Sloan-Kettering Cancer Center**, New York City, 212-639-2000. Memorial is strong in the diagnosis and treatment of testicular, bladder and prostate cancers.

●**Parkland General Hospital,** Dallas, 214-590-8000. Parkland, which is affiliated with the University of Texas Southwestern Medical School, is tops for urological surgery.

●**UCLA Medical Center,** 310-825-9111. UCLA provides inpatient and outpatient evaluation of urological disorders, including kidney transplantation, treatment of kidney- and gallstones, male infertility and male and female sexual dysfunction.

HOT SPOTS

●**CHRONIC PAIN.** Chronic pain includes pain caused by diseases such as arthritis, cancer and diabetes, as well as migraine headaches or back trouble. You can find a pain program or center in almost any major city in the country. Some of the oldest programs include those at the Hospital for Joint Diseases in New York City (212-598-6000), Johns Hopkins Hospital in Baltimore (410-955-5000), Lenox Hill Hospital in New York City (212-439-2345) and Massachusetts General Hospital in Boston (617-726-2000). For headache treatments, call Montefiore Medical Center in New York City, the first such center (212-920-4636),

the National Headache Foundation (800-843-2256) or the American Council for Headache Education (800-255-ACHE).

●**EATING DISORDERS.** Almost all the psychiatric hospitals listed in that section have eating disorder programs.

●**GENETIC COUNSELING.** Most of the hospitals listed under obstetrics/gynecology provide these services. St. Barnabas Medical Center in Livingston, N.J. (201-533-5280), is especially strong; Mount Sinai Medical Center in New York City (212-241-6500) has the world's only center for Tay-Sach's and other Jewish genetic diseases.

●**LYME DISEASE.** One of the major research centers, the State University of New York at Stony Brook, has a Lyme disease hot line: 516-444-3808. Lenox Hill Hospital in New York City (212-439-2345) and the New England Medical Center in Boston (617-956-5000) also have Lyme disease centers. Because Lyme is considered a rheumatic disease, most of the centers listed under that section can also be helpful.

●**OBESITY.** Weight loss programs are faddish and numerous, but they can be risky. Talk to your doctor or contact a major teaching hospital. Important research on the causes and treatment of obesity is currently under way at the Obesity Research Center of St. Luke's-Roosevelt Medical Center in New York City (212-523-4000).

●**SLEEP DISORDERS.** Sleep disorder clinics can now be found in almost every city. Among the best are those at Johns Hopkins Hospital in Balti-

more (410-955-5000), McLean Hospital in Belmont, Mass. (617-855-2000), Montefiore Medical Center in New York City (212-920-4841), the National Jewish Center for Immunology and Respiratory Medicine in Denver (303-388-4461) and the University of Chicago Medical Center (312-702-9200 or 800-289-6333). Most of the psychiatric hospitals listed can also help.

●**UNDIAGNOSED ILLNESS.** People struggling with an illness that seems to stump their local doctors may want to consult Johns Hopkins Hospital in Baltimore (410-955-5000), Massachusetts General Hospital in Boston (617-726-2000) or the Mayo Clinic in Rochester, Minn. (507-284-2511). These centers see many patients who believe their doctors have failed to diagnose or treat them correctly. One organization that may be able to refer you to help is the National Organization for Rare Disorders in New Fairfield, Conn. (203-746-6518); another is the National Institutes of Health in Bethesda, Md. (301-496-4000), which coordinates and funds much of the medical research in this country.

●**WOMEN'S HEALTH.** Because most medical research has focused on men, several organizations, including the National Institutes of Health, have started programs concentrating on women's health problems. Brigham and Women's Hospital in Boston has more than 250 research projects devoted to women's health, including the Women's Health Study assessing the effects of vitamins and aspirin on cancer and heart disease. The hospital has a menopause center and recently established a free women's health telephone referral line (800-522-8765). The Menninger Clinic in Topeka, Kan. (800-351-9058), has a separate women's program specializing in psychiatric problems.

Credits/ Acknowledgments

Cover design by Charles Vitelli

1. America's Health and the Health Care System

Facing overview—United Nations photo by John Isaac. 24-25—Illustrations by Jared Schneidman and Guilbert Gates.

2. Contemporary Health Hazards

Facing overview—U.S.D.A. Soil Conservation Service photo.

3. Stress and Mental Health

Facing overview—WHO photo by Jean Mohr.

4. Drugs and Health

Facing overview—American Cancer Society.

5. Nutritional Health

Facing overview—WHO photo.

6. Exercise and Weight Control

Facing overview—State of Minnesota Department of Economic Development. 143, 145, 147—Photos courtesy of Consumers Union of U.S.

7. Current Killers

Facing overview—Dushkin Publishing Group, Inc., photo by Pamela Carley. 184—Diagram by John Karapelou.

8. Human Sexuality

Facing overview—WHO photo. 192—Photo by Wisconsin Pharmacal Company. 195—Graphics courtesy of Time Inc. Magazine Company.

9. Consumer Health

Facing overview—Dushkin Publishing Group, Inc. photo. 210—Illustrations courtesy of FDA Consumer. 215—Photo courtesy of FDA Consumer. 217—Illustration courtesy of FDA Consumer. 231-232—Photos courtesy of FDA Consumer.

ANNUAL EDITIONS ARTICLE REVIEW FORM

■ NAME: _____ DATE: _____

■ TITLE AND NUMBER OF ARTICLE: _____

■ BRIEFLY STATE THE MAIN IDEA OF THIS ARTICLE: _____

_____

_____

_____

_____

■ LIST THREE IMPORTANT FACTS THAT THE AUTHOR USES TO SUPPORT THE MAIN IDEA:

_____

_____

_____

_____

_____

_____

■ WHAT INFORMATION OR IDEAS DISCUSSED IN THIS ARTICLE ARE ALSO DISCUSSED IN YOUR TEXTBOOK OR OTHER READING YOU HAVE DONE? LIST THE TEXTBOOK CHAPTERS AND PAGE NUMBERS:

_____

_____

_____

_____

_____

_____

_____

■ LIST ANY EXAMPLES OF BIAS OR FAULTY REASONING THAT YOU FOUND IN THE ARTICLE:

_____

_____

_____

_____

■ LIST ANY NEW TERMS/CONCEPTS THAT WERE DISCUSSED IN THE ARTICLE AND WRITE A SHORT DEFINITION:

_____

_____

_____

_____

_____

*Your instructor may require you to use this Annual Editions Article Review Form in any number of ways: for articles that are assigned, for extra credit, as a tool to assist in developing assigned papers, or simply for your own reference. Even if it is not required, we encourage you to photocopy and use this page; you'll find that reflecting on the articles will greatly enhance the information from your text.

ANNUAL EDITIONS: HEALTH 94/95
Article Rating Form

Here is an opportunity for you to have direct input into the next revision of this volume. We would like you to rate each of the 54 articles listed below, using the following scale:

1. **Excellent: should definitely be retained**
2. **Above average: should probably be retained**
3. **Below average: should probably be deleted**
4. **Poor: should definitely be deleted**

Your ratings will play a vital part in the next revision. So please mail this prepaid form to us just as soon as you complete it.
Thanks for your help!

Annual Editions revisions depend on two major opinion sources: one is our Advisory Board, listed in the front of this volume, which works with us in scanning the thousands of articles published in the public press each year; the other is you—the person actually using the book. Please help us and the users of the next edition by completing the prepaid article rating form on this page and returning it to us. Thank you.

Rating	Article	Rating	Article
	1. Wasted Health Care Dollars		28. The New Thinking About Fats
	2. The Clinton Cure		29. Snack Attack
	3. Healthtown U.S.A.		30. To Be Active or Not to Be Active
	4. Unclogging the Drug Pipeline		31. Exercise Without Injury
	5. Keeping Score		32. Walk Off Calories and Get Fit
	6. The Mainstreaming of Alternative Medicine		33. Losing Weight: What Works, What Doesn't
	7. Beach Bummer		34. Chemistry and Craving
	8. Gut Reactions		35. Your Health History
	9. Dangerous Liaison		36. Cholesterol: Put Knowledge Behind Your Numbers to Lower Your Confusion Level
	10. Sleeping with the Enemy		37. The "Diseasing" of Risk Factors
	11. The ABC's of Hepatitis		38. Pressure Treatment: How Exercise Can Help You Control Your Blood Pressure
	12. What Every Woman Needs to Know About Personal Safety		39. From Here to Immunity
	13. Stress		40. Eat to Beat Cancer
	14. Slow Down, You Breathe Too Fast		41. Confronting the AIDS Pandemic
	15. Mind Over Malady		42. The Long Shot
	16. How Anger Affects Your Health		43. The Mating Game
	17. The Mindset of Health		44. The Female Condom
	18. Ordinary Medicines Can Have Extraordinary Side Effects		45. New, Improved and Ready for Battle
	19. Foods and Drugs That Don't Mix		46. It's Not Just AIDS
	20. Rx to OTC		47. How Do You Know If It's PMS?
	21. Placebo Effect Is Shown to Be Twice as Powerful as Expected		48. 'Nutrition Facts': To Help Consumers Eat Smart
	22. Saying Goodbye to an Old Flame		49. 'Daily Values' Encourage Healthy Diet
	23. Alcohol and Tobacco: A Deadly Duo		50. Full Sun Protection
	24. Alcohol in Perspective		51. The Purist's Guide to Tap Water
	25. How's Your Diet?		52. Patient, Treat Thyself
	26. Are You Eating Right? and Eating Right: It's Easier Than You Think		53. Preventing STDs
	27. To Salt or Not to Salt		54. Top Medical Centers

(Continued on next page)

ABOUT YOU

Name_____ Date_____

Are you a teacher? ☐   Or student? ☐

Your School Name _____

Department _____

Address _____

City _____ State _____ Zip _____

School Telephone # _____

YOUR COMMENTS ARE IMPORTANT TO US!

Please fill in the following information:

For which course did you use this book? _____

Did you use a text with this Annual Edition?   ☐ yes   ☐ no

The title of the text? _____

What are your general reactions to the Annual Editions concept?

Have you read any particular articles recently that you think should be included in the next edition?

Are there any articles you feel should be replaced in the next edition? Why?

Are there other areas that you feel would utilize an Annual Edition?

May we contact you for editorial input?

May we quote you from above?